The Truth About Cancer

GLOBAL
QUEST

A GLOBAL QUEST
COMPLETE TRANSCRIPTS
OF ALL 9 EPISODES

The **TRUTH** About
CANCER™
educate • expose • eradicate

THE TRUTH ABOUT CANCER
"A GLOBAL QUEST"
Complete 9 Episode Transcripts

DEDICATION

This book was created for and is dedicated to **YOU** the courageous person who is seeking to reverse cancer or prevent cancer while seeking a natural approach to healing.

Many blessings to you and your family.

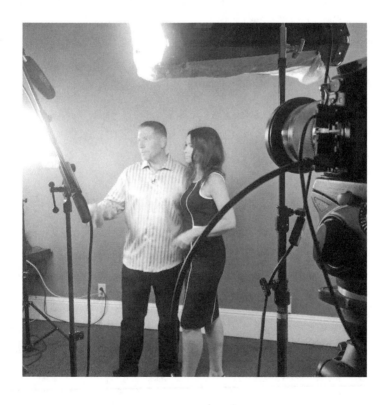

~ Ty & Charlene

Table of Contents

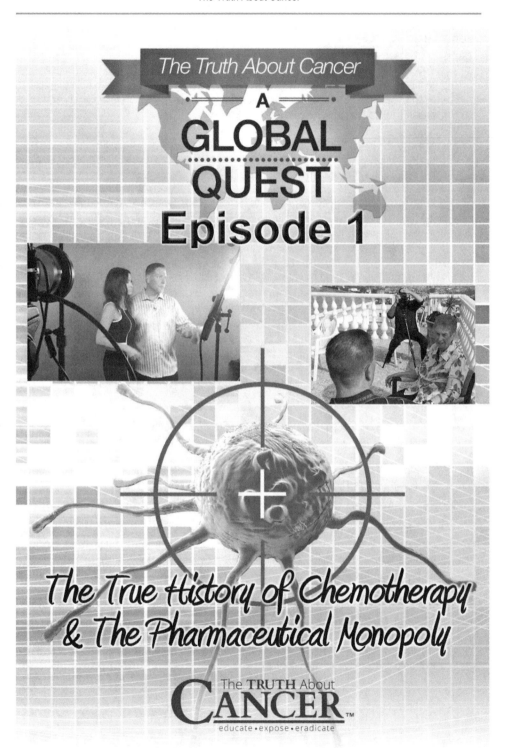

Ty: Welcome to the *Truth about Cancer: A Global Quest.* I'm your host, Ty Bollinger. Many of you may have seen *The Quest for the Cures* last year. We were able to travel across the United States interviewing doctors, scientists, researchers, and cancer patients to learn what they were doing to treat cancer.

It is only because of your support that we have been able this year to travel across the globe and to do over 100 new interviews with top scientists, researchers, doctors and cancer patients that are preventing, treating, and beating cancer.

What you just saw represents less than half of the total interviews that you will see over the next nine days. We traveled the entire globe to gather this lifesaving information so that we can empower you with knowledge. The hard part about this whole process was that I knew I would have to leave my family again.

The difference was that last year when I traveled for *The Quest for the Cures*, it was here in the United States. This year it was global. I was across the ocean from my dear wife and my four children. The consolation for me was that they support me 100 percent. This is our mission together as a family. So knowing that in my heart helped me to leave them again so that we could get this lifesaving information for you.

Please, tell your friends and family to tune in for the next nine days. This information is of vital importance. Dr. Ivars Kalvins, one of the 2015 finalists for the European Medicine Award, explains why.

Dr. Ivars Kalvins: It is calculated that the new generation, the generation of today... from this generation... each second man and each third woman will have this illness... cancer.

Ty: One in two men and one in three women that are alive today are going to face cancer. That's why we, at The Truth about Cancer, are so passionate about our mission to educate, expose, and eradicate cancer once and for all.

In order for us to educate, we felt that it was vitally important that we obtain the most cutting edge information about cancer preventions and treatments and that's why we traveled across the globe. We obtained interviews with over 100 new experts representing over 20 different countries.

A big portion of educating people about the truth is exposing the lies. And that's why, specifically in this Episode One, we're going to be exposing the lies about the history of modern medicine and the history of cancer treatments. So after the next nine days of educating you about the truth and exposing the lies, together we will be one step closer to eradicating cancer once and for all.

But let me ask you a question. Can someone educate someone else about something that they know nothing about?

Dr. Jonathan Wright: They gave us a whole hour on our nutritionals. A whole hour.

Ty: A whole hour.

Dr. Jonathan Wright: In four years of medical school.

Ty: Wow.

Dr. Jonathan Wright: And they told us, "There is vitamin A, and B1, and B2, and C, and D, and they are in alphabetical order and you can look them up." And then they told us some really basic facts. We got a whole hour.

Ty: So how much training did you receive on nutrition when you were in medical school? Because I know here in the States, it's almost none.

Dr. Gaston Cornu-Labat: Yes, not much.

Ty: Not much? Even in Argentina?

Dr. Gaston Cornu-Labat: Not much. It was close to—very little.

Ty: Close to none?

Dr. Gaston Cornu-Labat: Very little.

Dr. Suzanne Kim: Even in medical school they don't teach you—they don't teach you anything about nutrition.

Ty: So you see, doctors, while they're in medical school, they don't learn anything about nutrition. Then when they get out they are heavily influenced by Big Business, just like you and I are.

As a matter of fact, those of you that were alive back then, if you remember, in the 1950s there was a magazine campaign that used doctors to promote cigarettes. There was one ad that I remember seeing that said, "A pack a day helps keep lung cancer away."

The word doctor actually means teacher, so doctors should be educating their patients and teaching their patients. But unfortunately, the only thing that doctors are taught while they're in medical school is how to prescribe drugs.

Dr. Jonathan Wright: We got hours and hours and hours on how to use basically patent medicines which, as you know, are what usually goes on the prescription pad. It's a molecule that can be patented, which means it's not found in nature, because you can't patent it if it's found in nature and that's what we get educated in.

Dr. Irvin Sahni: Because they don't get paid to educate people. They get paid to write prescriptions. And you know, you can imagine the drug lobby made sure that's the case.

Dr. Garry Gordon: A doctor is brainwashed when he gets out of medical school because the medical school has too much subsidization of the professors who are being paid by the drug company. So the professor never teaches any student in medical school, "Why don't you try Vitamin C?" They're going to tell them the latest drug.

Dr. Joseph Mercola: That's by design, specifically. No, and that's by design, specifically. Over a century ago, there were foundations, the Carnegie and the Rockefeller Foundations, who sort of engineered the curriculum through their grants and donations.

Ty: Are you wondering what Dr. Joseph Mercola meant when he mentioned that the Carnegie and the Rockefeller Foundations engineered medical school curriculum over a century ago? He was referring to the Flexner Report of 1910, which we covered in our last documentary. Just in case you missed that important piece of this foundation that we're laying today, here's a brief recap.

You see, if we're going to change where we're going, we need to know where we've been. And that is why history is so important. Because as the old saying goes, "Those who don't know history are doomed to repeat it."

G. Edward Griffin: So I don't need to go any further. You can understand when the money is coming from a source, which has a vested interest in the outcome, now what's going to happen is the outcome is going to be what the donor wants it to be, generally.

So this is the problem. And that goes back even further in time to the turn of the last century when the Rockefeller Group and the Carnegie Group actually came together and they decided that they would "reform" medical education in America.

Dr. Robert Scott Bell: At the time of the late 1800s, early 1900s, 20th century, medical schools taught a lot of different things. There were homeopathic medical schools. There were naturopathic schools, there were eclectic herbal-type medicine schools. And so it was all there. There was not one way. What happened was that the Rockefeller and Carnegie Foundations were interested in establishing the one way.

How would they do that? Well, they would get ahold of the education system and create a medical monopoly by basically eliminating all competition to patent petrochemical medical education. That's the Flexner Report of 1910, as it became known. Abraham and Simon Flexner were hired to do this. It was a preordained commissioned report.

Dr. Darrell Wolfe: Not surprisingly the basis of the report was that it was far too easy to start a medical school and that most schools were not teaching sound medicine. Let me translate this for you. These natural health colleges were not pushing enough chemical drugs manufactured by who? Carnegie and Rockefeller.

The AMA, who were evaluating the various medical colleges, made it their job to target and shut down the larger respected homeopathic colleges. Carnegie and Rockefeller began to immediately shower hundreds of millions of dollars on these medical schools that were teaching drug-intensive medicine.

G. Edward Griffin: By the way, when they donated the money, the donors would say, "Now we've given you a lot of money, and we know you're going to do the right thing with it. But would you object if we had someone from our staff appointed to your Board of Directors. Just to make sure—just to see how our money is being spent?"

Well, that was really a condition of getting the money. So you know the university said, "That would be fine. Anybody that you would suggest would be, I'm sure, more than adequate."

So they began to load up the Boards of Directors of these teaching centers with people who literally were on the payroll of the donors. Once that was in place, the curriculum of the universities, the teaching centers, swung completely in the direction of pharmaceutical drugs and it has remained that way ever since.

Dr. Darrell Wolfe: Predictably those schools that had the financing, churned out the better doctors. Oh, wait a minute. Or should I say, the more recognized doctors? In return for the financing, the schools were required to continue teaching course material that was exclusively drug-oriented with no emphasis on natural medicine.

By 1925, over 10,000 herbalists were out of business. By 1940, over 1,500 chiropractors would be prosecuted for practicing quackery. The 22 homeopathic medical schools that flourished in the 1900s dwindled down to just two by 1923. By 1950 all the schools teaching homeopathy were closed.

In the end, if a physician did not graduate from a Flexner-approved medical school and receive an MD degree, then he or she could not find a job anywhere. This is why today MDs are so heavily biased towards synthetic drug therapy and know little about nutrition, if anything.

G. Edward Griffin: Now this whole medical field has been skewed in the direction of pharmaceutical drugs, which can be patented and produce great profits for the producers. Then the next step is that means that anything coming from nature is excluded, and that's where we think, some of us think, that most of the promise lies. In these very complex substances found in herbs and plants and trees and things like that, seeds. Some of us feel that it was probably meant to be that way.

You come out of all of this analysis and all of this history with the realization that the medical profession is really like a lapdog of the pharmaceutical industry and most of the doctors have no idea that that's the case. They don't understand this history.

Ty: It's so vitally important for us to understand this history if we're going to answer that question, "Why is modern medicine so drug intensive?" It's not because patent petrochemical medicine is superior. It is because of a monopoly medicine, which was created over 100 years ago.

Dr. Aleksandra Niedzwiecki: And the other aspect is also a monopoly on treatment. Only pharmaceutical, conventional medicine is the medicine that is officially approved and acclaimed. And people who try to find other solutions have difficulties when it comes to insurance coverage and other problems. So maintaining a monopoly on treatment is also one of the ways to protect and grow this business.

Dr. Jonathan Wright: And have you noticed that when a new drug comes out and they call it, "a blockbuster drug," they're not talking about, "It cures cancer." They're not talking about, "It's blockbuster for health."

They're talking about how many bucks you can make and that's what it always is. It seems that the number one goal of a lot of health care is to make money. And if we happen to do some good with it, that's fine, but our number one goal is to make money.

Dr. Matthias Rath: Very few know that the birth hour of the pharmaceutical industry is actually a deliberate decision by a handful of people on this side and on the other side of the Atlantic Ocean to define disease as a marketplace and build what has now become the largest investment industry upon that simple thought.

So cancer is just one element of this unspeakable business of defining diseases as a marketplace. Everything else that you see today around the pharmaceutical industry— the tremendous profits, the inability to eliminate diseases, the propaganda war from that side that they are actually making progress in any disease—all of that comes from the fact that it's a business model, an investment industry, that thrives on the continuation of existing diseases and the launching of new diseases.

Ty: Yes, modern medicine is a business. And just like any business, the goal is to grow this business and also to eliminate competition and to maintain the monopoly. Even in 1913, the American Medical Association developed an internal department that they called the Propaganda Department and its main goal was to eliminate quacks. But what exactly is quackery?

In the United States, our first President, George Washington, died as a result of blood-letting and that was an approved treatment of the day. Ignaz Semmelweis was called a quack because he suggested that doctors actually wash their hands before surgery. And physicians today that do not use chemotherapy, they're considered to be quacks.

But very few people know the real history of chemotherapy and its origins.

Dr. Sunil Pai: How we first discovered chemotherapy, the first chemotherapy agents in the early 1940s, was because in Italy, when they dropped nitrogen mustard gas on one of these missions and they were doing the post mortem autopsy of the bodies, the lymphocytes of these patients dropped down.

And then some of these doctors got an idea. "Well guys, if someone has leukemia or lymphoma where these lymphocytes are producing too much, it was suppressed in these people that were dropped with mustard gas." So the chemotherapy agent comes from the history of actually making—

Ty: Mustard gas.

Dr. Sunil Pai: You said it.

Ty: As shocking as this may be, the first chemotherapy agents, and even some of the agents that are still used today, are derived from the mustard gases that were used to kill soldiers in the World Wars. This explains why many people, including myself, would never touch chemotherapy. It's just too darn toxic. But it's not just me. As you're about to learn, and we learned from previous interview, 90 percent of oncologists won't do chemo either.

Dr. Sunil Pai: And there's a study came out that about 90 percent of physicians, particularly in oncology, would not prescribe the drug that they give to their patients to their wife or their child. Right? So what does that tell us?

Dr. Steven Klayman: He's probably not going to do his treatment, why would you?

Ty: In 1971 US President Nixon declared a War on Cancer, but are we really winning this war in light of the fact that 90 percent of oncologists won't even take their own treatment? Is the cancer industry any closer today than they were then in finding a cure? Why is this perpetual war on cancer continue?

Dr. Aleksandra Niedzwiecki: One of the reasons why this war continues is the money that is being made in this war. This refers to the treatments, so called treatments that are being used in cancer, namely chemotherapy and radiation.

Chemotherapy uses the most powerful toxins known to humans and these toxins of course are being sold to us as substances that can kill cancer cells. But these substances also kill, annihilate, healthy cells in the body and damage its organs, which makes the recovery from cancer almost a miracle, impossible.

And also the very substances that are being used to fight cancer are cancer causing chemicals. So instead of eliminating cancer or curbing cancer, we are inducing, generating new cancers.

Ty: That's pretty interesting, isn't it? Maybe one of the reasons that 90 plus percent of oncologists won't do conventional treatments like chemotherapy is that they actually *cause* cancer. Let's listen to Dr. Veronique Desaulniers, who actually cured her own mother and herself of breast cancer, talk about Tamoxifen, which is the most popular drug prescribed to treat breast cancer.

Dr. Veronique Desaulniers: Tamoxifen is a drug that most women are put on when they have breast cancer, but they don't tell them that it is classified as a carcinogen by the American Cancer Society and the World Health Organization. Does it make sense to give women a carcinogenic drug that will cause cancers in other parts of her body to "prevent" cancer?

Ty: That's really shocking, isn't it? Tamoxifen, the number one drug prescribed to treat breast cancer, it actually causes cancer. What about other chemotherapy drugs? Is Tamoxifen alone?

Dr. Ben Johnson: It's estimated that by 2020 more than half of all cancer in America will be medically-induced from drugs or radiation. So our medical establishment itself will soon become the leading cause of cancer in America.

Dr. Rashid Buttar: It's not the cancer that really hurts people. Statistically, 42 to 46 percent of patients will die – that have cancer – will die of cachexia, which is basically wasting of protein. They basically lose all their lean body mass. So that leaves between 58 and 54 percent of patients that didn't die of cachexia. And the joke, which is only maybe half funny, is that the rest of them die from the treatment.

In other words, really nobody dies from the cancer. If you think about it, when a patient gets immunosuppressed and they have cancer, what actually takes them? Liver failure, kidney failure, pneumonia, sepsis—but all these things are usually associated with also the person getting chemo and radiation.

Dr. James Forsythe: Then I went into practice in San Francisco as an oncologist with a group of oncologists that began to notice that my long term survivor list was pretty short. And I began reading in the literature that everyone was, that after five years of chemo, in their own literature they recorded only a 2.1 percent survival rate.

Bob Wright: We know that 97 percent of people who undergo chemotherapy are dead in five years. That study was placed in the 2004 edition of the *[Clinical Oncology] Journal*. It was the cancer doctors telling on themselves.

Do I know this study to be true? It was a massive study done by epidemiologists who themselves were doctors. I interviewed the lead of that study just within the last six months and I said, "Is this still true today? This was published in 2004." And he says, "It's absolutely as true today as it was when we published it back in 2004 and it may be getting worse."

When they tell us that chemo is our only chance, it's the first lie you hear. And then you have the surgery. The second lie is, "We got it all." You can't get it all if you're focused on tumors. You simply can't. The cancer is probably already metastatic. Surgery spills it.

Radiation – proven not to kill the stem cells, but to enhance them. Well we always hear, "Well, the cancer came back." It didn't come back, folks, it just never left.

Ty: But chemotherapy is not only incredibly ineffective, it's also hazardous material.

Dr. Rashid Buttar: Let's look at chemotherapy, for example. Chemotherapy – yes, it can kill cancer cells, possibly. It can kill any cell. Here's the issue that I have with chemotherapy. When I see somebody that is handling chemotherapy, making chemotherapy, and they have to wear hazmat suits and gloves and, you know, "Can't touch it because it's toxic!" Then why are you going to give it to a person who is already sick? Does it make any sense?

You ask a three-year-old child this question, I would bet you that 90 percent of the three-year-old children would get it. "If that looks dangerous then I shouldn't touch it." That's it.

It's almost like sending in napalm because you've got an ant problem. Yes, you'll take care of the ants, possibly, but then you're going to take care of every other form of life, including the grass and you're going to level the site just to try to get the ants. The collateral damage are the people that live there in the same house as the ants, meaning that the normal endogenous healthy cells are also going to get massacred.

Just from a common sense standpoint, does it make any sense to take a therapy – let's use radiation as an example. To take a therapy that we know is dangerous under any circumstance—you break your leg, you break your hand, you go to the hospital, they take you in to get an X-ray, they've got the skull and cross-bones, they've got the universal triangular radiation sign as a warning. Why is there a warning there? You tell me.

Ty: Because it's known that it's harmful.

Dr. Rashid Buttar: And how is it harmful?

Ty: It damages DNA.

Dr. Rashid Buttar: It damages DNA and what is the consequence of damaging that DNA?

Ty: Potentially cancer.

Dr. Rashid Buttar: Bingo! So then why would we take something that we know has a very high propensity to create cancer and use that to *treat* cancer?

Ty: It does seem insane to treat cancer with chemotherapy and radiation that actually *cause* cancer, doesn't it? But doctors are required to do this. As a matter of fact, they suffer adverse consequences if they do not prescribe chemo and radiation. They can even lose their license to practice medicine.

Dr. Grinblat: There was one good doctor who was allowing some natural treatments when the parents were asking to introduce them. But he could not offer it himself, and when I asked him why, he said, "I couldn't do it, I will lose my job."

So it means oncologists here and in many other countries I'm sure, they are very restricted in protocols. They are not free to offer good treatment. They are very restricted in their protocols.

Dr. Joseph Mercola: There are many physicians who are truly, authentically motivated to want to help people. But there is this pervasive fear that they are going to be discredited and ostracized in their own community when they start to embrace some of these alternative philosophies. That's a strategy that is used to suppress this type of information. When you've got tens of billions of dollar of revenue, there is no limit to the clever and sophisticated techniques that you can acquire to manipulate the masses.

Dr. Badakhshan: It's against the law in California for oncologists to recommend integrative.

Ty: Is it really?

Dr. Badakhshan: They cannot tell you, "Go to integrative medicine."

Laura Bond: So unfortunately, doctors in America, Australia, the UK, they can risk losing their medical license if they recommend anything other than the gold standard, which is chemotherapy and radiotherapy.

In my mind those treatments are substandard. We know that chemotherapy and radiotherapy cause cancer, which is the very thing that they're supposed to prevent. I mean, you look on the back of certain chemotherapy drugs like doxorubicin and you'll see a listed side effect is leukemia.

Ty: And doxorubicin is a pretty popular chemo drug.

Laura Bond: Absolutely. And you know as well as I do that the latest research from Harvard Medical School and UCLA is showing that chemotherapy actually stimulates cancer stem cells, which are the germ cells from which new tumors arise.

Ty: Investigative Journalist Laura Bond just mentioned the fact that chemotherapy stimulates cancer stem cells. But what's a stem cell and what does this have to do with cancer? "What is a cancer cell and what does it come from?"

Dr. Russell Blaylock: Well we used to think that any cell could become cancer except for a few limited ones. We thought that if you irritate a cell enough and damage its DNA enough it'll become immortal and just keep growing.

Now we found that's not true. Only stem cells seem to be the source of cancers. Stem cells are cells that haven't decided what they want to be yet. They are very primitive cells so they can be anything – a heart cell, a brain cell, lung cell. So these stem cells are all through your body just sitting quietly.

But if you damage the DNA of the stem cell enough through free radicals or whatever, it will become immortal and then it just keeps producing more and more cells. It wakes up and is producing lots and lots—thousands, millions, billions of cells and it becomes a cancer. But it's the stem cell that's pouring it out. Kind of like a water hose, it's pouring all these droplets of water out.

The trouble with chemotherapy and conventional treatments is they have no effect on the cancer stem cells. They only kill the daughter cells, the cells that are produced by it. So the tumor will shrink and they'll claim success, but you haven't killed the stem cell so it all just comes right back. And what they found is when it comes back, it comes back infinitely more aggressive than it did before.

Ty: And why would that be?

Dr. Russell Blaylock: It's kind of complex chemistry, but it has to do with the chemical changes in what we call the micro environment of the stem cell. What you're doing you're producing a lot of cytokines around those stem cells. These are inflammatory chemicals. Those inflammatory chemicals produce even greater DNA damage so the cancer that comes back is more malignant that the one that started.

What they are finding is, when you treat a patient with chemotherapy and radiation and you don't cure them, then you make the cancer infinitely more aggressive and the patients usually die quicker.

You have a room full of oncologists listening to the latest drug and they'll say, "Oh, this one. We're getting incredible responses with this drug." Well, as they claim, what happens with that incredible response is it causes dramatic shrinkage of the tumor initially because it's just killing the daughter cells.

And some are not even non-malignant cells, but it's not affecting the stem cell. So then the cancer grows tremendously. But they can say, "Oh, we get good response from this chemotherapeutic."

Ty: And when they say, "good response" they mean the tumor shrunk.

Dr. Russell Blaylock: They mean initially it shrinks the tumor, but they don't say, "Well, six months later (or less), it actually is going to grow a lot faster and it is more likely to metastasize."

Dr. Badakhshan: One of the problems with chemo is because when your patient does chemo, those circulating tumor cells, cancer cells that we have, once you have the primary tumor, they can mutate and they become more resistant to other treatments.

Ty: Sayer, talk to us today about chemo and radiation resistance.

Sayer Ji: Okay, great. I feel the word itself is almost like a euphemism for something really terrible, which is that when you are exposed to radiation that's based on gamma radiation, it is basically ionizing, it will cause damage to whatever basic tissue it's being exposed to. So, in the same way chemotherapy is also designed to be genotoxic. You're trying to target fast replicating cells and by doing so, it is by definition also carcinogenic.

Really, when we talk about resistance to chemo and radiation, it's really just a way of blaming the victim because we're all, when exposed to conventional chemo and radiation, we are going to be harmed and it is actually going to have a carcinogenic effect and it will often cause secondary cancers.

Technically, I think people need to be aware that this isn't truly a cancer therapy. At best, it's palliative in the sense that it might shrink a tumor. But really, the main thing I would like to get across is that it is going to cause an enrichment of the actual mother cell that's beneath the tumor, which is known as the cancer stem cell.

Technically you are shrinking the tumor size, but you're enriching the population of the tumorigenic cells at the very same moment. Again, the idea that some people are resistant to chemo and radiation is really a false concept. Everyone exposed to radiation and chemo will have secondary adverse effects, some of which are worse than the original condition they're being treated for.

Ty: Stem cells are the key, and chemotherapy and radiation actually enrich stem cells. Now, we will get back to this topic a little bit later on. But that last statement from Sayer Ji really shook me. *Everyone will have secondary adverse effects from chemo and radiation.*

Despite this fact, as we've already learned, many doctors from countries across the globe might even lose their license if they do not prescribe chemo and radiation. Are you beginning to see the way that Big Pharma has its tentacles throughout this medical cartel? Especially when it comes to chemotherapy?

But that's not all. Chemotherapy also creates side effects that can then be treated with more drugs. Let's listen to Dr. Aleksandra Niedzwiecki elaborate on this issue.

Dr. Aleksandra Niedzwiecki: Chemotherapy business is also a wonderful example of multiplicator. Because the side effects that chemotherapy produces is bone marrow transplants. This is the result of chemotherapy. Bleeding from the intestines that requires drug, anti-nausea drugs, and many others. Changes in the brain. There is even a term for it. It is called "chemo brain" because the chemotherapy affects so many organs in the body and it's the reason for prescribing more drugs. So chemotherapy multiplies the business. This is why it lasts until this day.

Chris Wark: Chemotherapy destroys your army, destroys your immune system. Not only that, it causes secondary cancers in the body. It makes existing cancer stem cells more aggressive, and it causes a host of lifelong, potentially lifelong, damages to the body.

From brain damage, to hearing loss, to neuropathy with loss of the use of your hands and feet, to kidney and bladder damage, bone damage, heart damage, lung damage. It's just total collateral damage from chemotherapy.

A.J. Lanigan: We didn't know 50 or 60 years ago the role that the immune system played like we do today because we didn't have the technology to measure it and identify it.

But today, a person who is paying attention will see more and more medical articles. They'll see more and more stuff come out on the investigative news shows talking about breakthroughs in immunotherapy. And how they are, in fact, tapping and harnessing the immune system to ferret out cancer and kill it in a very specific manner, instead of this global napalming of the body with chemo and radiation. Which, I don't know that it's ever been successful at any level except to provide more money for the administration and, I guess, the folks that are coming out with that.

If the money had been poured into immunotherapy over the last 50 years as it has been these other attempts that ended up failing, I'd have to believe that the results would be a whole lot better. There would certainly have been a lot less suffering. I think anybody who has met or been close to someone undergoing chemo and radiation will admit that it is a suffering instead of a treatment.

Dr. Matthias Rath: In order for having a maximum chance of fighting and overcoming cancer, we need an intact immune system. That, too, makes the current approach of chemotherapy so unethical. It destroys – the chemotherapy – the first organ that is affected, actually the target organ, is the bone marrow.

The destruction of the generation of the defense cells, leukocytes, etc. are built in the bone marrow. From the very onset, from the very planning of chemotherapy from the very scientific approach, it is a deception. It is an unethical, deceptive business that creates illusions for millions of people and every scientist involved in it.

I'm not blaming the doctors because they sometimes don't have the education to go at that length of it. But every scientist knows that it is a huge fraud. Those who say they don't, they should quit the job of being a scientist.

Ty: I appreciate what Dr. Rath just said, that doctors are not educated about this. They don't understand that chemotherapy is a huge fraud, but that every scientist that doesn't understand and admit that chemotherapy is a huge fraud, they should quit the job of being a scientist.

Now, Dr. Rath and A.J. Lanigan, an immunologist, just both addressed the same topic: that the immune system is the key to fighting cancer and to health. One of the interesting things about chemotherapy is that it totally destroys and devastates the immune system.

Another unique thing about chemotherapy that many people don't know is that oncologists can actually make kickbacks from prescribing chemotherapy drugs. This is a unique characteristic to the cancer industry that does not apply anywhere else in pharmaceutical drugs.

Dr. Sunil Pai: Cancer is a big business. It's over $127 billion that is being spent on cancer care. A majority of that is in the pharmaceutical drug costs of the care. The average patient now, according to a study that came out by Kaiser Health last year, was that they spend between $10,000 a month and $30,000 a month. So $10,000 to $30,000 a month just for the chemotherapy agents that they are using.

This price keeps on going up higher and higher, so the average person has a three to four months of treatment. Some people have continuously ongoing treatment so they suppress the cancer, but we're not curing the cancer for example, and that can go up to 12 months or more. They keep coming back for "tune ups" they would say.

Most people don't realize that in cancer treatments that the facility, or more importantly the physician that is prescribing some of these medications, say if the person is a Medicare patient, the Government allows the physician to charge the cost of the drug plus a percentage. Medicare, for example, gives six percent on the cost of the drug as a reimbursement for de facto aspects of overhead costs, whatever it was.

What happens is, if I was a physician and I was in that system for example, I would prescribe a $100 drug, I would get $6.00 back. If I prescribe a $10,000 drug, I get $600 back. Right?

Ty: In other realms that would be called a kickback. But in this realm, since it is legal—

Dr. Sunil Pai: It's a reimbursement.

Ty: It's a reimbursement.

Dr. Sunil Pai: Right. The thing is this is the only field, in oncological care, that gets that type of reimbursement.

Dr. Irvin Sahni: Oncology is an unbelievably lucrative field of medicine especially when you are running the business side of it.

Ty: Oncology is an incredibly lucrative business. Maybe it's because of this fact that we see stories like the story of Dr. Farid Fata in Michigan. He was an oncologist that over the last several years—he was recently convicted of prescribing chemotherapy drugs to patients that didn't need it. Many of whom didn't even have cancer, and sadly, many of whom died from the chemotherapy.

Dr. Irvin Sahni: You know when I hear about this guy, you start thinking about Charles Manson. You start thinking about Ted Bundy. You start thinking about Adolf Hitler, Stalin or any of the many, many people that have hurt large groups of people. Mass murderers, rapists, whatever you want to call them, people that are tyrannical.

This guy in one sense is worse than, say, Adolf Hitler because at least if you were a victim of Adolf Hitler you knew when the SS was coming or you knew when Adolf Hitler was coming, you better run. Or if you're one African tribe attacking another African tribe, when the guys are coming down the road with the machine guns, you know to run.

But in this case you're trusting this person with your life. You are going to him asking for help. And even in cases where people really did have cancer, he was inappropriately continuing to administer chemotherapy to them when they didn't need it or even worse, or just as bad or worse, giving chemotherapy to people who simply didn't even have cancer. To me that's just unbelievable. It really is mind boggling, that someone could be that evil and that greedy.

Mike Adams: He's been sentenced, I believe, to 45 years in prison. But the most disturbing thing about this is not that he was caught and that he has been sentenced to prison. The disturbing thing is that there are hundreds of other cancer doctors out there doing the same thing and they haven't been caught and they get away with so much deception, violating medical ethics, lying to patients.

Most patients never question their doctors because they think the doctor is the sole authority. Most patients don't even get a second opinion. Most patients believe the explanations, the diagnoses that the cancer doctors give them. "Oh, this shadow on this X-ray, this means you have cancer. We have to start now or you're going to die." The fear tactics that these oncologists use are highly unethical and really should be criminal.

It is completely unacceptable that oncologists profit from the treatments that are justified by their own diagnosis. It's kind of like taking your car to a greasy mechanic somewhere that's not very honest and he says, "Well, yeah, your carburetor needs to be replaced or car is going to blow up down the road."

But he's just making that up because he wants the business, and if you believe him, then you're going to have to pay all this money for a procedure that your car didn't need. The same thing happens in the cancer industry every day in America.

Ty: I agree with Mike Adams. As he just mentioned, we must question our doctors, we cannot place blind faith in them. We must be educated and that is why we are on this mission with *The Truth about Cancer* to educate you on these issues.

Why are we addressing chemotherapy at such length? Because you must know the history of chemotherapy. You must be informed about the dangers of chemotherapy if you are going to make an informed decision. Knowledge is power and people are dying because they don't have this knowledge.

It seems to me that the FDA in the United States and the TGA in Australia and other regulatory bodies across the globe should be actually protecting us from chemotherapy drugs and other toxic substances. Burton Goldberg, the voice of alternative medicine, gave us this telling quote.

Burton Goldberg: The agencies that were designed to protect humanity are protecting the industry they are supposed to protect us from.

John Rappaport: Well, any drug that is on the market available through prescription that has serious and widespread adverse effects, as they say, was previously declared safe and effective by the FDA. That's the only reason that drug reached the market. So if, after approval, it suddenly has opposite effects, very dangerous, that's fraud. Fraud at the level of the FDA for not investigating the drug properly or *concealing* the truth.

Ty: And the FDA, on its own website openly admits that 100,000 plus people die each and every year from properly prescribed prescription drugs. What does this mean, the term "properly prescribed prescription drugs?" This means, according to John Rappaport, these are drugs that were previously declared to be safe and effective.

But what does it mean to be declared "safe and effective"? What is the drug approval process that would declare a drug safe and effective?

Sayer Ji: The real interesting thing, Ty, is that what they do is drug companies pour literally a billion dollars into the research needed to get FDA drug approval. That starts with finding lead compounds to produce a synthetic chemical that then they go through phase one, two, three, human trials with. But when they do this, they pour inadvertently a billion dollars or more – all of these drug companies – into looking at turmeric, resveratrol, green tea, and literally thousands of compounds and they find all this research showing it's superior to chemotherapy.

Those studies are there and people don't know about them. But they also can't expect those studies on things you grow in your backyard that cure cancer to receive a billion dollars of capital because the whole game is based on producing a synthetic analog to get a patent, to get FDA drug approval. And then, of course, more than 50 percent of FDA approved drugs, before the patent life expires, get pulled off the market because of the devastation and death that they cause. So the whole system is rigged.

Ty: I would have to agree with Sayer Ji. The system is rigged. But oftentimes so are the articles that would validate the safety and efficacy of a particular drug. Let's listen to Dr. Russell Blaylock as he describes the way that even doctors are duped with ghost-written articles.

Dr. Russell Blaylock: What happens sometimes, in fact it's happening more often than we would like—and there's a lot of stuff being written by the people that look into medical journal articles. But these pharmaceutical companies have written for them "ghost articles" they call them.

And what they'll do they'll get this company that writes articles that look just like beautiful medical articles with all the graphs and charts and numbers and references. They'll write this article without any authors for the study, because they wrote it, and then they'll go to an oncologist that is very well known and say, "Wouldn't you like to put your name on this article? If you do it's going to be in a very prestigious journal – *The New England Journal of Medicine"* or some oncology journal that is very prestigious.

A lot of these people are tempted because this puts their name even further out front. So they'll say, "Yeah, put my name on there." So they'll put a string of names on the article who had nothing to do with writing it, had nothing to do with the study, and they'll end up in a very prestigious journal.

These journals they choose are the ones that affect how doctors behave, how they treat patients. They'll read this article not knowing it's a ghost article and they say, "Gee, they've got tremendous responses and there's hardly any complications."

So they'll order the drug and then they'll tell the patient the same thing they got out of that article. There's hardly any complications, patients are doing very well, and it's a good chance that this could cure you.

Ty: And it's not an independent article.

Dr. Russell Blaylock: It's not an independent article and the doctors have been tricked and the patients have been tricked.

Dr. Robert Gorter: It also briefly was a big scandal, but nobody really paid attention. That the FDA approved about four years ago, approved an antibiotic. The data was submitted by a French company. But it turned out the study was never done.

Ty: Falsified completely.

Dr. Robert Gorter: It wasn't even done.

Ty: This next physician asked that we not show his face, but listen to what he has to say about the way that money has corrupted the drug approval process.

Doctor (Identity Obscured): I was actually groomed to become a person in one of the most successful clinical trials companies in the country. They picked me for medical—this is how it's like *The Firm*—they pick you, they help you through, and then you're supposed to join them. That's what you're supposed to do. You're like "Great, I get to join the FIRM. I get the big car, get the big house, and then you start realizing, once you start to looking at data and how we're manipulating data and this and that. And the are people behind these drugs.

But that's the standard now, right? So I can get any drug passed. I can get any study manipulated. It's a pay to play game. We sat in rooms where we had CEOs of the top companies come in and say, "This is what it is." The FDA would say something like, "It doesn't work."

And then within an hour we can have a phone call with six different universities and statisticians, $3,000 each person to work on two hours of crunching numbers, flip the numbers out, three editorial reviews and then in three months the perception of that has changed. "It's the greatest and best miracle drug ever," although they didn't ever show anything to support it but they make billions of dollars. As long as we put a black box warning everybody makes money.

And the physicians, through no fault of their own, a lot of them are just doing what they are told. But we can go back in history where did we hear that, "I'm just following orders." That's not a good way to do it.

Ty: But falsifying research and producing toxic prescription drugs, that's only the tip of the iceberg when it comes to Big Pharma. Let's have a the listen to Dr. Matthias Rath as he describes the way that three big pharma companies – Bayer, Hoechst, and BASF – they were responsible, directly, for creating the concentration camps of Birkenau and Auschwitz.

Dr. Matthias Rath: We were in Auschwitz because we have a friendship with some of the survivors that are still alive from that time. And since you asked me this question I may just spend a moment on something that is very little known about Auschwitz.

We've been told in the history book it was a camp that was built to annihilate Jewish people and Slavic people and people that the Nazis didn't like in the conquered countries. But what made Auschwitz the mega death extermination camp was actually the decision by Bayer, Hoechst, and BASF to build the largest industrial plant of wartime in Europe. It is called IG Auschwitz, 100 percent subsidiary of Bayer, Hoechst, and BASF.

The plant was eight kilometers long, about five miles long and two miles wide. So it's a giant industrial area. And the Birkenau concentration camp, the huge camp that was featured in *Schindler's List*, in that movie, was a deliberate decision to supply slave labor for the construction of this industrial plant.

So without the interest that we just touched upon that put profits over lives, Auschwitz would never have had this meaning. The decision of Wannsee, which was the decision by the Nazis to exterminate the Jewish people, was taken roughly one year after the decision of IG Farben to build this plant.

So the Nazis used the death apparatus that was already existing because of the slave labor camp being in existence. The chimneys were burning. IG Farben was "taking care" of the sick people. After three months on average, the people were emaciated and so they were just put to the gas chamber and shot up in the chimney.

So I used a few more sentences than normal to exemplify. If we are talking today that there is an industry among humanity that sacrifices millions of lives or puts them at risk for profit—we are sometimes, you included, being attacked as being out of this world, conspiracy people.

Now we turn around, we look at Auschwitz, we look at the industrial plant. We look at the concentration, extermination plant being built, initially built, to serve as slave labor camp for that purpose. And we can say, "They've done it before."

Ty: I'm literally speechless. Millions of Jews were annihilated during World War II and those concentration camps were built by Big Pharma to provide slave labor. As Dr. Rath said, they've done it before, they'll do it again.

We must understand that people's lives once again are being sacrificed for the almighty dollar. Did you learn this in history class? I certainly didn't. But please keep an open mind as we're approaching these subjects. We *must* understand history if we're going to understand the current state of modern medicine.

Dr. Matthias Rath: I'm a German. I didn't learn anything about that. I was 35 years old when I learned about Bayer, BASF, the largest pharmaceutical companies at that time were actually building, or responsible for, the extermination camp at Auschwitz. Then I wanted to know more and there was nothing.

So we finally found in the archives of the US, in Washington, the US National Library [Library of Congress], the records of, case numbers, six of the Nuremberg War Crime Tribunals. We are told that it was only one tribunal against the main war criminals, but in fact there were 12.

Number six was against Bayer, BASF, and Hoechstat the same. At that time they were forming a cartel by the name of IG Farben. And that whole case lasted an entire year against 24 managers of these pharmaceutical and chemical companies. It showed that they were largely financing the rise of the Nazis to power. That they supplied 100 percent of the raw materials so that the Nazis could lead the war including 100 percent of the synthetic gasoline, rubber, 100 percent of the explosives.

The report came to the conclusion, the US prosecutor said, "Without IG Farben, World War II would not have been possible." In other words, we have to redefine history. Even if we talk about cancer today, we need to know those things. That these interests for expanding patented product markets worldwide—they were risking, eventually they were responsible for the death of 60 million people in World War II.

That shows you the dimension of the topic that we are talking about today. There is nothing, absolutely nothing that these interests will not do if the profit is high enough, then and now.

Ty: Did you know that one of the 12 Nuremburg Tribunals was actually against Big Pharma? World War II actually could never have happened without the involvement of big pharmaceutical companies, specifically IG Farben.

Dr. Rath mentioned patents. The cancer industry – yes, it is an industry – is part and parcel with the multinational pharmaceutical companies. And the way that multinational pharmaceutical companies make their money is through patents.

Big Pharma patents drugs and they call that medicine. But do patented molecules, this medicine that they've created, does this have a place in modern healthcare? Or I think maybe the bigger question is, can we, as mortal men, improve on nature?

Dr. Jonathan Wright: Patent medicines do not belong in human bodies and I know I keep saying "patent medicines" and people aren't accustomed to that. They think of the 19th century. I'm sorry, but all the giant pharmaceutical companies are, are holders of patents for molecule after molecule after molecule that is *sort of* like what belongs in the body. Just sort of enough to do something, but enough to cause a lot of damage, too.

So if we're going to be as healthy as we can in the bodies we now have, we have to use only the substance and energy that belongs in the body. It makes no sense using patent medications. Patents are wonderful for certain things, protection of intellectual property rights and so forth, but patents have no place in healthcare.

Dr. Nalini Chilkov: You can't patent nature, which is why we don't get a lot of money for research in plant medicine, but then they'll make a molecule that looks like the molecule from nature and then that pharmaceutical company can own it. But that's not really the same animal.

Mike Adams: You cannot take and isolate every chemical out of a plant and expect that plant to have the same healing powers. This is why chemical cancer medicine fails 97 percent of the time. Whereas plant medicine, being holistic, is safer, it's more efficacious (in other words it works better), it's more affordable, readily available, and you don't have to pay patent fees to Mother Nature.

Dr. Patrick Quillin: Francis Bacon was the founder of the modern scientific principle in 1600. He said, "Nature to be commanded must be obeyed." What we're doing in modern medicine is saying, "We don't care about the rules, we're going to change the rules. We know that you need vitamin D and sunshine, but we're going to say we can't patent that so we're going to try and come up with a drug that bypasses all of those pathways." Nature to be commanded must be obeyed.

Ty: I love that quote from Dr. Quillin, "Nature in order to be commanded must be obeyed." And I think that's where big pharmaceutical companies fail because they try to take nature and maybe a molecule from nature and tweak it and change it, but then it never works as well as the original molecule.

Why do they tweak and change it? So that they can patent it. We've already seen about the greed in this patent medicine industry, this cancer industry. Remember early in the show we talked about the war on cancer. I have a question for you. What if the real war on cancer was actually a turf war aimed at protecting its profits?

Dr. Stanislaw Burzynski: This is a total war. The Texas Medical Board is going after my doctors, is going after my assistants. They are suing everybody because of using the treatment which is non-conventional.

Ty: According to Dr. Burzynski, the real war is actually being fought against doctors who dare to step outside the box and use any kind of non-conventional treatment that is not approved. Dr. Burzynski has been persecuted heavily for decades.

Another doctor that has been heavily persecuted is Dr. Jonathan Wright. His crime? Using natural medicine that was outside of the Standard of Care and was not an approved treatment.

Dr. Jonathan Wright: And on May 6th, 1992 they raided our clinic with guns drawn.

Ty: No kidding?

Dr. Jonathan Wright: No kidding. Yes. They told the King County Sheriff that we were selling drugs. Because remember they called feces a drug and so vitamins are drugs, anything used for treatment is, according to them, a drug. Okay, we were selling drugs. So the King County Sheriff's Office was expecting drug dealers and, they raided with guns.

One of them came in and stuck his gun within a few feet of the receptionist's face. One thing though, they didn't have jack boots. You've heard of the jack boots and all that. They had on regular shoes, and even though they had guns, they wore regular shoes and kicked the doors in with their regular shoes. The doors were locked. You see they had the raid shortly before 9 am. And how do we know they kicked the doors in? Because somebody was sitting outside in a wheelchair waiting for his appointment and he saw these guys come and kick the doors in.

They came in with guns and what do they do? They herded all the employees into a corner of the reception area and they proceeded to start seizing equipment, and medical records, and payroll records, and banking records, and everything. And they told the King County Police it was because we were dealing drugs.

So anyway, that's what they did and they empaneled a grand jury. Eighteen months later, nothing. They empaneled a second grand jury, another 18 months, nothing. No indictments. After the second grand jury failed to return any indictment and the first one did, too, they then announced to the newspapers – not to me, they did not call me or my attorney – they announced to the newspapers they were closing the investigation. And both my attorney and me, we read about it in the newspaper.

Never got the patient records back. Never got the banking records back. We had to reconstruct as best we could on the banking records. On the patient records, we just had to ask people to tell us what they told us before. But no, that never came back.

Ty: So Dr. Wright lost all of his patient records and in the end he was never convicted of anything. This almost sounds like there is a conspiracy, doesn't it? People are afraid to use that term "conspiracy" because people might think you're nuts. But what if I told you that the United States Senate concluded that there was a conspiracy to suppress natural cancer treatments. Would that matter to you?

Now people hear this and they may say, "You know this sounds conspiratorial." Right? You've heard of the Fitzgerald Report. Right?

Dr. Jonathan Wright: I have a copy of some of the conclusions over here. Should I read them to people?

Ty: Absolutely, yes. The Fitzgerald Report. Tell the viewers what the Fitzgerald Report was.

Dr. Jonathan Wright: I'll tell them. Or you can tell them and I'll just read it.

Ty: You go ahead and tell them.

Dr. Jonathan Wright: The Fitzgerald Report was published in the *Congressional Record*, folks, the *Congressional Record*. Actually, it was an appendix to the *Congressional Record*. And Fitzgerald was an investigator for the Interstate Commerce Commission. Now, I'm going to read this because I've got to read you the citations because people will otherwise think it is conspiracy theory.

1953. He was investigator for the Interstate Commerce Commission, a Senator whose grandson had been cured of cancer by natural means, and had a lot of trouble getting that cure done, asked him to investigate. Now here's just one quote. Fitzgerald says, *"My investigation to date should convince this committee that a conspiracy does exist."* This is testimony before Congress by a Chief Investigator for the Interstate Commerce Commission. *"A conspiracy does exist to stop the free flow and use of drugs."* He calls it all drugs because, I'm sorry, but most people in conventional medicine call even vitamins drugs. If it's a treatment, it's a drug.

And you do know that FDA declared stool a drug some two years ago. And then they got so much ridicule from the academic centers that were doing these fecal transplants that they undeclared stool a drug. But for a while, feces was a drug. How do you like that? Anyway, back to Fitzgerald. I know. It just seems weird.

Ty: Insane.

Dr. Jonathan Wright: Okay. *"...to stop the free flow and use of drugs in Interstate Commerce, which allegedly have solid therapeutic value. Public and private funds had been thrown around like confetti at a country fair to close up and destroy clinics."* Notice he uses the word *destroy*.

What he's talking about is the occasions when an FDA went in with sledgehammers and broke up Royal Rife equipment in the office of Dr. Ruth Drown where they made someone throw all of his books that he had written on one aspect of energetic medicine. They were all burned in a bonfire in New Jersey.

Book burning. Sledgehammers. Now Fitzgerald didn't say that. You can find that other part. I'll go back to Fitzgerald, but that's what he means by "destroy." That's why he used the word "destroy." Okay. *"To destroy clinics, hospitals, and scientific research laboratories, which do not conform to the viewpoint of medical associations."*

It's got nothing to do with the law, it's got to do with a viewpoint of medical associations. *"Benedict Fitzgerald, Benedict S. Fitzgerald,"* excuse me, *"Junior Special Counsel, United States Committee on Interstate Foreign Commerce, 1953."*

And his report goes into a pages-long report of suppression of natural treatments and it's in the *Congressional Record*. And did anybody ever do anything about this? No. And part of what he says in that report is that the collusion, the actual conspiracy, is between *Los Federales* at FDA, the patent medicine companies, and the AMA. That's where the conspiracy that Fitzgerald identifies is.

Ty: The Fitzgerald Report of 1953 which concluded "there was an active conspiracy to suppress natural cancer treatments in the United States" was due to the suppression of laetrile. More suppression of laetrile followed over the next couple of decades.

Dr. Joseph Mercola: First of all what is laetrile? Laetrile is also called amygdalin and vitamin B17. And there actually have been investigations showing that it has some benefit to the use of treatment of cancer, and it may be because cyanide is a component of laetrile and that may also be a nutritional deficiency. It provides some benefits that are nutrients that the body needs to fight these malignancies.

But anyway, there was a Japanese researcher at Sloan Kettering who was studying this and Dr. Ralph Moss was an investigative journalist there at the time and he started covering it. He appeared to have beneficial results, but then for some unbeknownst reason the information was suppressed and that information was not allowed to be disseminated and Dr. Moss wrote extensively about it.

It was about mid-1970s. I'm not sure how beneficial laetrile is. I have no experience with it, but it is an interesting example of how this type of—these alternative approaches are routinely suppressed when they are opposed to the traditional, conventional approaches. Because there is such a significant amount of funding that is involved.

The big agencies, the FDA, of course, the AMA and American Cancer Society which are all in some way influenced by the drug cartels. They are funded to oppose these and essentially classify them as quackery. It's a common strategy that is used for many alternative treatments. Laetrile being one of the earlier ones where they targeted, but there are dozens and dozens since then.

Dr. Stanislaw Burzynski: There is merciless harassment by the authorities of doctors who are inventors. So now in going through three years of harassment by Texas Medical Board. And one of the reasons why I am going through this is I use a treatment which is not standard treatment for pancreatic cancer.

I use this for the type of incurable lung cancer, like malignant mesothelioma, the patient is surviving now five years. He would be dead a long time ago. And these results were evaluated by outside oncologists. Amazing results, okay? I am being harassed because the Texas Board is saying, "You use a treatment which is not standard."

Dr. Rashid Buttar: If you do the Standard of Care and you give chemo and people die, it's okay. If you don't do the standard care and people live, that's not okay. It is politically incorrect. So this is the amazing thing: you take a poison, you give it to people, they die, it's part and parcel of the normal status quo or modus operandi, this is how it's supposed to be.

Now you break that. You actually do something that's not toxic, you help patients, they live. "Hey. We don't care whether the patient lives or not. That's irrelevant, it's not part of the Standard of Care.

Dr. Tullio Simoncini: The risk of reprisal, the risk of the jail, and the persecution. It is unbelievable. They tried to shut me down in any way. Yes. Because, you know—tell me one big revolutionary discovery that it was not shut down. Tell me one. There is no chance, no possibility to escape. Because when you see something that is very new and people cannot think about it, you are persecuted because you destabilize all the system. So any discovery, big, true discovery, makes the old system useless. That's why you are shut down. Because we live in a medieval status. This is the real reason why cancer is still killing millions of people.

Dr. Stanislaw Burzynski: It's not easy to treat these advanced patients because you are continuously being harassed for doing this. It is incredible. We should be rewarded. We should be set as the example. We are saving the lives of people who have been sentenced to die. No! We are unmercifully harassed by lawyers, by people who know nothing about treatment, who are stupid puppets of the guys behind who know very well what we can offer, whether they're acting these guys like in Nazi Germany and they are simply obeying orders because they are programmed this way.

I think maybe with time they will do some type of Nuremburg trials. All of these white collar nicely dressed lawyers and clerks who are chewing the money of taxpayers may be held accountable for what they do. Because many people died because of their actions. They do it secretly. They are not exposed. That feel that they are beyond any punishment and they can continue to do this type of work.

Dr. Rob Verkerk: If you look at someone who has cancer—and you've had for a long time in Europe this notion that, if you're using a natural approach, you run the risk as a doctor of having your license revoked. If you're a nonmedical practitioner, you can be basically put into jail as the Cancer Act 1939 in the UK to deal with you.

This is utterly wrong because an individual that has cancer is just another individual whose body needs nourishment and support more than a person who is healthy. And yet to have that denied to those individuals is a real loss of fundamental rights of freedoms and that needs to be changed.

Ty: It's a crime.

Dr. Rob Verkerk: It is a crime, indeed.

Dr. Stanislaw Burzynski: Maybe we need to be awakened because, obviously, this is killing people.

Ty: If you withhold treatment that can save someone's life, isn't that the same thing as murder? I would have to agree with Dr. Burzynski and Dr. Verkerk. But this is not the only time that the medical industry has been guilty of conspiracy against natural physicians.

Dr. Patrick Vickers: In 1987 four chiropractors from Illinois, particularly Chester Wilk – he was the head chiropractor that took the AMA to court – they actually took the entire American Medical Association to court. Accusing them of having a branch within their organization designed to eliminate chiropractic as a profession, a licensed profession they were trying to eliminate through the use of propaganda.

A Federal District Court judge in Illinois, Susan Getzendanner, in 1987, found the AMA guilty of conspiracy. That was the judgment. So if anybody tells you when you're talking about these things, "Oh, you're just a conspiracy theorist," you can lead them straight to the Wilk versus the AMA, the court ruling of 1987, and the judgment was *guilty of conspiracy*.

Ty: Are you beginning to get the picture here? This is *not* conspiracy theory, this is conspiracy fact according to the courts. Now, why are we sharing this with you? Because you must understand the belly of this beast if you're going to believe the truth.

One of the many victims of this conspiracy to suppress natural cancer treatments is a man named Jason Vale. Last year I had the privilege of interviewing him and he shared with me the true story of how he was arrested, convicted, and spent five years in federal prison – not for murder or rape or assault – but for selling an unapproved cancer treatment, namely apricot seeds, which contain laetrile, on his website.

But Jason is not alone. Almost 80 years ago a scientist named Royal Raymond Rife faced jail time for using an unapproved treatment.

R. Webster Kehr: In the 1930s, Royal Rife, Dr. Royal Rife who was a microbiologist, knew that there were microbes inside the cancer cells. And he came up with an electro-medicine device, a couple of them actually, which was designed to do nothing but kill the microbes inside the cancer cells.

Dr. Jonathan Wright: He did something very smart, taking from Einstein the cue that everything has its own vibratory frequency – molecules do, people do, everything has its vibratory frequency. He determined the vibratory frequency of those microorganisms and then he sent in a beam, which is why the machine is called a beam ray – he sent in a beam that had a dissonant frequency.

What's that? Have you ever tried to tune your radio and you tune it just right and it's nice and clear, crystal clear, but you go a little bit off and it's (making buzzing sounds) in addition to the talk? That's dissonance. You are almost on the right frequency, but not quite.

So he sends in a dissonant frequency that is *almost* what these bacteria do, but they can't stand that because they are vibrating and are really close. So basically they rupture and die, all the bacteria do. He beamed them, and the cancers were cured.

Now, it's more complicated than that. He had to follow certain doses of rays and certain days and so forth, but the cancers were cured and it was celebrated in the *Los Angeles Times*.

He reports that he was visited by two people, one being Morris Fishbein of the AMA, who was President at the time, and another person. I believe him because I have read that same report in a doctor's book from Alabama who was curing cancer with intravenous hydrochloric acid. I'm not kidding you, it's published for three years, I've got all of his reports.

He was visited by two men from the AMA saying that he should sell them his treatments or he would never be published again. He refused to sell and he was never published again. I have the three years' worth of reports. I can't get any more, there weren't any more. Rife had the same visitation and so did other cancer-treating practitioners. Visitations from AMA telling us, "You sell us your stuff or we'll do you."

R. Webster Kehr: He developed this technology. The American Medical Association tried to buy him out and he refused because he did not trust them. Good for him. So the Food and Drug Administration went down and destroyed his laboratory, his equipment, and destroyed all of his inventory.

Ty: In the end, Dr. Rife's lab was burned, his records were stolen, his life was ruined, and he eventually died of a drug overdose.

Harry Hoxsey is another example of a man who was treating and curing cancer naturally that was heavily persecuted. Now, this is a story that is near and dear to my heart because in 1996 when my father, Graham Bollinger, was diagnosed with stomach cancer we were doing everything that we possibly could to take him to what is called the Hoxsey Clinic in Tijuana, Mexico.

Unfortunately, Dad died before we could get him to the Hoxsey Clinic, which is now called the Biomedical Center. That's why it was so exciting to me and *The Truth about Cancer* Team to travel to Tijuana, Mexico and visit the Biomedical Center to learn more about Harry Hoxsey's Treatment, which is still being used there. It's called the Hoxsey Tonic, and the rest of that protocol.

Another exciting thing for me personally was to be able to meet Liz Jonas. Now, Liz Jonas is the sister of Mildred Nelson, and Mildred Nelson was Harry Hoxsey's Chief Nurse.

Liz Jonas: I'm Liz Jonas and my sister was Mildred Nelson. I have no medical background. Mine is business. Mildred was the medical one in our family.

My mom had cancer – ovarian and uterus – and they had planted radiation in her body and burned her very bad and then told her to go home and die. My dad heard about Harry Hoxsey who was in Dallas, Texas and we lived in Jacksboro, which is about 90 miles. So my dad called my sister. She was the oldest in our family. There were seven of us and asked her to come drive for him. He was an old-timey rancher.

She said, "What are you going to Dallas for?" She said, "To get parts for the tractor?" And he said, "No. I'm taking your mother to the doctor." So she came and drove. And through the day, Hoxsey found out she was a nurse and offered her a job. And my dad told him, "No, she doesn't want to work for you. She thinks you're a quack."

He offered for her to go look in all his files, but she didn't. She couldn't talk my mother and daddy out of this, so she decided to go to work for him to prove he was a quack and to save her mom. Our mom lived to be 99 years old.

Ty: What a great story. Liz's sister, Mildred Nelson, wanted to prove that Harry Hoxsey was a quack. But she ended up becoming his chief nurse and their mom lived to be 99 years old. Now the head of the AMA at that time was Morris Fishbein. He was the same man who was head of the AMA when Royal Raymond Rife was destroyed. And the AMA wanted to buy out the Hoxsey Formula. The almost signed the paperwork, but...

Liz Jonas: They got to the point of signing the papers and he said, "You have to make this available to everybody." And they said, "We may not make it available to anybody. We may not use it even." And he said, "No, then I won't sell it."

Ty: So they basically wanted to buy it and bury it.

Liz Jonas: Bury it, yes.

Ty: Harry was arrested numerous times.

Liz Jonas: Numerous.

Ty: What were the charges?

Liz Jonas: All different kinds. Just whatever they came up with, you know. But the patients sometimes—he always carried a roll of bills in his pocket with him, a big roll of bills. And he made his money, in my understanding, in penny stock, all. Penny stock.

But he carried a big roll of bills with him and sometimes he'd bail himself out. Sometimes he'd just stay in jail. The patients would come and bring food and they would circle the whole block. So they would just let him out to get rid of the patients.

Ty: Wow! If that's not a testimony to Harry and the treatment, then nothing is. So the patients would surround the jail.

Liz Jonas: Yes. Surround the jail. Can you imagine?

Ty: No, I can't. I mean not today. But this was back when, 40s, 50s?

Liz Jonas: In the 40s. But his patients were very loyal to him because the AMA and FDA, if they would find out they were going to mail medicine to a patient and they would be standing at the patient's door and take the medicines so the patients couldn't have it.

When Mildred moved the clinic to Mexico, he told her, he said, "You have to drop the Hoxsey name." And she said, "I can't do that." And he said, "Yeah, you have to. That's what they're after. They are mad at me. They're after me."

So that is where the Biomedical came in. But then the patients wouldn't drop it. We're still known as the Hoxsey Clinic. And that's what we're put on this earth for.

Ty: It is.

Liz Jonas: Really. If you really stop and think about it, we're supposed to help each other.

Ty: That's right.

I have to agree with Liz. One of the main reasons that we are put here on earth is to help other people and I commend her and the doctors there at the Hoxsey Clinic, the Biomedical Center, for doing this. One of the doctors there at the Biomedical Center that we interviewed, was Dr. Elias Gutierrez. Here is some of his interview.

Dr. Elias Gutierrez: Basically, what everything spins around is what is known as the Hoxsey Formula. It's a liquid made with a combination of several herbs and minerals. And because of the way that it's put together, it's selectively targets only the malignant cells. Any cell with bad DNA or bad metabolism, those are the ones that are going to be destroyed.

Of course, there's a few vitamins. There is diet, which is not a difficult one to follow and we also use a lot of herbal, both occidental and Chinese herbal formulas.

Ty: The formula that you're using, is this pretty much the same formula that Harry Hoxsey used 80-100 years ago?

Dr. Elias Gutierrez: Exactly the same. It was passed down from Hoxsey over to Mildred and then Mildred brought it into the clinic and then she passed it on to Liz who is the owner now. She is Mildred's sister. And we still use basically exactly the same formula as it was being used in Texas.

Ty: So if somebody comes into the Hoxsey Clinic here and they want treatment, how long does treatment typically last?

Dr. Elias Gutierrez: This is a clinic that does something in a different way than most of the regular things. We try to do everything on a single day. People come in in the morning. They get registered. They go through the laboratory, they go through the X-rays, they get their consultation, a very thorough physical examination.

And then we have to wait until we get the reports from the laboratory X-rays, which takes a couple of hours. And then we call the people up for a second visit in the afternoon and we explain all the findings to them. We give them their instructive, their treatments, and they just pick up their supplies and make their payments and go home.

This is something you can do at home. You don't have to be necessarily hospitalized to do it. They stay on the diet and they come back for a checkup every three, every six months, every year. Eventually they just come back every two or three years.

Ty: Being a one-day treatment, the Hoxsey Treatment is relatively affordable?

Dr. Elias Gutierrez: I think so. And we're the cheapest clinic in town.

Ty: Are you really?

Dr. Elias Gutierrez: Oh yeah.

David Olson: Eight and a half years ago, back in August of '06, I couldn't lay down. As a matter of fact Zack was with me on a motor car trip on the railroad. The seat belt starting hurting on the way back from the trip. We went about 300 miles, and the seat belt started feeling tight. The next week I had another trip and coming back the seat belt was also tight. And shortly after that I couldn't lay down.

I went to Mayo Clinic and was diagnosed. The first time they said I didn't have cancer and in a two week period they found out I did have cancer pretty bad and it was non-Hodgkin's lymphoma. I had it in the esophagus, the liver, the kidney, lymph nodes all under the arm and in the groin. I had a tumor bigger than a volleyball in the stomach and then in the bones, Stage 4. And the doctor gave me three days to three months.

One doctor says, "You know the last guy we treated like you made it three days." So it was not a very good forecast. The day I found out that I had it in the bones, I found out about it at two o'clock up on the tenth floor of the Rochester Mayo Clinic, at the Gonda Building.

Things looked very bleak. On the way, after we left Rochester, for instance, we had to be at a flight in Minneapolis at four o'clock that day and didn't find out till after two and we made the plane by 13 minutes to get down here.

It's just no chance of living afterwards. But here it's been eight and a half years later and I've not had cancer for eight years and three months. They have not found it. The Mayo Clinic could not find, they haven't found it here. There is no cancer that is visible anymore.

We started at the Mayo Clinic, had 13 doctors at Mayo Clinic. And they gave me the same forecast of three days to three months. And I went up to the University of Minnesota and then to Fairview Hospital and Masonic Cancer Center.

I received a death sentence from 17 doctors, and the 18th one that was down here, Dr. Gutierrez, and it was no big deal to him. It was bad, yes, but nothing special. And, as far as I know, I was taking more medicine, more tonic than any other patient I ever talked to so far. I've talked to a lot of patients that I have sent down here and other patients.

I was taking the strongest dose they had, but I never missed a day of work. It never affected my ability to do whatever, but it made the total difference in life. And this life is fantastic. I mean, I've got three grandsons, but the only one that can come with me once in a while, the other two are very busy.

This one here gets to come with me. We do a lot of things together including come down for Jeep rides and stuff. We would never have been able to have that if I hadn't been here so I could get some help, a lot of help. Life. Life is great. Life is great.

Ty: What an encouraging story from Dave who has been cancer free now for eight years due to the Hoxsey Formula, and who was told by 17 traditional doctors that he had no hope and that even the toxic chemotherapy drugs couldn't save him.

I want to be clear. We are *not* saying that everyone that works in the medical industry, the cancer industry, or the pharmaceutical companies are bad people. Not at all, that is not what we're trying to say.

There are a lot of *good* people that are working in the medical industry, the cancer industry and for those at alphabet agencies, even the FDA. We're not criticizing everybody that works for those agencies.

What we are saying in this documentary, and we're trying to communicate this fact, is that the entire medical system has been hijacked. If a plane is hijacked it is not the pilot's fault that it's hijacked. In the same manner, the fact that the medical industry has been hijacked is not your doctor's fault that that's happened.

The fact that the pharmaceutical companies, their sole purpose is to make money. That's not the fault of any person that works for the pharmaceutical companies. The sales reps and other people that work for those companies, it's not their fault. We want to be clear that we communicate that.

The problem is that *the system* is broken. Money is driving the decisions of the people that are the leaders in those industries and not the health of the people that take their products. The number one goal, for big pharmaceutical companies at least, is shareholder profits. They are publicly traded companies and the bottom line is their bottom line.

Over the course of our travels, we were privileged to meet a couple of people that had previously worked for pharmaceutical companies. But once they realized that the number one driving force behind those decisions in Big Pharma is making money and not necessarily getting people healthy, both of them got out, to their credit.

Dr. Subrata Chakravarty: I would hear a lot in our meetings and the town hall meetings that it was all about making the shareholders happy. And I'm like, "You know what? I don't want to make the shareholders happy. That's not the point of what we are doing. We want to be able to solve bigger problems than to see how much money goes into the shareholders' pockets."

Tara Mann: In 2011, I just, kind of by chance, found a documentary and the title caught my eye. It was called *Dying to Have Known*. It was one of the documentaries about the Gerson Therapy. I remember watching it. It was almost stages when I was watching the video.

First it was, "What in the world are they talking about?" They were talking about people that had late stage cancer and they had somewhere to go and they were surviving. And I'm like, "I have never heard of this." So I keep watching and, as a pharmaceutical representative, the doctors teach us very well that we practice evidence-based medicine.

Ty: Right.

Tara Mann: Evidence-based medicine. So I'm watching it and I'm thinking, "This all sounds really good, but I wonder what kind of evidence they have." So they switched to the physician and, I believe it's China that is doing the Gerson Therapy, and I just remember him sitting in front of this huge filing cabinet. And the person that was interviewing him told him, "Just pick files." And he just started opening these drawers of all these files of patients, all this evidence.

All this evidence. So I'm going, "Wow. How is this possible, there is evidence?" Then the documentary goes on to talk about Max Gerson, the way that the therapies were suppressed. And that—I remember sitting up on the couch, on the edge of the couch like… You know, it was like the band aid being ripped off, that moment of just disbelief.

My whole life. My mother's a nurse. I mean, we grew up at the doctor's office and at the nursing home. I had no idea. I worked in a hospital, I was a phlebotomist. I worked in a lab. My whole life was medicine. And so it was just shocking in a really impactful way, immediately. Immediately it changed my life.

So I wanted to research, but I really thought that my research would disprove it. I thought, "This is really awesome, but it's hard to believe." So I started researching and I felt really strange. I felt like I was alone and I'd go to work every day in this industry and I'm thinking, "Do they know this? Do they know what I know?"

Ty: Now to her credit, Tara Mann used to make a ton of money working for big pharmaceutical companies. But once she realized that they weren't healing people, that they were actually harming people, she got out. And then she and her husband Steve began a nonprofit called Cancer Crackdown. That's one of the charities that we at *The Truth about Cancer* are happy to donate to.

Tara just mentioned the Gerson Therapy. We will learn a lot more about the Gerson Therapy in Episode Eight so be sure that you tune in for that one. But in the meantime, we are about to hear of some telling quotes from doctors about the absurdity and the arrogance of trying to force treatments on people against their will.

Dr. Gaston Cornu-Labat: If I tell you, "You have to do this," which is very typical of conventional medicine, "You have to do this." There is a degree of arrogance in that statement. "This is what you need." Given the complexity of the human experience, for me to presume that I know what you need, that is a tremendous arrogance. That's common in medicine, it's very common. "This is what you need to do, and if you don't do it of course, I'll force you. I'll have somebody force you." And that happens, we know that.

We know that when somebody doesn't choose for their kids the exact path, we'll have somebody enforcing that so that they choose that because that's what they need. Oh my God, what arrogance. What a humongous arrogance.

Mike Adams: It was best called by John Rappaport, a "scientific totalitarianism." I think it's a great term for it. Some people call it "medical fascism." It means that the so called science, which is really just corporate driven fraudulent science, but the so called science-driven medicine is being forced upon you now in absolute violation of the American Medical Association's Code of Medical Ethics, which says that the patient must be given the choice. The patient must be informed. They talk about informed consent.

This is supposed to be a pillar of the ethical practice of medicine in the United States of America and really all around the world. That is now being stripped away. Parents are being told, "You *must* submit your children to these interventions whether you like it or not." That's a violation at every level, of human rights, of human dignity, of parental rights.

Chris Wark: Parents need to know and they need to prepare because if you are in a situation as a parent and your child is diagnosed and you don't want them to have chemotherapy, you need to prepare to run. Because if not, they are going to come take your kids.

Ty: Was Chris Wark exaggerating? Will the government really come and take your children?

Jay Matthews: I'm a pharmacist by my profession, so I have been practicing now for about 20 years. When my daughter was diagnosed about three years ago, we decided the whole treatment was just huge and barbaric and the options were just very limited. I think I ran that by you at that time. The prognosis was less than 20 percent, amputation was almost definite.

When the swelling happened, that was mistake number one. We went to the emergency room. At that point I thought, "Well, look, if they didn't have significant successes with that…" And I thought that in an ethical standpoint if you don't have very much you shouldn't be doing that much. That's what I thought.

I didn't think that they would pursue such an aggressive means to get it. At that point, the doctor was – again, depending on who you get – we had a physician that was very stubborn and thinks that he has all the answers, didn't know anything about what we were approaching.

Ty: They kept Selena.

Jay Matthews: Selena. They had armed guards at that point because they knew where my mind was at.

Ty: They had armed guards in the room.

Jay Matthews: In the room. They knew where my mind was at because my mind was to take her back to the facility of my choice. And a facility that would give her a chance at having some sort of a normal life.

They came with their lawyers and they said, "If you don't sign consent, we're going to take custody of the child. You're going to lose custody of the child." Ultimately, the judge said, "You're not an expert, he is." The oncologist, he's the expert. There's nothing he can do and the custody was given to the state.

Ty: So they took custody of Selena.

Jay Matthews: Correct. And then they started aggressive chemotherapy at that point. This is documented. They knew that but they continued with the chemo. And I think that any adult would have been just saying, "Hey, look. My arm's deteriorating, every dose you give my arm is opening up. It's just opening up and the wound is getting bigger."

I pleaded with the physician. I had no way of even getting second opinions at that point because the State's got custody. Nor can I go to her physician and say, "This is wrong, you've got to take a look at it." Because they wouldn't approach us because we don't have custody. "You're not the legal custodian."

Ty: You don't have custody of your own child.

Jay Matthews: Correct.

Ty: The State of Illinois did.

Jay Matthews: The State of Illinois. So I pleaded with him. I said, "The arm's not going to stand it. It's not going to make it." And every time, a bunch of about eight white coats come into the room, look at her wound getting bigger and bigger with every dose. As much as I pleaded with them, as much as they saw. The wound got so big, got infected with MRSA.

They didn't need all these cultures at that point. And the wound, if you see it, it's horrific. It's so graphic you will not believe that's a human arm, the way that it deteriorated over time. It was just incredible. It was graphic for her. That's post-traumatic stress for her. For us certainly it is.

Then in the end, an amputation was required. After that point we still didn't have custody after the amputation for another six months. We have custody of her now. We have custody now. We had the best insurance and I think, really, it's the worst thing you can have. We had the best insurance. To have the best insurance means every drug that is covered will be used and was used. Every drug that wasn't covered...

I mean, he would have used Avastin. Avastin is another $400,000 drug. He would have used it if it was covered, but ultimately I was in a position where I could have dropped her from my insurance. The State didn't pay for it. All this $2.2 million was paid out to the hospitals.

Ty: $2.2 million.

Jay Matthews: Yes, $2.2 million and it was all paid from *my* insurance.

Todd Jones: It's something where everything just blurs. Your energy leaves your body, you're in shock. It's traumatic and you just look at each other and you don't know what to say. I called my boss. I was supposed to be at a trade show and I was bawling. I said, "Man, we just got some bad news."

But after the first month, and I shared this with you too, we made a decision that we wanted to—since the cancer was so far down and in remission as they say, and they told us themselves. That we were like, "Okay. You know what? Thank you for your business. We're good now. We're going to go ahead and build her up naturally now that the cancer and half of her system has been "chemoed," chemically cleansed, we're going to go in and put in the natural good stuff now and see how we can get her to respond there."

Well, the hospital didn't like that. When that happened, it wasn't three days later and there was that very, very, very loud aggressive knock at our door. I'm thinking, "That doesn't sound like anybody I know. Nobody knocks like that." It almost sounded like a boot.

So I went to the door and it was the Office of [Children's] Services and they came and they said, "Look, the hospital called. You have taken your child out of treatment and you need to bring your child right back to treatment."

I'm like, "Well, we're finished with that treatment. We're just going to continue on with another treatment." Right? I'm the parent. I even looked up the Alaska statutes. Parents have a legal right to decide how their children get treated. What I didn't know is it doesn't matter what the statutes say, and the administrative truth about that is that the child is a ward of the State.

Cassandra Callender: The Department of Children and Families was called because we were wasting time according to the doctors. They wanted me in for chemotherapy a week after my biopsy was done at Hartford and they came in and they took me because they said that I had to get the chemo.

Ty: What do you mean when you say, "they took you?"

Cassandra Callender: They came into my house in October around Halloween and they said that I had to go with them.

Ty: And who is "they?"

Cassandra Callender: The DCF workers.

Ty: Okay. They actually came into your home and took you from—

Cassandra Callender: Yes. They had about 12 police squad cars surrounding my house and the block and they basically just came into my house and said, "We have to go." My mom wasn't even home. I was hiding in my closet upstairs because I had no idea what was going on.

Ty: Were you the only one at the house?

Cassandra Callender: Yes. I called my mom crying and she came home immediately to police and DCF workers surrounding our house. After about two weeks of being in the hospital, going through courts and judges, they got the order that they could force me to do the chemotherapy.

At that point I was in the hospital. I couldn't leave my room. There was a guard sitting outside of my door. I couldn't use my phone. I couldn't contact my mom. Basically, it came down to one morning they came in and they strapped me to the bed and they sedated me for surgery.

Ty: Really.

Cassandra Callender: Yes, because you have to have a port to have chemotherapy, which is why I have a scar.

Ty: And you didn't want a port.

Cassandra Callender: No, because I didn't want the chemo and the idea of having an object inside of me grossed me out and so they came in to insert an IV and I said, "No." So they had to have the officers and the security guards and the staff come in. And they brought in a bed that had straps and they had to tie me down by my wrists and my ankles.

And a woman came in and they put a needle in my neck to knock me out and the next thing I knew I woke up and I was in the recovery room.

Dr. Rashid Buttar: Well, I would like to know how is that any different from Nazi Germany, when people were put into concentration camps and experimented on or forced to do certain things? I don't know what the difference is. Because we live in the United States, the land of the free, the home of the brave, so that makes it different?

It's amazing to me that the entire population of the United States doesn't know about this and the reason they don't know about it is because it's shushed up by the media. Nobody wants to talk about it. But this is no different than what was done in Germany or when people are basically raped and pillaged. To me that's the same thing.

Mike Adams: This is unacceptable. This is incompatible with a free society. And frankly the doctors that engage in that kind of activity and the hospital staff that strap people down and force chemotherapy into these children, they should be arrested. They should go to jail just like this other oncology doctor who's serving 50 or 45 years in prison now.

Dr. Rashid Buttar: When people allow a government to dictate the foods they put in their mouth and the medicines they take into their bodies, their souls will soon be in the same sorry state as those who are ruled by tyranny. As much as I would like to take credit for that phrase, that was uttered by Thomas Jefferson over 250 years ago.

Dr. Matthias Rath: We talked about concentration camps. They are surrounded by a fence. If someone tries to escape, the fences of the modern concentration camp, the ones that confine the cancer patient within the perimeter of conventional thinking, of chemotherapy thinking, they are being hunted.

How many court cases have been filed around the world for withdrawing custody of parents who went into natural health as opposed to staying within the confines, within the fences, of conventional chemotherapy treatments?

It's nothing else. The dimension of a child dying in a concentration camp or dying from leukemia that is being intoxicated by chemotherapy as opposed to choosing natural paths are the same. The parents are losing a child. The family is losing their future.

That's the deeper dimension of what we're talking about. That the same interest groups that have proven again and again in the past, namely the pharmaceutical investment business, how ruthless they are, are still around trying to fool us. Trying to tell us, "Well, believe us." Why should we?

If we don't have the courage to liberate ourselves, then we will not make progress among all diseases. The one disease that the status quo, meaning the pharmaceutical, the investment business, needs most to continue its business, to stabilize, to cement its system... is cancer.

They can afford to allow, let's say, advances in osteoporosis that decrease the number of bone fractures without major damage to its future existence. They can't allow progress in this and that disease to mask their principle business. But they cannot allow, they cannot allow cancer to disappear or be identified as a disease that can be regulated or prevented.

Long ago, they have initiated what Dr. Niedzwiecki mentioned, the fact of fear. In fact, it's more than that. It's a psychological warfare on humanity that the pharmaceutical industry is leading with the tool of cancer. Keeping cancer as a death verdict is the platform, is a precondition, for this entire investment industry to continue.

Ty: Big Pharma may need this cancer investment industry to continue so that the money keeps flowing in, but our goal with *The Truth about Cancer* is exactly the opposite. We want to eradicate cancer once and for all. That's why we've shared these truths with you today. Maybe they've been a little bit difficult to believe, but they are the truth.

Has your perspective changed on this? I hope that it has because the perspective that most people have when they hear "cancer" is that cancer is a death sentence and our message is exactly the opposite. Cancer is not a death sentence. There's always hope.

Pamela Kelsey: My name is Pamela Kelsey. I was diagnosed with cancer of the pancreas in 1975. I was told that I had a year and a half to live, at the most. If I did chemotherapy, possibly chemotherapy, radiology, the different treatments that conventional medicine has. I chose not to do that after finding out about the clinic in Mexico and I chose to go on their regimen.

I thought my life was over, but it was too soon to be over. I was only 34 years old and my husband and I have started a business called "Leading Estates of the World." We traveled the world. We saw the most beautiful properties all over the world and I enjoyed the business very much. I wrote and designed for the magazine. We were in a very happy relationship and I just wanted a solution. I was always proactive to try to—if there's a problem, I'm going to fix it. So a friend of mine—

I had this horrible pain, just terrible, terrible pain. I was in bed, off and on, for about a year with low blood sugar, abdominal pain and then it got worse and worse to the point where I felt like I had a knife through the middle of my chest and out my back.

So a friend said, "I know a friend who was cured. She had inoperable cancer of the colon and she went to a clinic in Mexico and she's five years clear of cancer." So my husband and I didn't waste any time. We came right down to Mexico and we had the—

We went through the physical. And I was still very nervous about everything, but we talked to patients down here. There must have been 40 patients down here with similar stories. So I began to gain hope and confidence that this was something that would really work.

So I took the medicine home, the tonic, and the supplements. I was very diligent, religiously so, about sticking to the diet, doing everything the doctors told me. And within a year – well they told me that within three months I would start to feel better – and so it was almost three months to the day that I was able to start not having so much pain.

My migraine headaches were not so frequent, not so intense. And I gradually stopped—I gradually, month by month stopped having the pain in my abdomen. I could start digesting my food and I got better. And within a year I was clear of cancer of the pancreas.

It was just so amazing because I knew that very few people survive cancer of the pancreas. Over the years, of course, since then I don't know of anyone that has survived as long as I have.

And then, we had another episode in our life because in 2011, I came to the clinic. I had been under a great deal of stress. We had had a lot of situations that were challenging. So I came to the clinic for a physical and I didn't expect anything bad, but I just wanted to come and have the doctor help me with some of the stresses. I wasn't reacting very well to stress.

So we went to St. John's Hospital. They did a CT scan and they detected lesions in the liver up to 3.9 centimeters. They were hypoechoic, and they said so liver neoplasm cannot be excluded. That meant that – as I was told – that the density of the tissue was so dense that that's what is normally from cancer.

I immediately came down to the clinic then and had another CAT scan and that confirmed that I did have cancer. I had 22 focal lesions on the liver and they put me on the treatment. I felt like I had been totally blindsided because I had been free for decades of cancer and here I had this terrible diagnosis. It was so surprising to me because pancreatic cancer was much more painful. This was very subtle. It was just this full feeling in my body and a little bit of pain.

They asked me to come back in three months. I couldn't wait three months. I was wanting to come back sooner and see what was happening. So I came back in two and a half months and all but three of the lesions were gone.

It was an unbelievable feeling. It was just so unbelievable that here 50 percent, they said, of my liver had been affected by all the lesions on the liver. So 50 percent of my liver was bad and had cancer and here I had only three small spots remaining and then the next physical shortly after that showed that there was no more cancer.

I'm the longest, to my knowledge, the longest living cancer survivor of the pancreas and I'm alive and well 40 years later. The doctors have confirmed that there is no longer any trace of cancer in my body. And I'm just radiant with happiness because I know that this treatment works and I know that had I done the conventional treatment I wouldn't have lived.

Pamela Kelsey: [*Speaking to Liz Jonas*] Bob and I just owe my life to you and to your sister. And yet you've carried on. It was her life work, she was totally devoted. She moved from Dallas to here and went through—she could have had a totally different life, but she was so committed. [*Pamela and Liz hug*].

Ty: Here's a summary of what you've come to understand during this episode. You've seen the heartbreaking truth behind why cancer is so rapidly spreading. And why the false cures have been perpetuated. I hope this side of the history equation helps you understand the foundation of why things are the way they are.

You've seen the shocking decisions concerning the Nuremburg Trials, where the vilest of crimes were praised, and that evil intent opened a floodgate of deception that led to the creation of a system that sought not to eradicate disease, but rather amplify it through disseminating false solutions for the sake of perpetual monetary gain.

You've seen the doctors who, rather than being praised or rewarded for their heroic deeds in healing their patients, have been persecuted, slandered, threatened, and, in some cases, have even had their patient records destroyed, their practice shut down, they've been imprisoned, even run out of a country, and have had their families undergo harassment and heartache for their loyalty to the cause. You've seen the children that have been forced to chemotherapy against their wishes and their parents wishes, regardless of their level of expertise or the effectiveness of their desired natural, proven protocol.

You've seen the proof that corruption, greed, coercion, deception, and fear have been tools employed to create a system that leaves people confused and afraid, rather than empowered. The great news today is that we have won the battle in your life as you have discovered the truth. And as it's said, *"The truth will set you free."* I'm so happy that you've experienced this and that through you, your loved ones too will know the truth about cancer.

I know you felt the hope and courage in the stories of the survivors that have recovered taking a natural approach, achieving feats unheard of by conventional methods of treatment. Isn't it wonderful to see real life proof? It warms my heart to see lives restored. I hope that you've enjoyed learning these things. And while they may be difficult to hear, it does bring us to the central truth that cancer, is in fact, NOT a death sentence. In light of this truth that we have established, you can give yourself one of the greatest gifts in this moment and that is the peace that results when you are free from fear. You do not have to live in fear. You *can* prevent and beat cancer, 100 percent naturally.

Ty: Wow! That's a lot of information that we covered tonight. I hope you've learned a lot from it. I know that I actually learned a lot traveling and getting this information for you. This information, these truths, that we've shared tonight are fundamental in the rest of our journey these next eight days.

I can't wait for the next episode, folks. We're going to travel all the way down to Australia and we're going to learn from a practitioner and a couple of cancer survivors what they have done to treat cancer naturally.

We're going to learn about essential oils and the role that they play, not only in preventing, but also in treating cancer. We're going to also discover some interesting knowledge about hormones and the role that they play in diagnosis and prevention and even treatment of cancer. But the biggie in the next episode is breast cancer.

This is Breast Cancer Awareness Month and there are a lot of lies and deceptions that are associated with treatment and diagnosing breast cancer. There's a lot of truths that are not commonly known. We're going to discover all of those in the next episode. I'm really pumped about it and I hope that you join us there.

I thank you for watching tonight's episode and I can't wait to see you for the next one. In the meantime, get some rest and we'll see you tomorrow. Thanks for tuning in tonight. God bless all of you.

[*Credits roll*]

[Sign: *In Loving Memory. Rest in Peace Dr. Nicholas Gonzalez*]

Dr. Robert Scott Bell: I'm most grateful not only for participating in this Global Quest, but that you all have been able to watch a great man. A tremendous healer who has passed from this plane much too soon. Dr. Nicholas Gonzalez, a good friend, a dear friend of mine. His legacy of healing, of empowering you to heal, to bring in that power to heal back where it belongs with you, will continue long after.

But I continue every day that I breathe and speak and communicate through radio and through this Global Quest to acknowledge the great works of Dr. Nicholas Gonzalez and what he brought to us all. And a passion and a dedication to really learn and to teach about nutritional ways to prevent and reverse cancer, detoxification protocols. And I hope that he has inspired you as he has inspired me to continue to learn and never stop learning and never stop helping and never stop working to help others who are genuinely in need.

This is why we do what we do and this is why the Global Quest is also greatly honoring and greatly appreciative of all the efforts of Dr. Nicholas Gonzalez. And his works will not perish because of this and because of what you are doing and watching and supporting this Global Quest. Thank you, Dr. Nick. We love you. We appreciate you.

Charlene Bollinger: He supported us from the very beginning and it means so much to have had his support and the world is just missing a great star and, of course, heaven's gain, our loss.

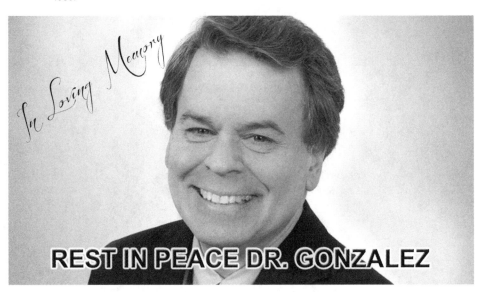

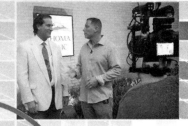

The Truth About Cancer

A

GLOBAL
QUEST
Episode 2

Cancer Facts and Fictions, Breast Cancer, Hormones, Skin Cancer & Essential Oils

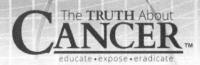

The **TRUTH** About
CANCER™
educate • expose • eradicate

Ty: Welcome to the *Truth about Cancer: A Global Quest*. I'm so thankful that you've tuned in to the show. Just in case you missed the last show, here's a recap for you.

[*video plays: Summary of Episode One*]

In this episode, we're going to cover a lot of ground. We're going to travel to Australia and get some survivor stories and some treatment protocols currently being used there. We're going to learn a little bit about hormones, we're going to dive into essential oils, and we're going to tackle a biggie, breast cancer.

October is Breast Cancer Awareness Month and there are a lot of lies and deceptions associated with breast cancer. We're going to try to get to the truth. But first of all we're going to take a step back. We're going to answer the question, "What is Cancer, and why does it spread?"

What, exactly, is cancer?

Dr. Bita Badakhshan: Basically cancer is abnormal growth of cells. Basically they lose their apoptosis, programmed cell death. They don't die, they become immortal. Your body's immune system usually takes care of the abnormal cells in your body.

We all have about 10,000 to 100,000 abnormal cells every day, but our immune system's job is to get rid of those cells. If your immune system is perfect, if you don't have a virus that it is already trying to fight, if you don't have too many chemicals or other stuff going on in your body. Then they keep growing and growing, increasing in number and then you get a tumor.

Ty: So the tumor really is the result of a lot of years of things going wrong.

Dr. Bita Badakhshan: Suppression of the immune system, exactly.

Dr. Linda Isaacs: Cancer is a condition where some cells in the body are no longer responding to the signals that tell them when to quit. In other words, most cells that have a purpose for developing, they develop to a certain point and then they stop.

Cancer cells keep reproducing, so they keep growing and they can spread to other places. That's what's called a metastasis. Cancer cells have escaped the normal controls for regulation and how big a set, a bunch of cells is supposed to become.

Dr. Aleksandra Niedzwiecki: Cancer is a process that occurs in our body all the time. As we are sitting and talking, there are cancer cells that are constantly created in our body. They do not always lead to the development of cancer because our immune system finds them as abnormal cells and eliminates them.

A cancer cell is a cell that escaped biological control to which all normal cells in our body are subject to. A cancer cell divides indefinitely.

And also, cancer cells are immortal. They never die because the genetic program that regulates the life and death cycle in those cells has been damaged.

Cancer cells also have another ability. They are not happy sitting in one spot in our body. They invade our organs and also they metastasize, which means that they escape to other organs. Metastasis is the most dangerous process of cancer, because nine out of ten patients die of metastasis, not of primary cancer.

Ty: So cancer results from a failure of the immune system, and the majority of cancer patients do not die from the primary tumor, they die from the spreading or the metastasis of cancer. It seems like we ought to be focusing on how to stop the cancer from spreading, doesn't it?

If our army wants to stop the invasion of foreign troops, it must be able to communicate with each other. Otherwise we can't stop the invasion. The same goes for our own personal army, the immune system. If our immune cells cannot communicate, we cannot stop the invasion of cancer.

Dr. Irina Kossovskaia: Cancer, by nature of the thing, is the major breakdown of systemic communication. What happens with the cancer, as you probably know, is the body does not see the growing tissue. We all grow a little cancer in our bodies many times a year, maybe sometimes once a day.

However, this growth is always controlled by the general regulation and management system of the body. The body is computerized, so when the communication is running correctly, our lines of communication are open. Then the body detects that growth at an early stage and suppresses it.

However, when the lines are broken that's when it happens that the body does not see the developing tissue until it is too late. If the body is not aware of the growing tissue, if the communication is broken, burning the cancer out of the body is not going to help because if it's burned in one place, it will come up somewhere else—

Ty: Because the communication hasn't been fixed.

Dr. Irina Kossovskaia: Of course! You've probably met many cancer survivors or sufferers who have had cancer several times. Treated conventionally, it will come up somewhere else because it is a systemic thing.

Mike Adams: Cancer is a failure of the body's own cells to communicate with each other properly. Genetics plus intercellular communication. Cancer is the mal-expression or the inappropriate expression of your DNA.

It is not something that has invaded you from the outside so you cannot look at cancer with a paradigm of carpet bombing your body, declaring war on an invader. It is not an invader. It is something internally that is not communicating correctly at a cellular level. So you need to become whole. You need to heal, not destroy, in order to overcome cancer.

There may be extreme cases where there is a tumor that is so large that it is pressing on an artery or a nerve or something like that where it has to be physically removed. I understand that.

I'm not saying surgery doesn't have any place at all; it can have its place. But even then, the surgery is only a temporary solution. You still have to address what has led to that tumor in the first place.

G. Edward Griffin: The present orthodox view is that cancer is a lump or bump. That's the cancer. If that is the assumption, if that is true, then to get rid of cancer all you have to do is get rid of the lump or the bump.

Hence, we have surgery. Well, that gets rid of the lump or the bump. Or we have chemotherapy which poisons the lump or the bump and we got rid of it. Or we have radiation which burns it and got rid of it.

You undergo these three therapies and if you get rid of the lump or the bump, the doctor will say "It looks like we got it all." That famous line, "We got it all." But did they? No. Statistics show that in most cases, it comes back. They didn't get it all because that was never the cancer in the first place.

If you're a farmer and you see all these little black spots on your corn leaves, you think, "Well, those are black spots, that's the disease," and you get the scissors out and you cut all the black spots off and you say, "Well we got it all alright." No, you didn't, because that wasn't the disease. What caused those black spots is still present.

Dr. Ben Johnson: There are so many things that cause cancer. Number one, you'll never have an oncologist ask, "What caused this? Let's get rid of what caused this." You'll never hear that question. They only have one thing and that is, kill cancer cells.

What caused the cancer cells? Why did this occur in the body? Obviously the immune system was suppressed, so are we going to unsuppress the immune system? Are we going to stimulate the immune system back into action? Are we going to lower nagalase counts from viruses and cancer cells so that the body's own defenses, the macrophage activating factor, can work? There are many things to do other than just give a poison to the body to kill cancer cells. We have to orchestrate healing here.

Dr. Bita Badakhshan: I think one of the main things is viruses. We do see a lot of different kinds of viruses in patients with cancer, not only HPV or herpes. You see mono, Epstein-Barr virus.

I have a handful of patients with breast cancer who have parasites. When they do a coffee enema or garlic enema, they can actually see the worms coming out. And what does a parasite do to your body? It suppresses the immune system! There are some doctors who believe you develop cancer because of the parasite. Some believe it's candida, fungus, yeast, but I think everything has to do with it.

Dr. Howard Fisher: We start to look at some other numbers. Eighteen (18) percent of all cancers are caused by infection. No one talks about that!

Ty: 18 percent?

Dr. Howard Fisher: 18 percent. 23 percent of all cancers are related to obesity. No one ever talks about that because obesity is running amuck right now. This year, overweight and obesity in the US alone will hit 75 percent with 41 percent being obese. They've already doctored the numbers, the body mass index, for declaration of that.

Then we look at the other environmental factors and they lump that into 41 percent of all cancers are due to environmental factors. So then we're looking at an unknown 18 percent.

This 18 percent that we're looking at could be genetics – small, 5 to 10 percent – or just other factors whether it's ambient environmental radiation, nonionizing, unlikely it's ionizing, but that can all be lumped in there into these same factors.

Ty: Is there a link between obesity and cancer?

Dr. Joseph Mercola: Well, I think it goes—

Ty: You mentioned insulin resistance as well.

Dr. Joseph Mercola: Yeah, I think it goes back to of insulin resistance. There are some studies that show correlation. Correlation of course is not causation. The central roles or whatever contributes to obesity most likely contributes to other diseases. It could be all the other chronic degenerative diseases like heart disease and Alzheimer's and diabetes. Cancer is just one of those. It's exactly what you'd expect when you're not giving your body what it needs. But insulin resistance is the core, absolutely the core.

I've known this for 20 years. I'm grateful to Dr. Ron Rosehill, the physician who taught me and helped me to appreciate and understand that. That has really been one of the primary focuses of the way I've treated patients, to understand strategies to address insulin resistance.

There is no question in my mind that the single most effective intervention I've ever seen to address insulin resistance is intermittent fasting – with the right foods ideally. That intermittent fasting… You might say, "Well I've got to eat every two hours, otherwise I'll pass out. I'll go with no energy." And yes, that's what happens because your body is used to that sugar high and you can't burn fat. But once you make that transition, it literally is nothing short of magical. Your body is not hungry anymore. It just isn't hungry.

We were never designed to sit down all day long. This is another problem. When you're sitting down it causes massive challenges in your system which it was never designed to do.

We were never designed to sit for eight or ten hours a day, so that's why I think it's really good to get up and walk a few miles a day, 7,000 to 10,000 steps a day or more in addition to an exercise program. It's not just exercise, it's movement that is so critical.

It doesn't have to be walking just as long as you're moving. We need regular movement throughout the day, not just one hour a day at the gym.

Ty: Wow, that's great information from Dr. Mercola on obesity and the link that it has to cancer.

Now, infections, parasites, viruses, fungi, and environmental toxins: these all are some of the causes of cancer. Why? Because they compromise the immune system. Again, the immune system is key.

But what about genetics? Isn't genetics the main cause of cancer? You've got bad genes, right? It's just bum luck.

That's what many oncologists would tell you, but the fact of the matter is, that's not true. Dr. Fisher didn't just pull that five percent statistic out of midair. He actually got it from the American Cancer Society's very own website.

Ty: Speaking of genetics, we've all heard stories about people that have the BRCA gene and they are afraid that they are going to get breast cancer because of this. Angelina Jolie is a prime example.

But was she misled? Was she misled by oncologists that told her that her only hope to avoid breast cancer was to remove both breasts? Did she choose this treatment because of a fear factor?

Dr. Nalini Chilkov: That's completely fear based and it's also because the media hypes that up, especially for a famous person like Angelina Jolie who has a double mastectomy. But the kind of cancer that she had is less than five percent of all women with breast cancers. So to remove your breast is, I think, barbaric. It's really barbaric.

Epigenetics, if people don't know what that means, means that something will act upon your genes. So epigenetics are like your software, something has to open it up and read it. You could have a toxic chemical in the environment that opens up some cancer genes and turns them on, but we could also turn those off with plant medicine. That is much more powerful that just trying to kill cancer cells.

Bob Wright: Doctors would like you to believe that cancer is genetic, that we've got genetic abnormalities and cancer rises from a genetic predisposition or a break in your DNA or whatever it might be. But it's not true. It's actually been proven that it's not true and doctors should in fact know this, but they don't.

Let's say that your body and your genetics is the computer. That's the hardware. People can understand this. The epigenetics is the software. The software runs the hardware. We know that from computers. We don't seem to understand that with the human body.

What we need to do is not dwell upon the genetics but on the epigenetics. In other words, what works that computer? If the software is working, generally the hardware is working.

Ty: Our last question. You wrote a book called *What Angelina Should Have Known and Didn't Know.* What should she have known?

Ard Pisa: I feel very sorry for her because she has removed healthy breasts. Can you imagine, Ty, you removed your manhood, your healthy manhood because of fear? It's crazy. But she thought this was the only way for prevention.

But there is another way for prevention because she should have known that our genes do not control life. You can activate genes and deactivate them. If we deactivate our genes with our healthy lifestyle, we do not get cancer. That's what she should have known.

Dr. Joseph Mercola: It's not so much that we're born with this gene that's going to give us breast cancer. It's that our epigenetic, our environmental influences – the food that we eat, the actions we do or don't do, the toxins we're exposed with – turns those genes on or off.

You don't have to worry about these inherited genes that may cause you to do a prophylactic double mastectomy. That's just insanity from my perspective and it's an irrational fear, if you appreciate and fully understand the amazing regenerative capacity that your body has if it's given the proper tools.

Dr. Rob Verkerk: One of the major problems that we have in terms of our old understanding of genetics is that people believed that if they were born, say as a woman with a BRCA gene, that might increase their risk of breast cancer, they have not been told and certainly wouldn't expect to hear from their doctor that the way they live their life will alter the expression of those genes and their risk of cancer.

Dr. Veronique Desaulniers: The BRCA gene scare was really quite a Hollywood hype last year and I'm not judging her. She saw her mother die a very horrible death, but there was a lot of misinformation.

The BRCA genes are actually cancer-protective genes. They help to repair DNA damage, so the BRCA gene, if it mutates, then it can cause a problem possibly, but what causes it to mutate? Look at the foods. Look at the radiation. BRCA genes are tumor suppressive, protective genes.

Ty: So do you inherit breast cancer genes? Is it inherited? Is it genetic?

Dr. Veronique Desaulniers: You know that's the big thing. "Well my mother had breast cancer so I'm probably going to have breast cancer."

But, we now know through the study of epigenetics, which is the science of looking into gene expression, and nutrigenomics which is the study of food, we know that we can change our gene expression by what we eat, how we sleep or don't sleep, how we manage or don't manage our stress, the foods that we eat. Something as simple as curcumin can help to really turn on the cancer-protective genes and change those gene expressions.

Ty: Wow, bet you've never heard that before, that the BRCA gene can actually *protect* you from breast cancer. It does not necessarily cause breast cancer.

Now, October is Breast Cancer Awareness Month. "Think Pink," "Run For the Cure." You see all of these different campaigns that are aimed at bringing awareness to breast cancer, which is not necessarily a bad thing. We want to bring awareness to cancer as well. However, let's look at the history of Breast Cancer Awareness Month through the eyes of Erin Elizabeth.

Erin Elizabeth: Yeah, so it is Breast Cancer Awareness Month and it's interesting how the whole story started with the pink ribbon that you were mentioning.

It actually used to be a peach ribbon and it was a woman named Charlotte Haley who had started that grassroots movement. Her whole objective was to get the word out that so little money was spent on prevention, first of all, not just research, but with prevention and that's still the case today.

Even with research not much of the money that they'll raise during the month of October is really even spent in research because of so much overhead. So yeah, it's a real shame.

But, what most people don't know is that back in '92 this little old lady started a grassroots movement with her peach ribbons, which she was giving out to people. She gave out five at a time with a little note and it really took off. She wanted people to be aware, not so much of just breast cancer itself, but of preventing breast cancer in the first place.

Then Estee Lauder and *SELF Magazine* came along and they wanted to use her ribbon. I think they were shocked when she said, "No, I'm not going to support these corporations turning my grassroots movement into this thing that really became more about making money."

And today, even when I was doing some research on it, I thought, "I'll try to find her name and pink ribbons," you keep getting these Estee Lauder ads selling their expensive—now they've got diamond encrusted ribbons you can buy. It really seems like it's been exploited. It's ironic that you have Susan G. Komen or Estee Lauder or Kentucky Fried Chicken and Susan G. Komen doing joint ventures with the pink ribbon, which really boils down to that these corporations that are not really healthy are—It's a bit hypocritical that they are trying to be out there selling the pink ribbon and saying they are all about curing breast cancer.

Jordan S. Rubin: We go around and celebrate wearing pink socks and pink ribbons and buying pink lemonade on the airline to contribute to cancer. It sure does! It's ridiculous. I coach youth sports. I won't wear pink! I won't put pink on. I don't believe in that. Why? Because the pharmaceutical intervention, conventional methods are not saving lives!

Dr. Darrell Wolfe: So now we're going to end the War on Cancer so we're going to get everybody involved. We're going to get them to run for it, we're going to get them to jump for it. We're going to get them to pray for it. We're going to get them to beg for it. So now everybody—you can't go anywhere without giving money at—I can't buy groceries without somebody wanting money from me.

Valerie Warwick, R.N.: With all the money that we're pouring into "Relay for Life," "The Komen" really hasn't helped change things for the patients.

Ty: You saw that first hand as an oncology nurse for 17 years.

Valerie Warwick, R.N.: I did.

Ty: It's not on the camera, but you got some really neon pink tennis shoes on. But what about the pink movement, right, the breast cancer pink movement? What's your take on the October "Get Your Mammogram"...?

Dr. Veronique Desaulniers: Its focus is on breast "cancer" awareness instead of breast *health* awareness, and the pink movement really has caused so much fear and so much misinformation when it comes to breast cancer in women. There are so many myths involving breast cancer.

Ty: Dr. V. just mentioned breast cancer myths. During Breast Cancer Awareness Month we always hear, "Early detection is your best protection." Everyone knows that, for breast cancer, mammograms are the best way to early detect – or *is this a myth?*

Dr. Martin Bales: There has been at least two studies, very large, that have come out on the limitations of mammography. One of them was a Canadian study, I believe. It was 20 or 25 years that they've watched in the past that found no benefit.

Also *The Lancet,* which is a large British Journal equivalent to our *Journal of American Medical Association* or JAMA, came out and said that there is really no benefit at all to doing, and possibly some harm. The harm being it is ionizing radiation, which we know isn't the best for us.

And also again with the pancake smasher, if you do have a cancer and you smash that wall that the body has put around it, are you spreading the disease that way? I don't know, but I don't want to find out.

Ty: Well yeah, and that's *The Lancet*, right? That's pretty reputable.

Dr. Martin Bales: Yeah it's pretty reputable and also the BMJ, *the British Medical Journal*, I believe, did a write-up as well. So that's two or three very reputable internationally published journals.

Dr. Leonard Coldwell: Early detection just means early death, because the earlier they find it, the earlier they start cutting you, the earlier they start treating you with chemotherapy and radiation, and the earlier you die.

Breast cancer grows seven to twelve years to a size in the breast that you can even diagnose it. So there is no rush. You know they find breast cancer – oh you have to go and get surgery tomorrow morning!

Ty: A lot of pressure.

Dr. Leonard Coldwell: A lot of pressure because they don't want you to get basically the time to get educated and educate yourself. So let's talk about this early detection.

Imagine your lymph system. You have four times lymph liquid more than blood. So your lymph system, your lymph nodes are there to neutralize poison. It's like when you have tonsillitis there are the big lymph nodes and then they are just working hard.

It's not a bad thing, it's a good thing showing, "Oh, the tonsils caught all these poisons and basically they are just diluting it and neutralizing it and then getting rid of it."

So when you have that, Ty… And imagine, like a pimple that is ready to burst, now the lymph node in the breast might be working hard and being inflamed and looks like a pimple that's getting ready to burst. So now they put 50 pounds of pressure on it…

Ty: That makes sure it bursts.

Dr. Leonard Coldwell: …that makes sure it bursts.

Dr. Ben Johnson: We as a medical society are *giving* women breast cancer with our demanding that they get mammograms. Mammograms cause breast cancer. Period. So mammograms are not healthy for women. Women should not be getting routine mammograms. That's crystal clear, published in the peer review literature.

And yet today, if a woman went to her gynecologist, her family doc, she would have this shoved down her throat, extreme coercion to go get this mammogram that is causing breast cancer.

Ty: Wow! What a telling quote from Dr. Ben Johnson that mammograms are actually causing cancer. Now in that respect, I guess they are sort of similar to chemotherapy, because chemotherapy actually causes cancer.

In last night's episode, we learned the story of Dr. Farid Fata that was diagnosing people with cancer that didn't even have cancer and then prescribing chemotherapy. I guess you could say he was over-diagnosing them.

What about mammograms? Is mammography prone to diagnose women with breast cancer that don't even have breast cancer? Are we being told the whole truth about this issue?

Sayer Ji: There has been a manipulation of the science and there has been a very dangerous thing called over-diagnosis that has really afflicted millions of women over the past 30 years, especially for breast cancer.

What they've done is that they convince women that if they were to basically subscribe to an X-ray mammography screening, even though they have no symptoms, that ultimately that would help them in the long run. They'd have a lower risk of cancer because they'd find it early.

Ty: "Early detection is your best protection."

Sayer Ji: Exactly. They even equated this meme with prevention when in fact you're exposing your breast to a type of radiation that is actually known to have a higher risk of causing cancer in the breast, especially if you have the BRCA 1 and 2 gene, mutations that everyone is so concerned about.

They make it harder for you to damage, radiate, to protect yourself from radiation-induced damage. So over-diagnosis, according to a recent study done in the *New England Journal of Medicine,* over the past 30 years in the United States resulted in 1.3 million women being diagnosed with early stage breast cancer that technically never had any type of cancer that would have caused harm.

This is called Ductal carcinoma in situ, or Stage Zero cancer, which they equated with actual cancer, which now we know is not. So what that basically meant is that they would give them the standard mastectomy or lumpectomy with radiation, with chemotherapy, things like tamoxifen, and then follow up hormone suppressive therapies like ARIMIDEX®.

Basically what we're dealing with here is a kind of medical holocaust of sorts. Those women now had to deal with being diagnosed with a cancer they didn't have, being treated for it, having the stigma and all the psycho-spiritual-emotional stress that is caused by that.

And then, statistically, the industry told them that they saved their lives, when in fact quite the opposite had happened. So they identify with the aggressor like a Stockholm Syndrome, and millions of people march in these Breast Cancer Awareness Marches not realizing that it is funded by the very corporations that make money off the drugs used to treat breast cancer.

We're talking about AstraZeneca, which is actually a derivative of Imperial Chemical Industries who started Breast Cancer Awareness Month in the '80s, and it has a patent or had the patent for tamoxifen and ARIMIDEX®. It's a vicious circle of brainwashing, and it is used to cover up really of what has cost the lives of hundreds of thousands of women ultimately.

Brenda Michaels: Well that's really what brought it all forward for me. I say to a lot of people when they have that disease that they don't realize yet what a gift that can be in their lives because it is a wakeup call, if you take it that way.

It's all how we perceive things, Ty. My perception was not quite there when I was diagnosed the first and second time, but the third time when I was told that I had about a year to live if I was unwilling to do the chemo, which I had been all along. And that the cancer would metastasize and maybe within a year, there would be no hope for me. That stirred something very deep inside of me and I began to awaken.

It was not an easy journey. I still had my fears. I still had days where I was just—I felt like maybe it was easier to die than it was to live. I went through all of that. But all along, underneath all that was this guidance that I had never opened up to before, but I was beginning to follow. That guidance just step-by-step, day-by-day, it led me, and it saved my life.

Ty: But they said—so it was late stage.

Brenda Michaels: Yes.

Ty: And supposedly terminal. You had less than a year to live.

Brenda Michaels: Yes. They thought they could maybe give me five years. That was a maybe. Maybe. But without it, they thought that within a year they were pretty sure it would metastasize and there would be nothing they could do.

I was learning to trust that information and trust my body, and my body was giving me signals. Because when I asked about chemotherapy, Ty, I would get this real deep clenching in my gut, sometimes almost painful.

And then when I would say something like – because I didn't know what to do, I had no idea there was an alternative out there of any kind – I would say something like, "If there was something out there better for me, would that be helpful?" and that clenching would just completely release. So I knew, even though I didn't know where to go and what to do, I knew I couldn't walk the path they were asking me.

Ty: You knew there must be a better way. Wow, that's an encouraging story from Brenda Michaels who healed her breast cancer naturally. And it is a stark contrast to a story that I saw recently on HBO.

It was a documentary special on cancer and a lady had been diagnosed with cancer in her left breast and she had had it surgically removed. You see her later in the show weeping. She's got a scar on her breast and she says she looks like Frankenstein, and then she says, "And now we're going to start radiation next week."

I was so saddened for her, because the lady did not know that she had options. She did not have the knowledge that you are gaining through watching this show. Much like Brenda Michaels, Dr. Veronique Desaulniers was aware of the options she had. Dr. Veronique was diagnosed with breast cancer and she treated and beat it, 100 percent naturally.

Dr. Veronique Desaulniers: As a woman, it was so shocking for me because I was the one that was helping my patients get well and reversing all these various diseases in my practice. So when I discovered that I had breast cancer, it was really a blow to my ego, for one, and it was also a big wakeup call for me. I thought I had the world by the tail and I realized that obviously, if my body allowed the cancer to grow, there was something that I was missing.

I had to really look at my life. I had to look at how I was managing my stress. I had to look at putting pieces of the puzzle together that obviously I'd missed. So it really led me down a path of soul searching and really digging deep.

There were a lot of tearful days, a lot of tearful nights, but like I tell my clients today, you have to transform the whole person. It's not just the physical lump or bump, you have to heal the whole body and that means heart, soul, mind, spirit – everything. Because if you keep doing the things you've always done, you're going to continue to get the same results.

You know, why? Why and how? If that could happen to somebody like me, who was doing so many things that were right, then how much more so could other women be vulnerable to this "dis-ease" in their body, and just helping them to understand that it's just the tip of the iceberg. Cancer is not the disease itself. It's just the tip of the iceberg that shows you that there's so many underlying things. Because you have to be sick in order to develop cancer. You know you don't get cancer and then you're sick. Your body's already sick and it's compromised. Your immune system's weak. You're toxic. You're stressed out. And that's how cancer develops.

So it's displacing that myth and that fear that cancer's just something that gets you. It's something that develops over a period of time. You're not a victim of it. You have a lot of control over it.

One of the reasons I'm doing the work that I'm doing is because there's so much information out there and where does one person start? Do I detox first? Do I do this? Do I do that? What herbs do I take? I developed a program. It's a seven step program called The Seven Essentials. It's so simple that anybody can apply it.

So the first one, Essential number one is "Let Food Be Your Medicine." We know that food has a huge impact on our genetic expression. We know that it can literally turn on specific cancer-protective genes, we know that through the science of epigenetics and nutrigenomics. Number two is to Detox. To reduce your toxic exposure. We live in a toxic world, we can't deny that, but there are things that you can do specifically to help support the detoxification pathways in your body and to prevent all the toxins from entering into your body.

Essential number three is to balance your energy. We are energetic beings, and so what can you do to keep that electricity and that energy flowing properly? Chiropractic care, acupuncture, exercise, proper sleep, making sure that your hormones are balanced, because hormones are very key in so many hormone-driven cancers.

Essential number four is to heal your emotional wounds. Learn to nurture yourself and to love yourself, to forgive yourself and others. Manage your stress better. Let go of the past, because if you keep stuffing those emotions inside, are going to grow a tumor. You either grow your life or you grow a tumor. So you have to change that emotional component. Essential number five is to look at biological dentistry because your teeth have a huge impact on your health. Your teeth are connected to your organs through your meridian system. What you have in your teeth affects your health, because if you have toxic amalgams in there it's causing toxicity in the body.

And then we look essential number six which is specific herbs and supplements and vitamins that can really reduce your toxic load, that can help heal the cancer, actually kill cancer cells, and boost your immune system.

Lastly, essential number seven in really practicing true prevention. Traditional medicine, unfortunately, does not really teach prevention and does not know about prevention. There are many, many ways and different technologies that can detect cancer when it's at the size of a pinhead instead of waiting until it's the size of a lump or a bump that you can detect on an X-ray or on a mammogram.

Thermography, for example, can read the physiological changes that are going on in the body. There are specific blood tests like the cancer profile which measures the HCG hormones, and the PHI which is a malignancy hormone, TK1 enzyme, the ONCOblot® test which can also determine cancer when it's just the size of a pinhead in the body. That's true prevention.

If you can stay on top of your health by monitoring, and not just guessing about your health, but making sure that you're moving in the right direction, there is no reason to fear cancer.

Ty: I agree 100 percent with Dr. V. There is no reason to fear cancer. She just shared with us what she calls her seven essentials.

1. The number one essential is Let Food Be Thy Medicine.
2. Number two is Detox.
3. Number three is Balance Your Energy.
4. Number four is Healing Emotional Wounds.
5. Number five is Biological Dentistry.
6. Number six is Specific Herbs, Supplements, and Vitamins. And
7. is True Prevention.

Now over the next few days we'll be covering all of these seven essentials.

The last one that Dr. V. mentioned was true prevention and she also mentioned thermograms. We're about to hear from Dr. Martin Bales whose father was a pioneer in the digital photography industry. That's what a thermogram is, by the way.

A mammogram is not necessarily the best way to detect breast cancer. There are other ways that are much better, they are superior. One of them is thermography. You're going to demonstrate a thermographic machine for us today and talk about that.

Dr. Martin Bales: I will. My father actually invented the first all-digital infrared camera in 1979, but it wasn't for anything with body or health. It was actually for our defense. It was used in missile detection back in Afghanistan.

Ty: So it was looking for heat.

Dr. Martin Bales: It was looking for heat, for missiles. It used to be that you had to track the missiles going across the sky manually. Now with our warheads it does automatically.

In the early 80s a group of doctors approached my father. "We've heard that the body obviously has circulation. We can diagnose a lot of diseases by seeing where there are hot spots or where there is cold." He said "Okay, I'll make a medical version for you."

Ty: Really? That's fascinating. But the first one was missile detection. Okay.

Dr. Martin Bales: First was missile detection. Yeah. Basically it can be used in any part of the body. Probably, as most people have heard, the breast thermography is the most popular. It is really limited as far as cancer to breast and possibly some skin cancer because it is skin deep. It doesn't look like for the liver or other organs.

It's a great way. It's completely painless. The ladies like because there's no pancake smasher, as they say. There is no ionizing radiation so it can be done as little or as often as one wants. It is just in a cooled room.

All cancers go through a process called neoangiogenesis, which is new blood vessel growth. Because the cancers grow faster than healthy tissue around them, they have to have their own discreet blood supply after they are a couple of years older.

It turns out that when most breast cancers – not all of them, there are a few that are fast growing, most of them are actually quite slow growing – to become the size of the pea, it's between eight and ten years.

So if we can catch them in year one or two when they are just getting that new blood vessel supply while the blood vessels are warm, that's how thermography is picking them up. Mammography is about two thirds accurate at finding them when they are pea size, so they are already eight years old.

We're going more from a prevention standpoint. If we find something early on, we can change diet and lifestyle, perhaps do some of the therapies you've discussed here as opposed to, "Okay, you've already had something for eight years and you're already in this bucket. What can we do?"

Ty: Thermography really seems to be a great way to early detect cancer, doesn't it? Dr. V. also mentioned essential number one, which was "Let food be thy medicine." Do you remember in *Mary Poppins* the song, "A Spoonful of Sugar Helps the Medicine Go Down?" Is this an oxymoron?

Dr. Veronique Desaulniers: If there is one food that women need to avoid if they are on a breast cancer healing journey, it's sugar. We know that sugar feeds cancer. Cancer cells have more insulin receptor sites than a healthy cell, so the first cells that get fed with sugar is the cancer cells.

Dr. Leigh Erin Connealy: Cancers like sugar, right, even though the doctors don't tell you that. I think the doctors tell you, "Oh you can eat anything." Well first of all, it's all over the world about how you treat illness whether it's cancer, heart disease, you've got to get off sugar! Sugar is a poison for all of us.

K.C. Craichy: So sugar we talk about as a big problem. Yes, it's a big problem. Sugar is wonderful, everybody likes sugar. I like sugar, but I choose not to thrive on sugar. See, sugar should have been in our FUN foods – building blocks, fuel, and fun.

Fun Foods that every now and then you have sugar. But these patients are often in an immunocompromised state to start with. Some of the treatments they are getting are taking their immunity down to almost nothing. And then they are throwing sugar in on top of that which directly feeds the problem but it also directly takes a whack at the immunity. It's a terrible cycle that people need to consider.

Valerie Warwick, R.N.: The key to overcoming cancer and getting your health back is in your gut and in your immune system. If you destroy your immune system, that's the very thing that you need to heal. So you may kill the cancer cells in your body with the chemo because, yes, it's going to kill those, it's going to kill everything. It's like dropping an A-bomb on your body and then expecting health to rebound, when really when you know in a garden, when you fill it with pesticides, all you're going to get back is weeds. So you need to rebuild your immune system and support your body in healing itself because it knows how to do that.

Ty: So the key to healing is to quit poisoning ourselves with chemotherapy, quit intaking sugar, because the truth is both chemo and sugar are oncogenic. They cause cancer. If an oncologist tells you otherwise, they're lying to you.

There are a lot of lies and misconceptions about bioidentical hormones. Have you heard that they cause cancer? Have you heard that they prevent cancer? I've heard both, but they both can't be true. Let's listen to Dr. Jonathan Wright explain.

Bioidentical hormones: do they cause cancer?

Dr. Jonathan Wright: Okay. Let's see. Did your own hormones cause you cancer yet? No.

Bioidentical hormones are no more dangerous, and no more safe, than a person's own hormones when they've got hormones.

We've got to admit that young women do get breast cancer in their 30s – occasionally, it's not very often, so there is a little hazard. That's from her own hormones.

I'm sorry. It is—estrogen related cancer is from her own hormones. But funny thing, there are lots of research papers that say that's because she's not metabolizing her hormones properly.

Dr. Veronique Desaulniers: Breast cancer myth number one is that women's hormones cause cancer. That's the biggest fallacy ever!

First of all, if our hormones cause cancer, then every 20-year-old on the planet would have cancer. So it's not our hormones, it's what we are exposed to.

Look at the xenoestrogens in the chemical estrogens in the environment – the chemicals, the pesticides, the herbicides, the metals in our teeth, the antiperspirants. Those metals are actually classified as metalloestrogens and mimic and stimulate estrogen production in the body. That's one aspect.

Secondly, if a woman has a problem metabolizing or breaking down her estrogens properly, then the more aggressive estrogens will circulate in the body. There is a way to support that methylation process, which doctors don't even talk about.

Ty: Dr. V. just mentioned xenoestrogens. What exactly was she talking about?

Dr. Roby Mitchell: Because of our exposure to environmental and pharmaceutical estrogens, that has the effect of throwing more gasoline on the fire. Some of the pesticides, fungicides that we use, they have an estrogen effect. These are what we call xenoestrogens, xeno meaning "foreign."

Dr. Nalini Chilkov: We're not designed to be ingesting or be exposed to molecules that aren't from nature. Some of those we can't even excrete them or some of those molecules in food growing, commercial food growing like the pesticides and the herbicides, they act like hormones. They are turning on hormone-like activities which are proliferative, which make cells grow.

This is one of the reasons we have so much breast cancer and prostate cancer, hormone driven cancers. People don't realize other cancers have estrogen receptors: colon cancer, pancreatic cancer, and lung cancer also have estrogen receptors, and so pesticides and herbicides will grow those cancers as well. You don't want that kind of signaling. Plastics also have this hormone-like effect.

Ty: Not only are breast cancer and prostate cancer driven by estrogen, but also colon, lung, and pancreatic cancer. Dr. Nalini just mentioned plastic. What many people don't realize is that in almost every bottle of water, in the plastic content there is the chemical called BPA. That's Bisphenol A and it is a xenoestrogen. In other words, it's a foreign estrogen and it is known to cause cancer.

An interesting thing that I've seen during Breast Cancer Awareness Month specifically is bottles of water that have a pink ribbon on it. In light of the fact that the plastic might be causing breast cancer, isn't that a little bit contradictory or ironic? Xenoestrogens, like BPA in the plastic, actually throw the hormone balance out of whack. What many people don't realize is that essential oils can balance the hormones.

Ty: What are essential oils? Let's go back to the basics.

Dr. Eric Zielinksi: Essential oil is a volatile organic compound and what I think what people need to recognize when it comes to an essential oil, there is no nutrition in it. There is no vitamin or mineral. It is a chemical that essentially God gave to the plant to protect the plant from outside threats, whether it's bacteria, viruses, fungus or even infectors like flies, bees, whatever that might attack the plant.

What it includes are organic compounds – not organic as we think meaning organic, having a carbon chain included in it – organic compounds like terpenes, alcohols, ketones, esters and you name it – is basically chemicals.

Ty: From the plant.

Dr. Eric Zielinksi: From the plant. Natural chemicals from the plant. God inspired the writers of the Bible long ago when he said "the leaves of the trees are for the healing of the nations." That's exactly what this is.

Ty: That's essential oils.

Dr. Eric Zielinksi: Exactly.

There is no oil for one specific issue. What we have found, and this is pretty fascinating, is that... let's use the Ayurvedic model, Indian folk medicine for example.

There is an abundance of lemons in India, so you'll find that the Indians use lemon essential oil for virtually everything: detoxification, internally, externally – whether or not you are going to clean the counter, or whether or not you want to clean your skin. They use the essential oils from lemon for everything from nausea to halitosis to diabetes to cancer.

When you go to Australia, they are using Melaleuca and tea tree and eucalyptus. You go to Oregon and Washington, they are using peppermint for everything. It's important to realize that these oils, a lot of them do the same things. When I report on research, it is limited because we've only done a limited amount of research, but as far as I know there is no essential oil that does not have a cancer effect.

I just recently read a report of over 130 research articles regarding essential oils, and what the researchers came about was: what essential oils do is they actually prevent angiogenesis, which is the growth of veins and arteries. It stops metastatic growth. It actually prevents DNA repair which is—that's pretty key.

That is really key, because there is one study that compared sandalwood and frankincense and they found that frankincense triggered that apoptotic effect where the cancer cell died, but sandalwood killed cancer another way, went around on the back end, in a sense and flanked it by triggering the actual DNA to not being able to repair itself so the cancer just died that way, too.

Dr. Josh Axe: Frankincense oil – if you look at the research today, it is probably the most powerful essential oil if not the most powerful supplement, period, when it comes to natural cancer treatment in my opinion.

Ty: What's in frankincense that makes it so good?

Dr. Josh Axe: Frankincense is really high on a compound called Boswellia or Boswellic Acid. It is highly anti-inflammatory. It is also a very powerful antioxidant. There are studies – there is actually a study that came out of the UK pretty recently, showing that frankincense oil is effective at shrinking tumors, it's effective against ovarian cancer, colon cancer and breast cancer. The Boswellia frankincense is a very powerful compound at fighting and treating cancer.

One of the most incredible things about frankincense is that the essential oils themselves are very, very small molecular compounds.

Almost everybody knows this, in cancer treatment, that chemotherapy is not effective at treating any sort of cancer of the brain because it can't pass through the blood/brain barrier versus frankincense oil. Those compounds are so small, they can actually pass through the blood/brain barrier and start to reduce that neural inflammation.

I'll tell you an incredible story. I was speaking recently and had somebody come up to me at the end, after talking about essential oils and she said, "I want—I can attest to what you're talking about with frankincense oil. My husband was diagnosed with a brain tumor six years ago and was given three months to live. We got turned onto frankincense oil, started using it every single day. We diffused it in the home. We rubbed it on the roof of his mouth. It has been six years and he is still alive and we really believe it's because of this use of frankincense oil."

But yeah, you look in the medical studies. It is effective against Alzheimer's. It's effective against any sort of brain inflammation and again four separate studies showing that it is effective at treating cancer.

Ty: Allison Huish was diagnosed with brain cancer at the tender age of 13, and she used frankincense oil to treat it. Here is her amazing story.

Allison Huish: I walked out of the waiting room about an hour later to see my mom who had just hung up the phone with tears in her eyes, and she told me, "Allison, you have a brainstem tumor."

I didn't know quite what that meant. You know, at 13 years old, I just started junior high school a couple of weeks prior. But I knew at that moment that my life would be different from there on out.

We immediately went to go see my doctor, to my pediatric neurologist, and he showed my parents what the tumor was. Basically it was a brainstem tumor, pilocytic astrocytoma is what it was, about the size of an egg and it rested on my brainstem. That next day, I was scheduled for emergency surgery and they were able to get rid of about half my tumor.

It was very interesting. My doctor told me, "eat all of the calories you can... If you'll eat pizza, if you'll eat ice cream," because I was very skinny, "just get calories in you, whatever you'll take."

But, in our research, we learned how nutrition was so important. I needed to give my body good calories to help support good healthy weight gain, support the cells so I would function better. Then we started doing research on what to do.

Of course, many people were pushing us to go see our radiologist and go that direction. My mom and I, we did go meet with our radiologist and I still, to this day, remember sitting in that room, the feelings that I felt in there.

Ty: What were they?

Allison Huish: It was very cold. It was very cold. It was not what I wanted to do and I actually left that appointment and I grabbed my mom's hand and I told my mom, "Mom, this isn't – this process isn't – for me." So she said she had also felt the same way.

But we left that radiologist's appointment knowing, "We need something else" and that is where we were really drawn towards these essential oils. They kept coming across in a lot of our research. We noticed how essential oils did incredible things. There's medical studies out there showing what essential oils can do.

In particular, with these essential oils we were really drawn towards frankincense essential oil. I love frankincense oil, a very powerful oil. I think there is a reason why it is called "liquid gold" or why it's one of the oils that the Christ Child was given. It's a very, *very* precious oil.

Ty: In the Bible the Wise Men gave Baby Jesus the frankincense and the myrrh. Maybe they weren't giving him just precious gifts, they were giving him medicine.

Dr. Josh Axe: Oh absolutely. Yeah. When you hear the story of the Three Wise Men bringing the infant Jesus gold, frankincense, and myrrh, I remember years and years ago not really knowing... Everyone knows what gold is, most people don't realize what frankincense and myrrh are, but those were the two main sources of medicine during that day.

Frankincense actually, at the birth of Jesus, would have been used because you look at children right after they're born, there is oftentimes bruising and sometimes it's a traumatic experience. So they would actually have rubbed frankincense oil on a child, which actually helps bring down the inflammation and swelling.

Also it is great for supporting and protecting the immune system. If he was exposed to different types of pathogens at that time, frankincense oil really protects the body, and so absolutely, Ty, frankincense oil was used. It was more than just a sweet smelling fragrance, it was a biblically-based medicine.

Frankincense was used along with something called the holy anointing oil, which was actually had myrrh essential oil, so when a lot of people hear frankincense also start thinking about myrrh. Myrrh is referenced over 160 times in the Bible.

Myrrh was also—actually there's a study in the *Journal of Food and Chemistry and Toxicology* recently that found that myrrh, another essential oil that's referenced in the Bible is also effective in treating cancer.

Ty: Really? Okay, because that was my next question. What about myrrh? You have the frankincense and the myrrh, so both were medicines. Both were sweet smelling fragrances.

Here's something interesting that Dr. Sunil Pai told us last year:

Dr. Sunil Pai: What we're looking at here is, historically the gold may be a reference to turmeric, turmeric or curcumin, specifically the part of turmeric. But turmeric was sold and cost more than gold at the time. This was during the Spice Trade, at the time of the Trade Route. We always nicknamed them golden spice.

Dr. Josh Axe: You could absolutely see that, that area in the Middle East uses turmeric today in cancer treatments. Talk about a powerful compound: frankincense, myrrh, and turmeric.

Ty: Yeah, triple play there.

Dr. Josh Axe: Oh yeah. But you look at something like myrrh and it's powerful because it really works on the hypothalamus in the liver. It reduces liver inflammation and also balances hormones.

What happens a lot of times these cancers are estrogen-based cancers. What myrrh can do is it really supports the body very similar... If people have heard of Indole-3 carbonyl, the benefits of indoles, fruits and vegetables.

Ty: Broccoli, right?

Dr. Josh Axe: It works very similar, but in even more potent way to where it really helps clear the body of excess estrogen or xenoestrogens that are found in things like soy and plastics and paraffins today. It really helps detoxify the liver and also to boost a very important antioxidant called glutathione, which supports detoxification. That's the way that myrrh essential oil actually helps in fighting cancer.

One of the things that I've had my patients do, including my mom over time, is start creating an at-home frankincense and myrrh body butter and body lotion. Basically, she takes ten drops of frankincense, ten drops of myrrh, along with some coconut oil and shea butter, and makes her own at-home body lotion, and rubs her entire body with that.

Really, those oils—the great thing about essential oils is those—they've been used as aromatherapy. So those small compounds coming off the body are protecting the body. They are fighting cancer. They are doing some incredible things there even topically.

All of my patients, or as I mentioned, my mom, take those essential oils and especially put it around that area of the neck. When you put it on the neck and the back of the head, you are constantly also breathing in those beneficial compounds.

Ty: So you are not only absorbing it through your skin, you are breathing it as well.

Dr. Josh Axe: Absolutely. And that's a good point. Your skin is your body's largest organ and this is why—this is the amazing thing about essential oils. We've talked about frankincense and myrrh. Other essential oils, as well, like lavender and sandalwood are so incredible at fighting cancer.

So many of these products people are using today, the body lotions, makeups, moisturizers, shampoos, conditioners – they are loaded with carcinogens. They are loaded with parabens, phthalates, and Sodium Lauryl Sulfate, and all of these different chemicals that cause cancer versus if people make their own, at-home, personal care products with essential oils rather than causing cancer they are fighting cancer.

Allison Huish: So use a lot of oils. I use a lot of frankincense oil. I also use clove oil.

Ty: How would you take it? Did you ingest it or did you rub it on your skin?

Allison Huish: Yeah.

Ty: Or did you do the aromatherapy? How did you do that?

Allison Huish: You know what? It was really interesting how we did it. I did do it back here, where my scar is. But I don't know how effective that was because you do have a very thick skull.

But, one way that I did and this was probably the way that was most consistent is, I always put a drop of frankincense oil on my tongue and raise the tongue to the roof of my mouth. I did that probably about every two hours because I figured, "Hey that's probably the closest way to get to my brain stem without interfering with the bones or things like that."

Ty: And a lot of blood vessels there, too, to absorb.

Allison Huish: Mm hmm, a lot of blood vessels, so just a lot internally. What happened was actually quite incredible. I started to gain health pretty quickly. Like I said, I started junior high school when I was diagnosed just three weeks later. I came home and started to regain health after my surgery. I was able to start school again with my peers the next semester. That was pretty incredible.

Ty: That's quick for a brain tumor.

Allison Huish: You know what? It was interesting. I was only in the hospital for about a week and a half. Most people are there for about six weeks. But once I had my tumor we started on good nutrition, we started on oils, and I just had an amazing recovery and that took about three years.

It took about three years and I would go see him. But every time I'd go see him, it just slowly was improving. It wasn't dramatic, overnight. It was a slow, gradual process, but it took about three years. I remember the point where I went to go see my neurologist and he told me, "You have no more tumor. It's completely disintegrated."

Ty: Wow. What did you feel like at that point?

Allison Huish: You know what? Words can't describe it. It was just like such an emotional relief. I had been praying and I wanted my tumor to go away and I was like "I need another chance at life."

So when those words were said, it was invigorating. It was like I had a new life again. I wanted to go to college. I wanted to become a registered dietician. I wanted to tell people my story. When I was told those words it was like, "This happened."

Ty: And that was at the age of 16 then?

Allison Huish: That was about–yeah, the age of 16-17 is when that happened. Ever since then, my health has just been improving.

Ty: Wow, what an inspiring story from Allison how she healed her brain cancer with essential oils. Another inspiring story is from Dr. Josh Axe who actually healed his own mother's cancer using essential oils.

Dr. Josh Axe: My mom has actually battled cancer twice. The first time was a little over 20 years ago. It actually came as a shock to her family. My mom was diagnosed with breast cancer at 42, and growing up, my mom was my gym teacher at school. She was a swim instructor, so always really fit, active, and healthy, but yet diagnosed with cancer.

My family lived in what I call the Medical Model of the Time. We were always taking drugs, my mom was always taking some sort of medication. But she went and had a mastectomy. She went through rounds and rounds and rounds of chemotherapy.

And, Ty, I can still remember to this day seeing my mom's hair fall out. I remember looking at her after the chemo treatments and thinking that she had aged 20 years in two weeks and saying to myself, "I never want to see anyone have to go through that again." That really drove me to being a physician, seeing how sick she was.

So she was diagnosed as being cancer-free and healthy but really, for the next ten years after she went through chemotherapy, she was really sicker than ever. She spent half of her days in bed, even after—I remember she'd get home from work at 3:30 and sleep till six every night. She struggled with depression. She struggled with chronic fatigue, anxiety issues, and leaky gut, digestive issues; just sick all the time.

Ten years later, I was actually working as a nutritionist in Orlando and finishing up my Doctorate and she called and said, "Hey I've been diagnosed with cancer again. What do I do?"

I flew home from Florida to Ohio and we sat down and prayed together and I just said, "Mom, I think we need to take care of you all naturally." So we started an all natural treatment program and she started juicing vegetables every single day. We had her start doing antioxidant-rich foods, loads of probiotics and using things like essential oils in helping her body heal.

We followed this treatment protocol for about four months, went back to the oncologist, and their first recommendation was surgery and radiation immediately. We followed it for four months. After four months, we went back to the oncologist, got a CT scan. He called us two days later and said, "This is incredible. We don't see this. The tumors have shrunk more than half. Keep doing whatever you're doing."

Ty: Whatever you're doing is working. Right?

Dr. Josh Axe: Yeah, he said, "Come back in nine months." We went back nine months later and, complete remission, and today my mom is in the best shape of her life. In fact, her and my dad just retired from Ohio down to Florida and she water skis every day. She has run three 5Ks with me in the past few years and gotten 2nd and 3rd in her age group.

She said she actually feels better now in her 60s than she did when she was in her 30s. She actually now teaches people how to use essential oils and make healing smoothies and juicing vegetables and how to ferment their own food. She just is a walking testimony of really what it takes to beat and fight cancer naturally.

Ty: That's awesome, man.

Dr. Josh Axe: Yeah. Thanks a lot.

Ty: Cool. Wow. It's truly amazing, the medicine we find in nature, isn't it? From essential oils to seeds to nuts to herbs to... eggplant? Hmm?

Dr. Jonathan Wright: Okay. BEC-5 is a compound derived originally from an Australian plant called Devil's Apple. It also is found in eggplant and it is found in green pepper.

Ty: Eggplant.

Dr. Jonathan Wright: Yes. It is one of the—any one of the things called Solanaceae, for those of you who are botanists. They all have some of this BEC-5 in them. The technical term for them is solasodine glycosides and all the glycoside means is that there's a sugar attached to something. It could be a string of sugars, too.

It was discovered by a Dr. William Cham. He likes to go by Bill, so we all call him Bill. He's a PhD. He is a brilliant guy and he was working at a university in Australia. Someone came out to talk to him.

Even though his major field is Lipid Chemistry they wanted to talk to him because they heard he was interested about why did their livestock, when they developed cancer in the eyeball – there's a certain kind of livestock that developed a lot of that – they go rub themselves up against the Devil's Apple plant with their eyes and, damn, their cancer would go away!

So they talked to Dr. Cham about that and Dr. Cham was intrigued. He went to research it and he isolated these things called solasodine glycosides. There are two or three of them but they are all lumped into the name in BEC-5. BEC-5 is Bill Edward Cham – that's his name – dash five.

So, here is what Dr. Cham found, very quickly. What he found is that there is a membrane change in the membrane that surrounds a cancer cell, and if any cancer cell – and as you'll hear later on from Dr. Gaston [Cornu-Labat], every cancer cell has this membrane change. But normal cells that are not cancerous do not have that membrane change.

The key thing is that the solasodine glycoside, the sugar that sticks down, has a particular type of plant sugar that connects with the cancer cell's changed membrane, and it connects.

And the cancer cell pulls that stuff inside the cancer cell where, it doesn't mess with the DNA of the cancer cell, it goes to little baggies called lysosomes, which are filled with enzymes, and they are the storage depot for enzymes that the cell uses. But this stuff, the BEC-5, it goes into the cancer cell, it goes to the lysosome somehow, it enters the lysosomes, and all the storage membranes are ruptured and this cell is flooded with digestive enzymes and digests itself to death. Seriously!

Now, if I had this skin cancer right here and I put it on there, it is not going to hurt the normal skin at all! That is the key thing. This is a beautifully targeted thing.

Dr. Gaston Cornu-Labat: So far is has been shown in all the animal studies and on the cell line studies that have been done, it has been shown that it has a very broad spectrum.

Ty: It works on lots of different cancers.

Dr. Gaston Cornu-Labat: So far the evidence is showing that it works on a very broad variety of cancers and sarcomas, and in other carcinomas, in squamous cell, basal cell.

So, BEC-5 went through a very interesting development phase with using it on skin cancers. Actually, it is still being used on skin cancer. This is a cream that is over the counter. In those jurisdictions where it's legal, it can be bought over the counter and you apply the cream. It starts getting, layer by layer, the cancer cells of the skin cancer – you know skin cancer is the most common kind of cancer – it just eliminates the cancer.

Ty: But just the cancer.

Dr. Gaston Cornu-Labat: It only targets the—at the beginning, it is very impressive because the characteristic with these early cancers is that the cancer cells are quite a bit more spread than what is evident. You start applying it, and suddenly redness starts spreading out and there is a lot of reaction. There's a little bit of an open wound in the first week or two that's a lot bigger and scary because it's bigger than what you thought it would be.

After the second or third week, that's when you start seeing normal skin coming in, coming in, coming in, and covering it up. And many, many, a majority of times, there's not even a scar left. What I have seen is it works consistently every time, every time.

Dr. Jonathan Wright: What happened to it? Well, Dr. Cham was in Australia and by the time the Australian Society of Dermatologists complained to the Therapeutic Goods Administration, which is the same as the FDA down there, down under, they had documented 70,000 people cured their own skin cancers with his stuff. And he was selling it over the counter! Can you imagine a cancer cure being sold over the counter and 70,000 people cured themselves?

Ty: We can't have that.

Dr. Jonathan Wright: We cannot have that, even if we're in Australia. So there was a complaint for the Australian Society of Dermatologists to the Therapeutic Goods Administration "Put this stuff on prescription! Only doctors should treat!" So the Therapeutic Goods Administration put it on prescription. There goes Dr. Cham's over the counter business. Guess what? Hardly any of the dermatologists have prescribed the stuff. They couldn't get it anymore.

Ty: This BEC-5 compound, which is selectively toxic to cancer cells, is contained in the Devil's Apple which grows freely all over Australia. While we're on the subject of Australia, let's have a listen to Dr. Manuela Boyle as she shares some of her treatment protocols and we're also going to hear from an Australian cancer survivor.

Dr. Manuela Malaguti-Boyle: I've been in practice for almost 20 years. I'm originally from Milan, from Italy. I worked for a number of years in London, a very big clinic in London. I used to see cancer patients over there. I worked in Singapore as well so over there, same thing, and in Australia.

Cancer is very much an international issue. There are some differences in perhaps obviously cultural backgrounds, beliefs, and diets. But at the end of the day, the patient who is undergoing chemotherapy at the local hospital here on the Gold Coast will be receiving exactly the same type of drug that a patient in Sri Lanka right now with breast cancer will be receiving. And the person in America will be receiving, and in South Africa will be receiving, which means that basically the conventional treatment is still one size fits all.

In terms of integrative approach, we know that this is obviously a very significant shortcoming. One size doesn't fit all, at all. We have the opportunity to use botanical agents and nutritional supplementation that is designed for each and every individual.

We have about 220 different cancers that have been identified, and those 220 different cancers are, again, different for each and every person. Individualized treatment is absolutely essential.

My team and I have the ability to use cutting edge technical, amazing machines which we have. We have a hyperthermia machine. Hyperthermia chamber. We have IV, Vitamin C, glutathione, alpha lipoic acids. We have dendritic vaccine injections. All this is absolutely evidence based. It is supported by human clinical trials, and it is very successful. Each and every time it is modified and tweaked according to the presentation of each patient. I'm very happy to be able to use all this knowledge and to help people.

Geoff Beaty: After multiple attempts, then they put a—I swallowed a pill that had a camera in it and that found it and I had a gastrointestinal stromal tumor. So, as soon as I found out, in a couple of days, I was like… Oh, they did another endoscopy to try and get to it to see more about it, that it had to go down a long ways. It was a difficult one.

A couple of days later, I was in surgery and they took out a foot of my small intestine and it was a gastrointestinal stromal tumor. And it was grown 10 centimeters so it was very— and I'm very lucky that it bled. If it hadn't have bled and it had got much bigger, I probably wouldn't have survived. So they took it out and I was put on chemotherapy and Clive Glivec. In America I think it's called Gleevec. That was hard. It just knocked the energy out of me. It was difficult to stand up for a year. I think that's something that—I think I got that second tumor some time later on.

That was probably a few years. I can't remember exactly, probably two years later, and that was in my neck. It grew very rapidly and I decided that I wanted to approach this not just medically.

Once I got the diagnosis for that and then had a think about it, treatment would have been chemo and radiation and—but, I just didn't want it all coming back again. I knew if I did just straight medical stuff if was not necessarily—you know this was the second time around.

I then had the treatment that was involved, but I went and approached Manuela and Manuela put me on a regime of things that... During the treatment – because I got Western medical treatment, but I also got Manuela's treatment and I did much...

There were a whole lot of people that I knew that were diagnosed at the same time, and I watched us all go through it, and the difference in me and the other people was amazing. I just coped with the treatments so much better. Less nausea, I didn't need to be fed by tube, which nearly all of them did that were going through at the same time.

You could see, just by looking at me, that I was coping much better than the others. It was still not a lot of fun. It was difficult to go through, but I did cope much better. I had much less burns from the radiation on my neck than the other people.

Once the treatments stopped, I just started picking up very quickly and within six weeks I could go back to work. Because we were cycled and going back to the doctors at the same time at the hospital, I saw a number of the others and many of them, four and five months later still not back at work, they were still not in a great shape.

What Manuela did for me made a huge difference. The herbs and the nutrients and the diet that I was on made a huge difference in my recovery. How can I repay her? How can I say enough about these things? I think she knows how much it has meant to me. I have a quality of life now that is great and life ongoing.

Now, three and a half years on, I'm back to full strength and I've been back to full strength for quite a while. Just amazing. Really, really good. It feels good. I feel confident that it's not coming back. I'm here to stay.

Ty: During this episode you've come to know about the true cancer facts and fictions. I'm so glad we could make it clear for you. You've learned how cancer spreads, and how the immune system is the answer to stopping cancer in its tracks. You've seen the alarming data on the hidden dangers of mammograms, which like chemotherapy, actually helps to spread cancer – the exact thing it is supposed to diagnose and prevent. You've also seen the propensity of mammograms to lead to over-diagnoses. All these facts leading to the conclusion that there simply *must* be a better way.

You've seen how thermography can actually diagnose breast cancer when it's as small as a pinhead, and how a life-threatening bout with cancer can be won before it even begins. The same goes for skin cancer. We've given you the most effective ways to prevent and beat skin cancer so you can make sure that your skin not only looks healthy, but it is healthy.

And as we will keep reiterating, nature itself will continue to give us answers as we tap into the amazing gift we've been given that surrounds us every day. You've heard the stories of how essential oils have helped to prevent and heal cancer like Allison and Dr. Axe's mother. And how these people will attest that their lives are indebted to gifts given in nature.

I trust this has not only been informative, but encouraging to you as you see that the answers are simple and there is a clear path to having a life free from cancer, pursuing a totally natural path.

Wow! We covered a lot of information in this episode, didn't we? I'm glad you joined us and I hope you'll make plans to join us for the next episode, because tomorrow we're going to travel across the Atlantic Ocean to a little country called Latvia.

We're going to learn about a virus that targets cancer cells and has been used in over 10,000 patients to completely eradicate cancer from the body, with no known side effects. You are not going to want to miss the next episode.

Thanks for tuning in to this one. Make plans to join us tomorrow and in the meantime, God bless all of you.

[credits roll]

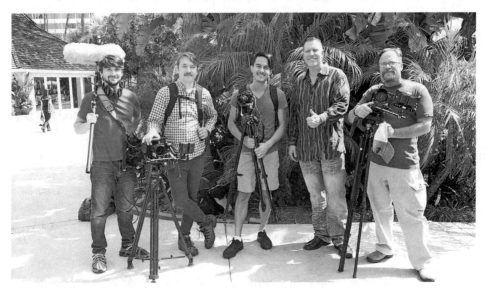

The TTAC Team in San Diego

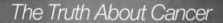

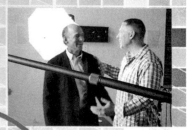

Ty: Welcome back everybody to *The Truth About Cancer: A Global Quest.* I'm really thrilled that you've joined us again tonight. But for those of you who might have missed last night's episode, here's a quick recap.

[Video plays: Summary of Episode Two]

As you can see, last night's episode was chock-full of information that's vital in keeping you healthy. Tonight's information will be just as important. So pay attention tonight as we travel over to a little-known country called Latvia, as we learn about the dangers of genetically modified organisms, and we learn about a little virus that can actually treat, and potentially cure, cancer.

In last night's episode, Dr. V's essential number one – let food be thy medicine. And tonight's episode is going to be chock-full of information about food and nutrition. But before we get there, we're going to explore some new discoveries about circulating cancer stem cells – or as they're now called, circulating cancer *tumor* stem cells.

Dr. Nalini Chilkov: Now, stem cells are a leading edge of research right now, because it's now thought that the stem cells, which are what we call pluripotent cells. They can turn into anything. They are floating around in the bloodstream of cancer patients, and chemo and radiation do not work on them. So it doesn't even touch them.

Dr. Russell Blaylock: The trouble with chemotherapy, and conventional treatments, is they have no effect on the cancer stem cells. They only kill the daughter cells – the cells that are produced by them. So the tumor will shrink, and they'll claim success, but you haven't killed the stem cells. So it all just comes right back. And what they found, is when it comes back, it comes back infinitely more aggressive than it did before.

Mike Adams: Again, chemotherapy is a chemical agent whose sole purpose is to kill – to kill cells. And the thinking, the medical justification, is well we're only going to kill the cancer cells. Well, even that doesn't work. If you shrink some of the cells of a tumor, you still have the cancer tumor stem cells that just regrow that same tumor. And then at the same time, you poison healthy cells in the body. So you've now reduced the ability of the body to fight future cancers and future insults and challenges to the immune system.

Dr. Bita Badakhshan: One of the problem with chemo is because when your patient do chemo, those circulating tumor cell, cancer cell, that we have once you have the primary tumor, they can mutate and they become more resistant to other treatments. Circulating tumor cells is formed from the primary tumor – and also, circulating stem tumor cells. And those can become bad cells, cancer cell, or may not. But circulating tumor cell as well, both of them will float in your body.

That's why when you do surgery or chemo or radiation, attacking one area, you're not getting rid of the cancer. What happens? You have these circulating tumor cells floating in your body. Circulating tumor cells keep adding up, adding up. And then what do they do? They go and metastasize, even vetrino that area, recurrence, or they could go to distant metastasis. That's why it happens. That's why patient is like, "Well I removed the whole both breasts. I removed all this. Why is it somewhere else?" It's because of the CTC.

Sayer Ji: The thing about it is, is because of the way that the cancer practice and industry really looks at the five year survival rate, is that they may "treat" somebody, give them chemo, radiation, see the tumor regress – go into remission. And then five years and two months later, when they get another cancer, they can just define it as a new cancer and not look at the root of it. Which is that it was just those remaining—those subpopulation of cancer stem cells, that were not only resistant to chemo and radiation, but were enriched. That then grew back slowly over time. Because as you know, a tumor or a cancer could take decades before you actually can get it to be surveilled.

The problem, of course, is that it's about the micro-environment of the "cancer" cell. We have to adjust and change things back, detoxify, we need to supplement with the right nutrition and information from the right foods, hydrate, oxygenate. Those are all the factors that will then re-educate that cell to say, "Oh, wait a second, I'm supposed to do this particular job as a hair cell, this job as a heart cell. I'm not going to go become a cancer and try to take over the whole body."

Jenny Hrbacek, R.N: So we took some blood. And he sent it to Research Genetic Cancer Centre over in Greece to do what was called a CTC count, which is a circulating tumor cell count. Which is what I now know, why all of those women had breast cancer when their breasts were cut off, in the trashcan – that tissue was gone – they would have breast cancer come back in their liver or in their lungs or in their bones. Because any tumor over two millimeters has blood perfusion, and those cells were circulating, and they took up shop in another place. I didn't know that, and I was a registered nurse. I was trained.

Ty: But the surgery did nothing for the circulating tumor cells?

Jenny Hrbacek, R.N: All it did was make sure these women did not get cancer in the tissue that was thrown in the trashcan.

Sayer Ji: Turmeric is probably the most heavily researched anticancer agent that has the ability to selectively target the root of the cancer, which again, cancer stem cells. And then leave intact the healthy tissue, but you have other substances such as resveratrol, green tea, quercetin – found in onions and other herbs, sulforaphane from cruciferous vegetables – especially broccoli sprouts. These are the heavy hitters that I'm sure you know a lot about. It's remarkable because really this category is often polyphenol category. And so things like catechin and green tea, resveratrol from red grapes, even peanuts, and curcumin from turmeric—actually that category of compounds is produced by plants when they're in distress.

And it turns out that organic plants are the only ones that produce these, really, in any significant amount, because they're not basically having pesticides to take care of their pests and PET (petroleum derived fertilizer) to burst their growth. They have to survive the elements like us. So they've developed these strong chemistries to protect them. When we consume those compounds, they activate longevity pathways within our body, similar to what caloric restriction does in fasting, as well as, activate things like anticancer mechanisms within the cell.

Dr. Nalini Chilkov: My first love is Botanic Medicine, because in plants there are so many, what we call, plant chemicals or fighter chemicals. And molecules from nature bind to many different cells and receptors. So, we get a lot of mileage out of using just a few things. So, many people know about curcumin from turmeric interacts with over 100 genes. If that was a drug, that'd be a blockbuster drug. Not only because it does that, but also because you can take it safely for long periods of time. We don't have medications like that. There happens to be plant chemicals that actually do work on stem cells. So we go back to some of our big levers which are resveratrol, curcumin, and Berberine. That's another one of my most favorite plant chemicals.

There's a famous Chinese herb called Huang Qin, and that is Scutellaria Baicalensis. And in China today – modern Chinese herbal medicine – you'll find Scutellaria Baicalensis in almost every anti-tumor formula. And it's got many, many phytochemicals, one of which is Berberine. And Berberine is very bitter, and it stimulates detoxification. Berberine also can control insulin. And so again, because that's a driver of tumor cells, and because in the United States over 40 percent of people are diabetic or pre-diabetic, this is one of the great drivers of cancer in United States today. So we look for plants and chemicals that do that as well. The Scutellaria Baicalensis also has baicalin and baicalein and wogonin, which are a flavonols group of chemicals that turn cancer growth off, turn inflammation off, turn apoptosis on, act on stem cells. So you can see that plants are multitaskers. We can do a lot with a handful of plants.

Dr. Russell Blaylock: For instance, you see in leukemia research. They have absolutely shown that leukemia is much more curable if you use quercetin. Most of the leukemias are very sensitive to quercetin. Lymphomas, all of these things – curcumin, quercetin, ellagic acid, resveratrol – all of these things inhibit the cancer stem cell. And that's what's interesting about, for instance, curcumin. It actually kills the stem cell – the cancer stem cell. It doesn't bother normal stem cells, but only cancer stem cells.

Ty: Curcumin?

Dr. Russell Blaylock: Curcumin. And that's the other thing about flavonoids in these plant extracts; they're very selective. They only damage, inhibit, and kill cancer cells. They have no effect on normal cells, except to make the normal cells stronger.

Ty: Wow. So they'll select the toxicity. That's a big thing. Because you don't want to kill the good cells. You want to kill only the cancerous.

Dr. Russell Blaylock: You see and that's what they always look for. We call it the magic bullet – something that will kill the cancer cell and not hurt the normal cell. Well this does even more. It kills the cancer cell, but it makes the normal cell stronger. And so what they found out, for instance, in radiation treatment – of breast cancers, colon cancers, and lung cancers – it actually makes the radiation much more effective and it protects the tissue that's being radiated that's normal around the cancer.

Ty: Really? And all of these do – the ellagic acid, the resveratrol, curcumin—

Dr. Russell Blaylock: It's a long list of them: auranofin, and ellagic acid, and resveratrol.

Ty: And they all—they affect the stem cells?

Dr. Russell Blaylock: They kill the stem cells, repress the stem cells growth, they kill the daughter cancer cells, they help encase the cancer, they suppress these invasion enzymes, reduce the metastasis, and they protect the tissue – the normal tissue – to help keep it from converting to this same process. Because what you see—when they did this study to see, well if inflammation is the cause of cancer, most people who have cancer should have chronic inflammation. So they did this large study, and that's exactly what they found. For instance, in certain people, 70 percent of them had definable inflammation – arthritis, chronic adenosis sclerosis, or some chronic infection. And that's what caused the cancer. If you stop the inflammation, you stop the cancer from ever forming.

Ty: So do these substances that you're talking about, these flavonoids, do they have any effect on the inflammation?

Dr. Russell Blaylock: They're powerful anti-inflammatory

Ty: So they're not only anticancer, but they're anti-inflammatory too.

Dr. Russell Blaylock: That's how they're preventing the cancer from occurring. And they have other mechanisms that affect the cell's signaling that kills the cancer – turns on the cancer suicide gene – Like B21, B53, and that'll make the cancer cell commit suicide, what we call apoptosis.

Ty: So Dr. Blaylock, in light of the fact that these flavonoids are so beneficial, why is not every oncologist using them to treat cancer?

Dr. Russell Blaylock: Well, because they don't read their articles. And they don't know what these flavonoids are because they don't know the chemistry. So they've never heard of it. They go to a meeting, and the meeting is about the latest protocol or the latest chemotherapeutic drug. And who sponsors the meeting? The makers of the chemotherapeutic drug.

Ty: Wow. So the meetings are sponsored by the pharmaceutical companies? So what kind of education do you think the doctors are going to get there? Of course they're going to get drug-intensive education. And again, this goes back to the premise for episode one. Doctors are not bad people. They're just not educated about these natural treatments for cancer.

A real popular natural treatment that does revolve around nutrition and food, is juicing – and specifically, wheatgrass. People are loving wheatgrass. And so we're going to learn a little bit about wheatgrass here from a cancer survivor that actually used wheatgrass in her protocol to treat her cancer and to cure her cancer naturally. Her name is Lourdes Colon. She's an actress from Hollywood. Let's hear what she has to say.

Lourdes Colon: Wheatgrass was a really big part of the things that I did in fighting cancer. When I found out that it's chlorophyll that's very similar to your blood, that it's just one component away from what your blood is. We have iron. That has magnesium. And magnesium helps build the iron. It's a win–win. I learned that it also had vitamin B17 in it. Well I knew that B17 fights cancer, shrinks tumors. So as much as I dislike the taste—

Ty: Yeah. Bitter.

Lourdes Colon: Yeah. And I meet so many people that love it. It's just it's so crazy. But, I will say that when I started doing a lot of wheatgrass, I would do between four to eight ounces a day. I did colonics every day. I would also do a coffee enema to detox the liver, which was very—it was immensely helpful on everything I was doing. And I would take the pulp of the wheatgrass, and I'd dip into wheatgrass juice. I place it on the tumors with tape, leave it on for an hour. I started seeing shrinkage that way. In fact, I did that for a couple days and there was a time when I couldn't lay on this side because of the pressure. But doing that, I was finally able to lay on my right side without any pressure. So it was that. It was wheatgrass. It was raw juicing. I did raw juicing for three straight weeks where I saw an immense amount of stuff that came out. There was this long – I can't tell you how long it was, but it was very long – parasite that came out. And this is just from doing the wheatgrass shots and doing the colonics daily that I would look and be like, "How is that possible that was in my belly?" But it was just this very long parasite that came out. And you see a lot of these dead cancer cells that came out. It looked like it was a web. And this stuff was coming out. It was tinted with the wheatgrass when they came out. It was interesting, but it pulled all that out.

Ty: Wow. That's amazing. Lourdes shared the story about expelling a foot-long parasite after juicing. That's pretty incredible to me. Most people think that the only way to get rid of a tumor is to surgically cut it out. But what if I told you that you could actually *juice* to remove tumors? Cherie Calbom is known as The Juice Lady. And in this next clip, she shares her personal story of expelling a tumor from juicing.

Cherie Calbom: Superior nutrition – just flooding the body with all of those wonderful nutrients that begin to feed ourselves and bring them to life – that's what we want to bring into our body. Live food.

Ty: And so, one of the ways we do that is through juicing.

Cherie Calbom: That's why I'm known as The Juice Lady.

Ty: The Juice Lady.

Cherie Calbom: Yes.

Ty: So talk about juicing.

Cherie Calbom: Juicing is my passion because we take these beautiful fruits and vegetables and mostly vegetables is what I recommend with maybe just a little fruit for flavor—

Ty: And I apologize. All we have here for props is a little bit of fruit [laughter].

Cherie Calbom: But imagine there are beautiful leafy greens here, and maybe some carrots, and cucumbers, and celery, and some ginger, and a little lemon. That's what I have for breakfast almost every day. So you juice all that up. You've got everything broken down so well that your body can begin to absorb it right away. So everybody is into fiber, fiber, fiber. Oh you've got to have all this fiber in your juice. But actually, when it comes to juice as a supplement, like a liquid vitamin, mineral, enzyme, bio-photon, vital nutrient glass of wonderful nutrients, it's even better when it doesn't have the fiber in there. Not the soluble fiber, yes. It's got soluble fiber, but the insoluble. Because it's going to go right into your system. It's estimated, guesstimated, that it's at work in your system in about 20 or 30 minutes. And that's bringing that life right into your body, and all those antioxidants that are binding up toxins and carrying them out of the body.

And when we're sick with cancer, it's even more important to do these kinds of things – to heal the body. Because as I see it, two primary reasons that people get sick – one is toxicity and number two is that we are undernourished in this country. People are not getting the vital nutrients that their bodies need. So again, back to the juice, broken down, you can get a big concentrate of nutrients like a great big bowl that it would take you maybe hours to eat. You can juice it all up pretty fast. It goes right into your system.

Ty: And it's so good.

Cherie Calbom: It's delicious.

Ty: Talk about your first five days of juicing a couple of decades ago – the story you told me.

Cherie Calbom: I was really sick in my late 20s, and decided that I better do something – this was more than a couple decades ago – I better do something because no doctor knew what to do with chronic fatigue and Fibromyalgia, and they still don't. And so I got an old Norman Walker book, and if you've seen the old Norman Walker juice books, it's not recipes. It's numbers one to 20-something or whatever, and it just lists the vegetables that you should be juicing for that condition. So I had to design my own recipes. The first stuff tasted and looked like motor oil [laughter]. You get too many greens and just the right mix and it looks pretty brown and nasty. But I didn't care. I was so desperate, and I'm just a very determined person. When I'm going to go for it, I'm going to go— completely jump in that pool and go for it. So I decided, I'm going to do a five day juice fast. On day number five – this is honest truth – my body expelled a tumor the size of a golf ball, about that big, with blue blood vessels attached to it. It looked like somebody just chopped them off. And that got my attention.

Ty: I bet it did.

Cherie Calbom: Like nothing else.

Ty: So five days?

Cherie Calbom: Five days, on day number five. So I thought, "Okay. I should just get well after this. Whatever was making me sick is probably gone now, and I should be well." No. I was detoxing. I had some good days and some bad days. I was climbing up that mountain, but it seemed like a couple steps forward and then a couple steps back as my body was getting rid of a lot of toxins. But there came a day when I woke up one morning and thought, "Oh. Somebody gave me a new body in the middle of the night." I felt like a brand new person.

Ty: Oh great!

Cherie Calbom: Yes. And so it wasn't just that one day that I had turned the corner. I was turning the corner the whole time. My body was healing and healing and moving in the right direction. I just didn't see the manifestation of that. And that's why I always say to everybody on their journey, "There is hope. I give you hope. As long as you're breathing, there's hope. And there's healing, and there's so much that can be done. Don't give up." Because just about the moment that you think, "This isn't working." You're probably about to turn the corner. And you could have a morning like I do, where you wake up and think, "Wow. I feel like a new person today."

Ty: That's really amazing. She expelled a tumor just from juicing. That shows you that there are other ways to get rid of tumors. Now, I asked Cherie, who's The Juice Lady, as I mentioned, "What's the best juicer?" because it's a very frequent question. I loved her answer.

Cherie Calbom: You know what the best juicer is on the face of the Earth?

Ty: The one that's in your kitchen that you're using.

Cherie Calbom: The one you'll use every day. If you won't use it, if it's too hard to clean, if it's too much trouble for you, it may be the most perfect one, but it's going to go under your counter. You won't use it. Get one that you'll use.

Henry McElligott: I was told that I had base of tongue cancer tumors that had spread to my lymph nodes on my neck. They were worried that it had already spread to the rest of my body and my organs. So, they put me in a room with about 34 oncologists at this major hospital and put a camera down through my nose to have a look at the tumors that were at the base of my tongue. And a copy of the tumors all appeared up in a screen behind my head. And my wife saw them. And she said, "They look scary." And the head oncologist came to us, and he said, "You need to start radiation and chemo immediately." Because they were worried about it spreading or else I would not survive.

And we were in total shock at the time. We were at a loss for words and we just looked at each other. A few days later, I went to see another group of 11 oncologists at another hospital near my home. And they said the same thing. They said, "Immediate radiation and chemo, or you will not survive very long. Because this is a very dangerous type of cancer. It's already spread to your lymph nodes. We don't know where it is at this stage without further PET scans, MRIs, things like that." So I went home with Joy (wife), just in total confusion, hopelessness, despair set in for a few days. We didn't know what to do.

So, I decided to start looking on the net. What are the side effects of radiation and chemo, and what exactly is chemo and radiation? I discovered on Ty Bollinger's *Quest for Cancer Cures*. I listened to all of his interviews with various cancer specialists all over America. And I was especially intrigued by some of them. I learned so much.

For treatment with chemo and radiation for the type of tumors I had, I would need a tube to breathe and a tube—they wanted to insert a tube in my stomach for food. So I rang the hospital and sent them an email, both hospitals, and I said, "I refuse the chemo treatment and the radiation. I'm going to do some research myself and seek a natural alternative to the chemo and the radiation." And that was it for a couple of days. And then they started ringing me, creating fear over the phone and saying things, "You won't live very long."

I went on total vegetarian food. I had a lot of fruit and nuts to eat. And I went on a three week fast – just water and taking these vitamins. And after the three week fast, I had lost about 10 or 15 kilos. However, I was feeling good. And what I noticed, after taking these products for about six weeks, the swelling at the left side of my neck would begin to decrease in size. And the swelling on my right decreased. And I was able to swallow much more easily. My tongue was not swollen so much. So I got really encouraged by this, because I was under no doctor's care whatsoever.

I continued this treatment until March. At that point, I decided, "Are these tumors decreasing, or has the cancer spread already?" That was my major concern. My blood test went to Germany at the end of April. I got a call from the doctor's secretary on the eighth of May. She said, "Your results are here from Germany. Would you like to come in and see them?" And I said, "Of course I do." I got really excited. When I got there, I had to wait in the room for about 20 minutes for the doctor to see me. It felt like the longest 20 minutes in my life. I just kept twiddling my thumbs. So eventually, he called me upstairs to his office, and he opened this envelope. And he looked at me stunned. I said, "Doctor, what's the result? I'm sweating. What is the result?"

And he said, "Henry, this is a miracle." He said, "I've been a doctor since 1979. You're the first person that has come to this clinic that hasn't been messed around with chemotherapy, radiation, or surgery as a cancer cure." And I said, "Am I?" He said, "These are marvelous results." And he said, "This report is a miracle." He said, "It says, 'Numerous fragmented dead cancer tumors floating all over the blood.'" And then he said, "It is the same result as if you've been having chemo and radiation treatment for the last six months." I was in total shock.

Ty: Wow. Very inspiring words from Henry. I don't know about you, but I love the footage of the kangaroos personally. Henry works really hard to create an anticancer lifestyle through nutrition and through supplements. And he didn't have to suffer through it. Let's listen to Mike Adams, The Health Ranger, address that topic.

Mike Adams: You can have an anticancer lifestyle that's actually very friendly – that's very enjoyable, and quite delicious – in terms of foods. Red grapes, citrus fruits, they're all anticancer. All these amazing things that you can eat, they're anticancer. Fruits and vegetables and even nuts and seeds, so many things, spices. Spices are anticancer. So you can have an enjoyable life and you can live an anticancer lifestyle at the same time. You don't have to suffer through it. The most delicious dishes are usually the most powerful anticancer meals, because they have all the colors and all the different tastes of all the plants that have anticancer properties. It's someone who eats a bland diet that is headed for diabetes, or cancer, or heart disease. Look at the processed food diet. It's high-fructose corn syrup, soybean oil, and—

Ty: Sugar and salt.

Mike Adams: Yeah. Sugar and salt and just garbage processed ingredients. That's a diet of cancer. And that diet tastes horrible. But that's what people have been trained to think is okay. And you know how the food companies make those foods taste good, is they add toxic chemicals to them – MSG, taste enhancers, whatever. So if you eat real food, you're eating an anticancer diet, just automatically.

Cherie Calbom: All your vegetables are going to be great.

Ty: It's hard to find a vegetable that's not anti-inflammatory and anticancer.

Cherie Calbom: Yeah. It is. Because God packaged them just right. They're our most important food in our fight against cancer. All the brightly colored vegetables, and there are hardly any that aren't, a few, and they're still good for us.

Ty: Eat the rainbow right?

Cherie Calbom: Yes. Absolutely.

Ocean Robbins: And there's two parts to healthy diet, I think. One is avoiding the bad stuff. The other is taking advantage of the good stuff. And avoiding the bad stuff is things like pesticides, and hormones, and chemicals, and antibiotics, and all of those sorts of things, and processed foods, additives, flavorings, and colorings, and the list goes on. And taking advantage of the good stuff is getting all the vital nutrients, and all the flavonoids, and all the beautiful things that fruits and vegetables and a balanced, varied diet provides to us. We need the fiber to help clean our colon out. We need the vital nutrients to give us that vitality and that energy and that ability to fight off cancer.

And it's incredible what can happen when you don't just eat a little less bad. When you actually make your food an expression of what you love, your body is more vital and more alive, and you have more bounce in your step. And you have more clarity in your mind. That's what I love getting to see happen in the work that I do. Every day I interact with people whose lives are transforming. Getting to see their smiles brighter, and their work more productive, and their energy stronger, and their lives longer as time goes by. It's thrilling.

Ty: We share Ocean's passions to see people's lives change through nutrition and through better health. And one person that's near and dear to my heart that loved to see people's lives changed as well, was Grandma Helen. She also, by the way, ate the colors of the rainbow as Cherie Calbom just mentioned. Now my Grandma Helen, I called her Mama Helen, was diagnosed with cancer in the late 1980s. And for over a decade, she took a product called Essiac Tea. And it kept her cancer at bay until she died. And, unfortunately, a couple of years before she died, she stopped taking Essiac Tea. In this next clip from Dr. Steve Klayman, you're going to learn a little bit more about the benefits of Essiac Tea.

Dr. Steve Klayman: One thing I got turned on to years ago was Essiac Tea. I read about this nurse, Renee Caisse, up in Canada, back in the 1920s. Many of the cancer patients who were referred to her were terminal. And she gave them this tea called Essiac Tea. E–S–S–I–A–C, Essiac Tea. It was a blend of herbs given to her by an Indian medicine man. And lots of people were getting cured.

About 15 years ago, 18 years ago maybe, my secretary said to me one day, "Dr. Klayman, my aunt has cancer of the spleen. What would you do if you had cancer of the spleen?" I told her I'd start drinking Essiac Tea. And she said, "Where can I get it?" I said,

"Go down to Whole Foods." So about a month later, she tells me her aunt has been drinking the tea and goes into her medical doctor. Medical doctor says, "I can't find any cancer in your body." I think you've had a healing. And she says, "Well, I've been drinking that Essiac Tea." And he said, "Oh that has nothing to do with it. You're in spontaneous remission." [chuckles] You've heard that term before right?

Ty: Many times.

Dr. Steve Klayman: That's a word that means, "I don't know why you're better." We call it spontaneous remission. So she goes on. Comes back to the doctor a couple of months later. And he says, "I'm sorry to tell you, the cancer returned. And I think you have about six to nine months to live." So when she goes home, Angie asks her, "Are you still drinking the tea?" And she said, "No. The doctor said that had nothing to do with my cancer disappearing." She (Angie) said, "You start drinking that tea." And she did. I spoke to Angie a couple of years ago, which is about 15 years after this incident, and she said that her aunt told her the next time you talk to Dr. Klayman, tell him, "Thanks, I'm still drinking the Essiac Tea. And I still have no cancer."

Dr. Murray Susser: Well I had a patient, who had a bowel obstruction, and they opened him up, and he had a cancer of the secum, where the appendix was. And to cut it out, but it had already spread to his liver. And so he was kind of doomed by conventional things. Instead of taking chemotherapy, he took Essiac Tea. He went for years under my care. The tumor never came back.

Ty: So that was just two people that we heard the stories of that successfully used Essiac Tea, plus my Grandma Helen, that's three. But there's literally thousands more people that have successfully used Essiac Tea to keep their cancer at bay and even completely turn it around. But according to mainstream medicine, Essiac Tea is quackery. According to the mainstream medicine, all of these natural remedies have no scientific basis. It's nothing more than snake oil. But is this really true?

Dr. Jonathan Wright: We have close to a hundred thousand references from scientific journals that tell us about diet, vitamins, minerals, botanicals, natural energies, and so forth, and their influences on health. Don't let anybody ever tell you that this isn't scientific. There's just tons of science. It's just that nobody pays attention to it. Because, I'm sorry folks, it isn't patentable. If you can't patent it, you can't make big bucks, and I think we all know that the trend in, let's call it, regular medicine right now, is for the newest patent medicines to be more expensive, more expensive, more expensive. What is it, $73,000 a year, $1,000 a pill, for Hepatitis treatment, that kind of stuff? You can charge that if you've got a patent and you've got a monopoly.

Ty: Right.

Dr. Jonathan Wright: And you cannot do that with unpatentable stuff. So that's why most medical doctors simply haven't even heard of it. It's not that they're, "I hate nature." It's just that they don't know the science is there.

Ty: Well that's really amazing. Over a hundred thousand references to natural medicine in the scientific literature. But the doctors don't know because they don't read the articles. They're too busy. And the only place that they get their education is from these seminars that are sponsored by big pharmaceutical companies or the medical journals that have 90 percent of their ads by the pharmaceutical companies. The deck is really stacked against them. But any kind of a successful treatment protocol for cancer must be focused around nutrition and supplements. But, what if there were a global effort to limit our access to nutrition and supplements? Let's listen to Dr. Rob Verkerk from England discuss that very topic.

Dr. Rob Verkerk: Governments out there don't want people to know about supplements. And they treat them much as they would want to treat medicines and basically as soon as you have a supplement, especially in Europe, that has a therapeutic effect, it's automatically illegal. Because, by definition, under the medicinal code of Europe that was evolved in 1965 to protect people from thalidomide. It basically said that any substance that has a pharmacological effect should be turned to medicine. So that leaves food as this thing that you can consume to provide energy, but not something you can use therapeutically.

So food cannot be medicine, which of course is contrary to what our dear friend Hippocrates said, supposedly said, many hundreds of years ago. So yes, we have major challenges with the food supply and also ingesting concentrated sources of nutrients. Presently, if you look at the nine essential amino acids, there's not one authorized health plan. We're not allowed to say, if you sell an amino acid, even though they're essential to life—

Ty: You can't say anything about it.

Dr. Rob Verkerk: —can't say anything positive about them. You can't say anything positive about glucosamine. And that's because again, the scientific lens that is being built in Codex.

Ty: So what exactly does Codex have to do with our access to vitamins and supplements?

Dr. Matthias Rath: During the first half of the 20th century, no less than nine Nobel Prizes were awarded for vitamin research for the benefit of vitamins for human health. In 1963, the German government, under pressure of Bayer, launched what is called a Codex Alimentarius Commission with a goal to make sure that vitamins and the benefits of vitamins for human health are being eliminated worldwide. So you can see, it's not just you and us talking about cancer. There's a century-long tradition of crime against human health. And when you follow that track, a lot of things we will be talking about today will become easier to understand for the people that watch this interview.

Ty: I don't know about you, but when I first heard that information from Dr. Rath, I was literally in shock. For several seconds, I did not know what to say. He said the Codex Alimentarius Commission was launched specifically to limit access to the benefits of nutritional supplements worldwide. That there's been a century-long tradition of crimes against human health. I wish that it stopped there. But unfortunately, the rabbit hole goes even deeper.

What if not only were we limited in our access to nutritional supplements that can heal us, but we were actually forced to eat foods that make us sick, without even knowing about it? That's the topic of genetically modified organisms or GMOs. We're going to learn more about this in this section.

Jeffrey Smith: Genetically modified organisms – you take genes from one species and force it into the DNA of other species. The GM crops on the market – there's nine of them – and the primary traits are either herbicide tolerance or pesticide production. So herbicide tolerance, Roundup Ready is the most popular. Roundup Ready soy, corn, cotton, canola, sugar beets, and alfalfa. They're engineered with genes from bacteria and pieces of virus etcetera, not to die – the plant doesn't die when it's sprayed with Roundup herbicide, which normally kills plants. So it makes weeding easier for farmers. They can simply spray over the crops and kill all the weeds, but not the Roundup Ready crops.

And the other genetically modified trait that's popular is pesticide production. They take a gene from bacteria in the soil called Bacillus thuringiensis, or Bt for short. They take that gene, which produces a known insecticide, and put it into corn and cotton. So when a bug – certain types of bugs – try to bite the plant, the toxin gets released and then it breaks open little holes in their stomach walls and they die. So now we eat that insecticide and we also eat the Roundup laden crops. So we're eating two types of poisons in these GM crops.

Dr. Ivars Kalvins: Now what we are doing with over modifying the genes in the plants to make them more resistant against bacterias. What is digesting the food in our stomach and intestines? Bacterias – two kilograms of bacterias in our stomach and intestine. And now you're serving them the food which they can't use normally because these are protected by a genetic approach, to avoid this destruction. And now new combinations of peptides are left in our stomach and our intestine and absorbed by our blood. And then we don't know their interaction with the systems in our body.

Dr. Nalini Chilkov: When we're making plants that are like Frankenstein that are not natural, that's where we get into trouble because then we're playing God with nature. We don't know what kind of monsters we're actually going to create, or if our body can actually metabolize them, or if those combinations of genes are going to turn on other disease processes. There's too many unknowns.

Ocean Robbins: We are all participants in a mass experiment. Pretty much unless you've been living in a cave somewhere or growing all your own food, you have consumed some

GMOs at some point. They're only in five major food crops, but those food crops are so wide spread. We're talking corn, soy, canola, sugar beets, and then of course cotton, which ends up in cotton seed oil. But all of our restaurants, virtually, contain genetically modified organisms in their ingredient supply. So, unless you never eat out at restaurants, you've probably being exposed to them.

We do know with certainty that genetically modified organisms are leading to vastly increased use of Roundup, Glyphosate, which has just been declared by the World Health Organization to be a likely carcinogen. We do know that they are leading to vastly increased use of 2,4-D, which is one of the two ingredients in Agent Orange, right? Which has been linked to a host of metabolic and health and neurological dysfunction – birth defects in large numbers. We do know that when we spray these chemicals on our crop plants, we wind up eating crops that have literally absorbed herbicide, which is unprecedented in human history. Because always before if you sprayed them on your crops, the crops would die.

Ty: But you got the resistant crops.

Ocean Robbins: Right. We have resistant crops. So they're absorbing the herbicide. So we're consuming the herbicide. What is the impact on human beings of consuming large amounts of Glyphosate and 2,4-D, and other toxic herbicides? I think it's pretty alarming.

Ty: Ocean just mentioned that Glyphosate has recently been declared a probable carcinogen by the World Health Organization. Now, Glyphosate's the main ingredient in Roundup. In this next clip from Jeffrey Smith, who's a renowned GMO researcher, and we recently learned on our quest, he explains why Glyphosate actually causes cancer.

Jeffrey Smith: Roundup can promote cancer in many, many ways. First of all, it's an antibiotic, and it kills off beneficial gut bacteria causing an overgrowth of the bad gut bacteria. This overgrowth of negative gut bacteria is linked to certain cancers, colorectal cancer for example. The overgrowth of negative gut bacteria can produce Zonulin, which can create leaky gut. It opens the gaps in the cell walls on the intestines. Leaky gut is linked to cancer.

Roundup also damages a set of enzymes called the CYP enzymes, which are part of the detoxification process. And CYP enzymes are linked to cancer. One of the problems with Roundup is, it can disable some of those enzymes that are involved with detoxification. So any toxic influence from the environment can be much more toxic when you're also exposed to Roundup or its active ingredient, Glyphosate. Through the gut bacteria overgrowth it can promote inflammation in the gut. And inflammation is also linked to cancer. So, Roundup has all these different ways, like a perfect storm.

Jefferey Jaxen: The other thing that no one really talks about is Glyphosate was patented in 1964 by a company called the Stauffer Chemical Company. And it was meant to be a chelator of minerals – trace minerals – magnesium especially. So what's happening is, every person tested has some Glyphosate typically running through them, depending on how they eat. But majority of people do, including mothers, including newborn babies. What you're looking at, is you're looking at going through your body as a sponge that pulls your minerals out of your body, pulls your magnesium out of your body. This is coming from, also, soil that has Glyphosate in it that takes up the magnesium.

So, there's a huge push for magnesium deficiency in people to supplement magnesium, and that's one of the reasons this is happening right now. That also affects circulation. And it's been shown that magnesium – go on that subject for a second – it's been shown that low magnesium levels is also a probable carcinogen – just having low magnesium levels. Supplementing magnesium with tumors shows tumor shrinkage. This is a huge thing when it comes to cancer. No one does this.

Dr. Ivars Kalvins: They irritate our cells and destroy their membranes. This is another cause for stomach or intestine cancer, or the colorectal cancer also.

Ty: It's amazing that we know that Glyphosate causes cancer, and it's the main ingredient in Roundup, which is used on all the GMO corn, and the soy. But the FDA does not require a single study to determine whether GMOs are safe. This is the result of a policy overseen by Michael Taylor in 1992 when he was at the FDA. He then moved on over to Monsanto that produces these genetically modified crops, and he was their chief lobbyist and attorney. He's now back with the FDA as the food safety Czar. Now, because of the policy that was developed by Michael Taylor while he was at the FDA, that GMOs are substantially equivalent to food, no testing is required. But is it really true that GMOs are substantially equivalent to food?

Jeffrey Smith: We have a situation where the claims in the policy, that they weren't aware of information showing that GMOs were different, was a complete lie. It was a total fabrication. The lawsuit forced 44,000 secret FDA memos into the public domain. It showed that the overwhelming consensus among the scientists working at the FDA was exactly the opposite. They said GMOs might create allergens, toxins, new diseases, and nutritional problems. They urged their superiors to require testing, complained about the drafts of the policy, and their concerns were ignored and even denied. And the test that they do, tobacco science, complete rigged to avoid finding problems, to catch them red-handed.

Ty: Tobacco science. Jeffrey Smith just mentioned that term. Another example of tobacco science was the Seralini study of 2012.

Dr. Howard Fisher: In the finding by Professor Seralini, who ran his same study that Monsanto ran, that recently came out – it was supposed to be for six months, but actually only for three months – in that study, when he ran it for two years on the *same* rodents, what did he find? Well he found liver and kidney damage beyond the control group. He found 50 percent shorter life for males, 70 percent shorter life for females beyond the control group. This is GMO corn. And he found 200 to 300 percent *increase* in tumors.

Ty: One of the popular theories is that genetically modifying crops is necessary in order to feed the world. We hear that all the time. But is that actually accurate?

Jeffrey Smith: GMOs are so inept at feeding the world that the biggest paper in the world – the biggest study, more than 400 scientists, sponsored by the UN, and signed on by more than 58 countries – concluded that the current generation of GMOs has nothing to offer feeding the hungry world, eradicating poverty, or creating sustainable agriculture.

Dr. Rob Verkerk: There've been so many studies looking at GMOs. There's very little science that suggests that, at the moment, there's any evidence that GMOs can play a realistic part in resolving world hunger. Yet, governments and the biotech industry are saying, "This is going to be the savior."

Dr. Robert Scott Bell: Do we need GMOs to feed the world? Absolutely not. In fact, there was a case a few years back we covered on the radio show out of India, where the farmers miraculously showed that they could double, triple, quadruple the output – the yield – going organically compared to GMO crops. This was supposed to not be possible. This family – on two and a half hectares, they said, two and a half hectares – 22.4 tons of rice.

Ty: Out of that? Wow.

Dr. Robert Scott Bell: Yeah, all organic. And that's supposed to not be possible.

Ty: 44,000 pounds of rice?

Dr. Robert Scott Bell: Yeah. You think you can't feed the world organically by doing that? Now the other aspect is growing our own food. Everybody should have a garden, as well. We shouldn't look to mass farm staff to feed the world, but we've got to rehabilitate soils. But there's a lot of evidence that shows, if you know what you're doing, organically, you can rehab the soils and you can grow abundant nutrient-rich foods to feed the world, without genetically engineered components.

Joel Salatin: At no time in human history has half of all human edible food been thrown away. That's never happened. The biggest lie of our time is that we're short of food. How are we going to feed all these people? Right now, we're throwing away enough food to feed the whole planet a second time.

Ty: Wow.

Joel Salatin: That's never happened in human history. And it's happened because of the inefficiencies in the industrial food system and the global food system where we have so much waste and spoilage, sell-by dates, dented, bent, crashed, whatever.

Ty: That's really startling to me that 50 percent of the world's food supply is actually thrown away. Now we hear that there's a food shortage, and that's why people are starving. It turns out, that's not actually true. They are starving. But it's not because of a food shortage. That kind of puts a little bit of a limp in the giddy-up of the people that are proponents of GMOs because they tell us that we need GMOs to feed the world. There's not a food shortage. While we're on the subject of GMOs, let's hear Dr. Steven Klayman discuss the very hot topic of GMO labeling.

Dr. Steve Klayman: In 1996, I ran for office—I ran for congress here in Texas against Lloyd Doggett, who's been in office for a long time. One of the parts of the platform is labeling GMOs. Even Obama campaigned on, in 2007. He said, "People have the right to know what's in their food." Of course, he turned around and signed the Monsanto Protection Act – like Monsanto needs protection from me, or you. Right? I've been on this issue for a long time, and I realized, back in the 1990s, as this issue was getting heated up, that the scientists were really playing God, and they didn't know what they were doing. And now, of course, you have a whole industry that's sprung out called gluten-free. They've so distorted the chemical makeup of the wheat that people can't digest it, or it causes illnesses.

Ty: Sure. And that's because the wheat used to be, what we call, ancient grains. And now it's not. Now it's been changed as well.

Dr. Steve Klayman: Correct. So it's just—you don't mess with nature. Man, in his attempt to improve on nature, is creating a disaster. This disaster, now, is banned in many countries around the world, because they recognize what it is. Unfortunately, in America, the politicians are paid off so that they won't ban it. Even though 90 percent of the people want GMO-free foods. They want them labeled GMO-free. Labeling hasn't taken effect yet.

Jefferey Jaxen: So essentially, we're fighting simply for the right to know. We're not even fighting to keep this stuff away from our body. We just want to know. So you have companies now that—I always say, I wrote an article, GMO food is the best product according to the manufacturers of GMO food, that no one knows where to buy and no one knows how to find. And it flies in the face of basic finance. If you're a company that has a product, you want people to know where it is. So they're spending millions fighting legally in the courts to keep people from knowing this.

Ty: That's a great point by Jefferey Jaxen. If GMOs are so good for us, why are the multinational companies spending millions of dollars to keep us from knowing if they're in our food. You may not be aware of it, but in the United States, there's current legislation, known as the DARK Act, which would stop any companies from being required to label genetically modified foods. These types of legislations, like the Dark Act and many others, basically legitimize the toxic poisoning of our food. They keep these toxic, poisonous, GMO foods in our food supply. And we're forced to continually eat them unknowingly, because they're not being labeled.

Dr. Connealy: Then you have nutrition. And it's not just that, are you ingesting foods that have nutrients and power and potential. Are you absorbing them? Okay, lots of us have gut compromise.

Ty: Why?

Dr. Connealy: Our gut is not good because there's loaded with chemicals, our food, the GMOs. We have now, in the wheat, Glycerol phosphate. We have all of our food today is challenged and compromised. Then, we're all stressed, so our sufficiency of hydrochloric acid in our stomach, which is naturally there to deactivate all the bugs, whether it's viruses or parasites, is compromised. Then, all of our food is laden with toxicity. We're eating dead food and we want to be alive. How is that possible? It's not possible.

Ocean Robbins: We've got this huge variety of flavors, and textures, and tastes, and cuisines, and opportunities – incredible opportunities. But, it's morally bankrupt. We've got a food system that is full of flavorings, and additives, and chemicals, and colors, and genetically modified organisms, and pesticides, and hormones, and antibiotics. All of these things together are creating this toxic soup. The tragedy, Ty, is that this toxic soup is killing us. It's killing our kids. It's leading to a two-thirds of our population suffering from obesity, a third of our kids expected to get diabetes in their lifetimes, massive epidemics of cancer, as you know, and so much of that could be prevented. It's not an exaggeration to say that in a society where toxic food is normal, and where illness and suffering and feeling like crap are increasingly considered normal, it's time for a serious change.

And so we're standing for a revolution. And we do that through education, through the Food Revolution Summit, through mobilizing with resources and information and knowledge. We want to empower people to put the food revolution into action. Now, the beautiful thing about the food revolution is that you don't have to wait for Monsanto or McDonald's or Coca Cola or the US government to be able to make changes. You can be an everyday food revolutionary in your own life. When you do that, you actually change the systems.

We are actually creating a demand for a whole new food economy. And even companies as big as McDonald's and Coca Cola are feeling the effects and are realizing that what made them food giants in the 20th century is going to make them food dinosaurs in the 21st century if they don't make some big changes. Because consumers are sick of being sick. We're tired of being tired. We're fed up with toxic food. We're hungry for a change. And we're demanding it. That's why we're seeing this massive change in sales of organic food, certified non-GMO food, natural food, local food. Farmer's markets have tripled in the last decade.

Ty: It's real, real food.

Ocean Robbins: Real food.

Dr. Joseph Mercola: The good news is that you can easily avoid it by eating real food. You don't have to worry about it. They're counting on the fact that you're not, that you're going to be the typical American that has 95 percent of his calories—95 percent of his calories is processed food.

Ty: Wow.

Dr. Joseph Mercola: 95 percent.

Ty: That's amazing. I didn't know it was that high. 95 percent processed.

Dr. Joseph Mercola: The typical American. That's not you and me. But the average American's 95 percent.

Ty: Wow!

Dr. Joseph Mercola: So they've got a long way to prevent—now, does it have to be 100 percent real food? No. You can have five to ten percent, that's probably okay – the lower the better, of course, and the less produced is the better. But that's the strategy is to eat as healthy as you can.

Ty: I think that's a great takeaway from this interview. Eat real food.

Dr. Joseph Mercola: Eat real food.

Ty: I love it.

Dr. Joseph Mercola: Keep it simple.

Ty: Yeah. Keep it simple.

Dr. Joseph Mercola: Our bodies weren't designed to be exposed to that type of food. So you have to be careful because it's easy—anyone could easily to do that today. And how do you avoid it? Just stay away from processed foods. There's three words that I strongly recommend. It's three easy words to remember that is: eat real food.

Ty: I love that. Eat real food.

Dr. Joseph Mercola: Eat real food. Because when you do that, you know what you accomplish? You avoid the artificial ingredients that are absorbed into your food. And most people are not aware that there's over 10,000 chemicals that are labeled GRAS (Generally Recognized As Safe) by the food industries themselves. And by labeling them as GRAS, they are able to penetrate a loophole that allows them never to be tested for human safety. Not just singly, let alone, when combined with all the others, so there's synergistic toxicity. So when you eat real food, you avoid the chemicals. You avoid the exposure to these untested chemicals that essentially is making the population a guinea pig. Because we have no idea what the chronic exposure to many of these combination of chemicals will be.

Ty: Because of the fact that many of these chemicals are generally regarded as safe, they're not tested.

Dr. Joseph Mercola: Right. Never tested. Because they've been labeled by the food industry.

Ty: So you're right. We are the guinea pigs on that.

Dr. Joseph Mercola: Yeah. And you can say, "Well that's okay. I'll just read the label." Well if you have the eyesight and the glasses to read the two point font, and the chemical understanding to read the label – because those are complex chemical terms – they're not even there. The loophole says, because they're GRAS you don't have to put them on the food label.

Ty: Really?

Dr. Joseph Mercola: Yes.

Ty: Wow!

Dr. Joseph Mercola: Yeah. So there's no way a conscientious consumer could possibly choose the right food in packaged food. So you just play it safe. Eat real food. Which means, you or someone you know or love or pay prepares the food. Now does that mean you have to do it 100 percent of the time? It's almost physically impossible to do that. Because you're going to go out eat in restaurants, and obviously you're going to delegate that responsibility. But your general pattern 80 to 90 percent of the time is to eat real food that's prepared by you or someone you know.

Ty: I love that – real food. Real food that God made, that's what we should be eating to nourish our body. And it's never too late to start eating good food. Don't be discouraged if you haven't eaten the diet that you should've up to this point. You can start now. And we're going to see evidence of that in this upcoming clip from Robert Scott Bell as he describes a study that was done in Sweden.

Dr. Robert Scott Bell: It was a recent study out of Sweden that was interesting. It was a two week analysis, very brief, but what it showed was just so profound. A family that was eating conventionally grown, non-organic foods, pesticide laden, who thought it was too expensive to eat organic, they did a test.

They said, all right, we're going to take urine samples when you start – eat your regular food. Then we're going to switch the whole family – kids, parents, everybody – to organic.

And over the course of even one day, and ultimately two weeks, the pesticide levels in the urine was extraordinarily high in everything. And each day it dropped to the point that in two weeks, it was almost undetectable. That tells you how fast the body can adapt once you stop putting the onslaught in, in other words, the things that put you into defensive posture.

I'm not saying they're out of the woods in two weeks. But the reality is, as the body then regains that strength that it used to defend against and detoxify from those pesticides, now it's got to relinquish the energy to go after the synthetics that have been bio accumulated in their bodies. And that's the long term recovery that's not always pleasant. But it was a very powerful visual for people to recognize how fast – especially in children – you can reverse ill health by simply stopping the inflow of things that put your body in a state of defense instead of growth and healing.

Ty: Sweden. This is a country right across the Baltic Sea from a small country called Latvia. Latvia is just west of Russia, and it's a country that I actually never learned about in high school geography class. I had to look it up on a map. Myself and the entire Truth About Cancer audiovisual team traveled over there to Riga – small city in Latvia, it's actually the capital of Latvia. And several things about Riga struck us. Number one, it's a beautiful city – a lot of historic monuments, and buildings, and cathedrals, and castles and dungeons are there.

Number two – another thing that struck us about the city, it's very, very clean for so many people there. Maybe the most important thing that struck us there – the most striking thing – was that all the food was clean. It was farm to table. They eat clean food, or real food, as Ocean Robbins mentioned. Almost every restaurant, that's what we found. The people there are extremely healthy, and there is almost no obesity in Latvia. If you remember in episode one, we learned about the war against cancer. But what if I were to tell you that there is actually a *virus* against cancer. Let's go learn a little bit more from Riga, Latvia as we explore this interesting topic.

Dr. Kaspars Losans: RIGVIR® is a live virus – live and frozen virus to keep RIGVIR alive. And it works as a live virus which finds, in the human body, cancer cells and destroys them.

Ty: So you could think of it as a good, or a healthy, virus?

Dr. Kaspars Losans: It's an exceptional, really good virus. We get used to that name, virus, meaning something bad. Here we talk about the opposite situation. We know at least one really good virus which helps patients to get rid of cancer cells.

Dr. Ivars Kalvins: There's only one medicine in the world, on the market, the live virus RIGVIR – Riga means virus, RIGVIR. This is constructed or discovered by Professor Aina Muceniece, and legislated or approved by Latvia FDA, let's say this European country. And is very, very successfully used to treat Melanoma, and not only Melanoma. Because this virus is human virus – native, non-modified virus. The main problem is mutation for all of viruses. This is a non-mutating the virus.

Ty: Dr. Kalvins was one of the three finalists for the European Medicine Award in 2015. He's also a distinguished member of the European Academy of Sciences. He holds 215 patents. He's published over 650 publications. Now let's go back to our history lesson on RIGVIR. Some of the initial experiments were performed on mice.

Dr. Peteris Alberts: They found that if you take a tumor from a patient, put it into a hamster, then it will start growing, or something like that. If you put [it] on the virus, it will just fade away. Do you know who did that observation first? Ms. Garklava, the lady you saw this morning.

Ty: Really?

Dr. Peteris Alberts: Yeah. She did that.

Dr. Jimenez: RIGVIR virus has the peculiarity of selectively targeting cancer cells, leaving normal cells untouched. That's called oncol-tropism.

Dr. Peteris Alberts: And you know who was the one that brought the first virus to the first patient? Ms. Garklava again. RIGVIR is an oncolytic virus. So this is a cartoon, but it shows how the cartoonist would display it. The virus infects the tumor cell. It replicates within the tumor cell. And it just destroys it – blows it up.

Dr. Antonio Jimenez: That's called oncolysis. As that cancer cell bursts, then these viruses that duplicated and replicated inside that cell, will go on and penetrate other cancer cells. One of the interesting things, Ty, about RIGVIR virotherapy, is that it also goes after the cancer stem cells. We know that even if some of the viewers of this docu-series have had chemotherapy or radiation and are considered in remission, or cured, there is a high possibility that they can have a recurrence or a relapse. And so with RIGVIR virotherapy, we can target those stem cells that chemo and radiation do not, and even make more aggressive.

Ty: I'm really happy to be here in Riga, Latvia this morning and I'm sitting across *from* a lady named Khrystyna. Thank you for joining us today. She is going to share with us her story of overcoming melanoma cancer.

Khrystyna Yakovenko: It all started in the end of 2012. When I contacted my doctor, he diagnosed melanoma of the fourth stage, with a metastasize of the liver. They prescribed the plan of chemotherapy and at that time, I even didn't understand what is what. I completely trusted our Ukrainian doctors and I trusted the methods they are using. I trusted this plan of chemotherapy. So I simply didn't realize—I didn't realize the effect of this diagnosis completely, entirely at that moment.

Ty: Okay. So you were diagnosed with malignant melanoma that had metastasized to the liver. So they did not offer you much hope as far as curing your cancer with chemotherapy. How many months or years did they approximate that you had left?

Khrystyna Yakovenko: Maximum of a couple of years.

Ty: Yesterday I saw you with your daughter, I think. Tell me about how it felt to you to have daughters that you may not be able to see. Take your time.

Khrystyna Yakovenko: I was not feeling afraid. I was not falling into panic. Simply, I understood that I had no right to leave it. I had to fight. When I first came to my therapy center, doctors didn't say, "Yes, we will do it." They said, "We will try." Because the stage was late. I think that sometimes on the earlier stages— on the initial stages people who have this very scary diagnosis, they sometimes are by themselves. They lose hope. They stop the fight. And they simply leave it. But, sometimes there are people who, even at late stages, they continue to fight, and continue to find the out of the situation. In this case, as the disease simply just is overwhelming.

Ty: Good for you. Because one of the very important parts about a successful cancer treatment is that you believe in it and you're ready to fight to save your life. That's exactly what you did. You determined that you were going to live and you believed in the treatment. That's a big part of the reason that you're healthy today, I believe.

Ty: Can you name the different lines of cancer – you mentioned melanoma – other types of cancer... [*that RIGVIR can be used for*]

Dr. Ivars Kalvins: There are at least ten different cancers, locations of cancer like renal cancer, like breast cancer, like stomach, lung, many others, also prostate cancer, which is very, very common for men. But, approved officially, it is only for melanoma now, but this is a very, very big success because we see that the people who use this virus for other indications of other types of cancers also can be healed.

Dr. Elita Shapovalova: In melanoma cases, in earlier stages when patients receive RIGVIR, the percentage survived is 92 percent. And later stages, for example, if they receive RIGVIR it's 60 percent. If they don't receive it, it's only 9 percent. There's no chemotherapy medicine that can treat melanoma, at least not found. In the beginning, we were using radiotherapy. But then, it got rejected. So we could not use it because it kills the immune system and it's very hard to fight. We come back to chemotherapy—the medicine in the chemotherapy field is not found to cure melanoma. And the second negative is that it has side effects, which simply destroys the immune system, which lowers the quality of life of the patient, and simply changes the whole life of the patient by these side effects.

Dr. Peteris Alberts: RIGVIR is the first real cancer therapy where you have an oncolytic virus which also has immunomodulating activity. That's the duel move to action.

Dr. Kaspars Losans: Then comes the second mechanism of RIGVIR. Whenever those RIGVIRs are attracted to cancer cells, those cancer cells become invisible for the human immune system. Until that time, they are invisible, they have the natural ability to be hiding from the immune system. And due to the RIGVIR guidance, because RIGVIR is attached, and attach to cancer, and RIGVIR is inside the cancer cell. So the immune system, due to RIGVIR, recognizes cancer and starts to react against this cancer.

Dr. Antonio Jimenez: Often times, in clinical practice, we focus on optimizing the immune system – getting the best immune system possible. And that's great. But still, cancer cells have now developed a way to bypass immune recognition. And the International Virotherapy Center here in Latvia, with the studies on RIGVIR, they have concluded that the RIGVIR is binding to the receptor site on the cancer cell surface, called the CD55. When it binds to this receptor, now the T-cells, the B-cells, the natural killer cells, will recognize the cancer cells and mount a specific immune response.

Ruslan Isayev: The only recommendation we have in Russia, in our country, after surgery, is chemotherapy. And doctors left me at home with seven months to live.

Ty: So seven months to live, there was really no hope that they offered you?

Ruslan Isayev: They said, "No. You're no hope. You can get ready to live the last period of your life." And when I got home, they prescribed chemotherapy and chemotherapy was prescribed. After the very first course of chemotherapy, I was feeling really bad. My condition was really, really weak. And I rejected to continue the chemotherapy, even though I had a very serious disease. Somehow, I survived for one year more without chemotherapy. After that, I decided to switch another—to find another treatment method. This is the one that saved me.

Ty: Tell us about your son, who's a miracle because of RIGVIR. I've heard the story, but go ahead and share it with us, please.

Ruslan Isayev: It's a very hard topic. I become very emotional.

Ty: Tell him to take his time.

Ruslan Isayev: We were sitting at home having dinner one evening and my wife said that she's pregnant. Before that, the doctors said that due to my disease, it would be very hard to have kids. Everyone said that, not even just too hard, it would be *impossible* to have kids. And the day when my wife told that we're having a baby after this very serious, difficult time, I thanked God and I gave my word that if were to be a girl, a daughter, I would name her after Aina Muceniece—after Professor Aina Muceniece, who was the discoverer, the great person, so Aina. And if it were to be a boy, then I would name him after the chairman of virotherapy, Jurgis, who is the grandson of Professor Aina Muceniece.

Ty: So Ruslan, you named your son Jurgis after the grandson of the inventor of RIGVIR. Do you have a picture of your son that you could show us?

Ruslan Isayev: Sure I have one. I will show it. See what RIGVIR does. [*holds up photo of son*]

Dr. Kaspars Losans: There's multiple studies performed before registration. Both proved efficacy and safety. Actually, you just talk about efficacy. But the safety profile is exceptional among all oncology treatments. Because in the field of oncology, all treatments are usually phrased like aggressive and full of damages. RIGVIR treatment goes mostly with no side effects. Since RIGVIR registration, there are no serious adverse events registered for RIGVIR.

Ty: There's no side effects to RIGVIR?

Dr. Ingrida Chema: No. I have not in my practice in oncology, since 1989, I have never seen side effects. I may never. No. What can be better if you have a medication with no side effects? It will help, but it will never harm you.

Dr. Kaspars Losans: We know the great ability of RIGVIR to destroy cancer cells. So we based on this effect, to prescribe to our patients why the therapy. They are getting great life expectancy due to RIGVIR. We know from clinical studies that efficacy is proven. But we are much more grateful for our patients who we saw with really bad stages, bad diagnoses, and we see them alive for five years, for 10 years, for 15 years. So they are cured.

Ty: Is RIGVIR approved in Latvia as an official medicine for cancer?

Dr. Kaspars Losans: Yes. Rigvir is registered in Latvia, in drug agency, as an official medicine approved for treatment. Actually, in Latvia, patients happy, for skin melanoma, Rigvir is compensated by country, so patients should not buy it. It's free of charge for them. So treatment is cure it in best possible way. Just today, I've seen patients from Ukraine, Lithuania, Russia, Latvia of course, Chechnya, part of Russia. I've seen patients from all over.

Ty: Is this becoming a place where people come from all over to get this treatment?

Dr. Kaspars Losans: Actually, here in International Virotherapy Center, we have largest experience yet accumulated for virotherapy with Rigvir, so patients today more than from 40 countries are coming to Riga to get this treatment and to be cured from their cancers.

Ty: One person who is alive due to RIGVIR is a lady named Zoya, she's from St. Petersburg, Russia, and she was literally given two weeks to live. Her family picked her up, out of the hospital, carried her to the car, and drove her all the way from St. Petersburg, Russia, to Riga, Latvia. Let's hear her story.

Zoya Sokolova: It was—the diagnosis was very sudden for me. It was after a very strong stress, and then after a month and a half, I was diagnosed with a third stage cancer. Already after the surgery I had my chemotherapy, then they assigned another six chemotherapy and a full course of radiotherapy. My condition allowed only for chemotherapy to be handles, and after the fourth, I wasn't able to stand up from the bed. I became a bed patient. Before these courses of chemotherapy I was told about a center, about a treatment, but I believed in our doctors and their treatment methods. So I decided to follow that path.

Ty: The doctors that treated you in Russia, did they give you hope that eventually the chemotherapy would cure your cancer and you'd be able to walk again?

Zoya Sokolova: It seemed that they wanted it to be so for me, but they couldn't give a warranty, they couldn't say for sure that I would [beat] this disease. That moment when I couldn't stand up from the bed on my own. I was so weak, and my relatives decided to take a van, to make a bed for me, and simply drive me to Riga, to the center. Before coming to Riga I made a blood test and a complete observation for the doctors here to have the full picture of my condition. When the doctor saw my blood test she was really astonished because all the blood tests was lower than for a live person. She was astonished how I managed to get here, staying alive.

Ty: So I understand this properly... your blood work was almost equivalent to that of a dead person. They were amazed that you were still alive at that point.

Zoya Sokolova: The doctor said exactly, "I'm not asking how you got here, I'm asking how you are still alive with this blood test?" From my feelings at that moment, I realized that I would not survive, and I felt how my body is fading from day to day. The doctors recommend me to take certain measures, to take certain indications – even before taking RIGVIR – to simply boost my immune system, to repair my immune system, my body, so I could be ready for RIGVIR. After a couple of weeks I started to take RIGVIR. It was really my family who made the decision because for me I was so weak, I was so done. I was ready to simply say goodbye to this life and my family took the decision. I simply accepted their decision and I thought "what shall be, this shall be." I followed them. After following the indications of the doctors for boosting my body, my immune system, after two weeks I was able to stand up and walk. Get up from the bed and walk around the house, and move so I was feeling better. After a month of already taking RIGVIR therapy my condition changed entirely. [Before] I was not even able to walk around, stand up from the bed. [After] I was even able to drive myself to Riga to receive the therapy.

Ty: After you began only a month of RIGVIR therapy, did you ever contact those patients that you used to know in Russia (when you were being treated with chemotherapy I'm sure you had contact with other cancer patients), did you ever contact them again and let them know that you'd found this place?

Zoya Sokolova: When I started to receive RIGVIR therapy I very quickly became a very healthy person. I started to travel, I started to have energy. I called them and I recommended to them to start this treatment. But for some reason they refused that and now they're all gone. It's a pity that all the great people are gone now.

Ty: Are you ever in contact with them today to see how they're doing?

Zoya Sokolova: But I'm happy, I'm healthy. I can't say at the beginning that I didn't trust this method, simply that I didn't know. I was so weak, but now, finally I don't have any more disability category. I'm a completely healthy person and I'm so much thankful to the people who helped me here.

Ty: Wow, if those testimonials don't touch your heart, I don't know what will. I can't believe it, but we're almost at the end of tonight's episode. But just in case you missed any of it, let's look at a quick recap of what we've learned tonight.

Wow! What incredible discoveries we've been privileged to learn from these experts today. We're accomplishing and fulfilling our goals to educate, expose, and eradicate cancer through covering these vital areas of discovery. Identifying cancer-killing viruses, learning the importance of cancer stem cells, the dangers of GMOs, the power of juicing, and the significance of eating the rainbow.

Had you ever heard of viral therapy before? Had you ever seen the documented evidence behind it? I know that seeing a virus that selectively targets and kills cancer without harming the body is truly encouraging. As you see the experts making scientific advancements, and survivors across the world are, in fact, winning the war against cancer.

I know you've been empowered by learning about cancer stem cells, and that this simply must be addressed in true cancer treatments and preventions. You may have been shocked to see that many conventional therapies are not even addressing this crucial origin of cancer. And consequently, the victims of false treatments are having their cancer recur and doctors and patients alike are scratching their heads and feeling trapped inside this cancer maze.

The Truth About Cancer is found in identifying and solving cancer's root causes. You've seen the horrifying poisoning of our major food supplies through GMOs, and how truly harmful these "Frankenfoods" are to our bodies. As well as how you can eat a diet which is GMO-free and prevent these harmful toxins from entering your body.

You've seen how bringing the right foods into the body is, in fact, medicinal, and that eating the rainbow (while a colorful metaphor) is an inspirational reminder to supply the body with its diverse needs.

Finally, you've seen how juicing can be an integral part of an efficacious protocol for beating and preventing cancer. And you've seen the inspirational stories of people that have trusted in nature's medicine to heal their body.

I'm so grateful we've been able to equip you with the keys of truth on these vital topics which affect cancer. And through the application of what you've learned, you can live free from fear, knowing that you can beat and prevent cancer in your life, as can your friends and family.

I hope you've learned from tonight's episode. Our desire is to educate and I really believe tonight's episode was jam-packed full of information that's vital to be healthy, and to prevent cancer.

In tomorrow night's episode we're going to fly down to Tijuana, Mexico. We're going to visit a cancer center that's curing patients all the way from Stage 1 to Stage 4 that have breast cancer, prostate cancer, ovarian cancer, thyroid cancer, and lymphoma, just to name a few. All using non-toxic therapies. We're going to also learn about the role of glutamate in feeding cancer cells. We all know about sugar being a primary cancer feeder, but almost nobody realizes that cancer has two fuels: one of them is glutamate. We're going to learn a lot more about that tomorrow night.

We're going to also take a tour through a very prominent doctor's garden, who grows much of his own food. We're going to learn about the medicinal properties in these amazing nutritional superfoods. We're also going to hear from a man who has started what's called the "Food Revolution Summit" as he gives us his take on nutrition, specifically as it relates to cancer.

I'm so excited to have been able to share this information with you tonight. I hope it's impacted your life. If it has, please share with your friends, share with your family, bring them back tomorrow for tomorrow night's episode as it will contain some life changing information. Until then, have a great evening. God bless every one of you out there.

[*credits roll*]

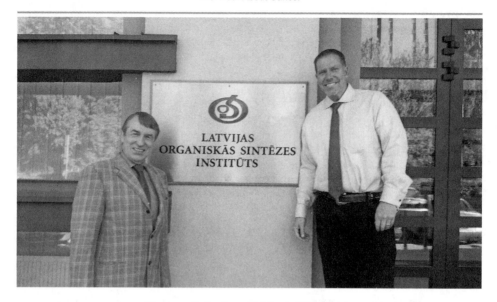

Above - with Dr. Ivars Kalvins in Riga, Latvia
Below – The TTAC Team in London across from Big Ben & the U.K. Parliament House

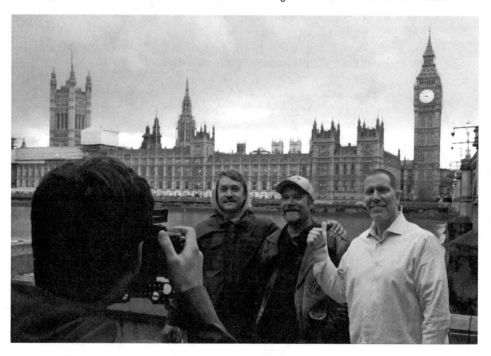

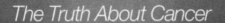

GLOBAL QUEST Episode 4

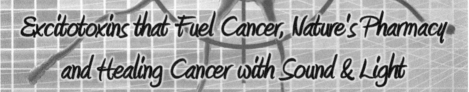

Excitotoxins that Fuel Cancer, Nature's Pharmacy and Healing Cancer with Sound & Light

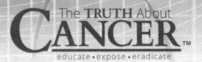

The TRUTH About CANCER™

educate • expose • eradicate

Ty: Welcome back to The *Truth About Cancer: A Global Quest.* I hope you really enjoyed last night's episode, but just in case you missed any of it, here's a brief recap for you.

[*Video plays: Summary of Episode Three*]

Ty: As you just saw, last night's episode was jam packed full of life saving information and tonight's will be the same. We're going to travel down to Tijuana, Mexico, to visit a cancer clinic that's treating and beating cancer naturally, all various types and stages of cancer. We're going to also learn about a class of chemicals that are called *excitotoxins*. They literally excite your brain cells to death. There's two very popular excitotoxins that we're going to learn about in tonight's episode.

Of course, nutrition is a huge piece of the cancer-fighting puzzle, so we're definitely going to address that again tonight. We're going to learn some valuable nutritional nuggets in tonight's episode. Before we get there, let me ask you a question. Last night's episode we learned that big pharmaceutical companies regularly buy off scientists and pay for studies to produce the results that they want in order to get their drugs approved. Is it possible that the nutritional industry also does the same? Let's listen to Ocean Robbins.

Ocean Robbins: Out of all the medical schools in the United States, less than a third of them have a single required course in nutrition.

Ty: Yeah.

Ocean Robbins: So it's possible for a doctor to go through six years of medical school, plus all of their residency and never have a single course in nutrition. We've got a food industry that pays no attention to health and we've got a health industry that pays no attention to food, and yet food is the foundation of health. We all know intellectually that an ounce of prevention is worth a pound of cure, and yet functionally the way we're living is the complete opposite of that.

Ty: Yeah.

Ocean Robbins: And that's not by accident. We have a lot of money being made by the food industry for selling whatever it can sell for the lowest possible price. We've got a lot of money being made by a medical industry that's now 19 percent of gross domestic product in the United States, and most of that money is being made off treating the symptoms of disease. Disease that we know how to prevent, but there's not money to be made in that. I'm not accusing every individual doctor of being out just to make a buck, I'm saying that we've got a system in place. That systematically causes us to be sick.

I'll tell you what else, even the Association of Nutrition and Dietetics, which is the major group for the dieticians of the United States. They have their annual meetings and some of their sponsors are companies like McDonald's and Coca Cola. They literally give away Coca Cola to everyone at those meetings for free. They will sponsor sessions, discussion groups on topics, but literally say in the program, sponsored by McDonald's, sponsored by Coca Cola. How objective do you think that information is going to be and how revolutionary do you think it's going to be? When you actually look at the data and what is the impact of these companies on the health of our kids, on the health of our population, then this isn't just funny, it's also scandalous.

Ty: Yeah.

Ocean Robbins: That nutritionists and dieticians whose job it is to look out for the public wellbeing and to help individuals to get on a path of health are being bought off, functionally speaking, by industries that are polluting the health of the people these folks are supposed to be serving.

Dr. Joseph Mercola: I didn't realize how nefarious the food industry was until I read Marion Nestle's book which will be out in October of 2015, called *Soda Politics*. They are every bit as evil as the drug companies with respect to their political lobbying, the revolving door between the industry and the federal regulatory processors. They've got the whole system stacked against you.

Ty: Money is oftentimes the deciding factor in decisions that directly affect your health and my health. It shouldn't be that way, but that's reality.

Dr. Patrick Quillin: Well, we have to admit that healthcare is a business in America. In fact there are vested interests in this business of healthcare; it's a $2.7 trillion a year medical industrial complex we have in America.

Dr. David Brownstein: The cancer medical complex is this whole monolith that's been set up to make money on cancer. And so let's take the young woman who has been feeling a breast lump, goes to her doctor, she goes for a mammogram, they pick up something. She's going to go for a biopsy, they pick up something. Now she's going to go for an excision, tell her she's got cancer, she's going to get chemo and radiation. It's this whole system set up to treat cancer and it's a multi-trillion dollar industry right now and the problem is, people aren't living longer from these therapies.

Ty: This cancer industrial complex that Dr. Brownstein just mentioned, where only certain *approved* treatments are covered by insurance, is alive and well in the United States, but it's not just here in the United States. This is a global thing. Let's listen to Ard Pisa as he describes the state of affairs in Holland.

Ard Pisa: It is by law, arranged in Holland, that a doctor must give chemo or radiation and surgery, but no natural treatment. Not allowed in Holland.

Ty: Natural treatments are not allowed.

Ard Pisa: No. You are going tomorrow, to Professor Dr. Alcott at the medical center at Cologne. You can't open the door for a medical center in Holland like that. It isn't allowed in Holland.

Ty: At least people in Holland have access to go the clinic in Germany. It's close.

Ard Pisa: Yeah, it's close, but you have to pay for yourself and that's a big problem.

Ty: Okay. Insurance doesn't cover it.

Ard Pisa: Exactly. Here in Holland they pay insurance for chemo, 50,000 euro; 30,000 euro for a natural treatment. In Germany, they won't pay it.

Ty: Wow.

Ard Pisa: It's crazy. It's the world upside down.

Ty: I agree with Ard the world is upside down. A prime example of this upside down world is in our food supply. Did you know that there are certain substances that may be in popular foods like Chinese food that literally excite brain cells to death? They're called excitotoxins. In this next clip Dr. Russell Blaylock, who is a neurosurgeon and a scientist describes the role of glutamate in producing and feeding cancer.

Dr. Russell Blaylock: MSG is monosodium glutamate—it's just a salt of glutamate. The damaging element is the glutamate. Not the monosodium. You forget that. Anything that says glutamate is an excitotoxin, that means they can destroy brain cells.

Now, when I did most of my research and writing about excitotoxins it had to do with the brain because that's where we thought all the glutamate receptors were. Now we found out that the glutamate receptors in every cell in the body. Not a single cell doesn't have glutamate receptors. What that means is, if you eat glutamate, now you don't have a blood-brain barrier to even consider protecting you. Because glutamate goes to all of these cells without any interference and your blood level rises very rapidly and very high over a prolonged period of time. Humans have a higher and more persistent level of glutamate in their blood than any animal that you experiment on.

The second thing once they found out glutamate receptors are everywhere is, they found out glutamate receptors trigger and stimulate the growth and invasion of cancers, of every kind. First they thought it was brain tumors only. They demonstrated that if you had high glutamate levels around the tumor, the tumor became highly invasive and grew twice as fast as a tumor that had low glutamate levels. They started looking at other tumors, lung tumors, colon cancer, breast cancer, prostate cancer, thyroid cancer. They looked at—every cancer they looked at, they found the same thing. Glutamate acted as a fertilizer if you will—a stimulant for the growth of that cancer. Made it grow extremely fast, made it highly invasive and less likely to be cured.

Now, the research has continued and we're finding that more and more. Now, the second corollary is that if you blocked the glutamate receptor, the tumor starts slowing its growth. It becomes less invasive. And the tumor will start dying. The cells start dying. It has no negative effect on normal cells. If you block the glutamate, normal cells reproduce, function just fine. It's only the cancer cell that starts dying when you start blocking glutamate receptors.

And then they found, well, if you take a patient who is getting chemotherapy, and you give them these glutamate blockers, the chemotherapy works a lot better.

Ty: So you take it along with—the chemotherapy.

Dr. Russell Blaylock: You can take it along with...

Ty: I know a lot of people that are watching are on chemo now.

Dr. Russell Blaylock: Right. This is a really hot area of research. The big question is, you don't want to block all glutamate receptors because the brain needs them—for its function. You wouldn't be able to remember—you'd fall into a coma. So you want to do a selective way to cut down that glutamate production. There's an enzyme in your cells called glutaminase, and its function is to convert glutamine into glutamate. That's how that cancer cell starts producing lots of glutamate. If you block that enzyme, that tumor starts shrinking.

Ty: Are there natural glutamate blockers that we should be familiar with?

Dr. Russell Blaylock: Fortunately there is a lot of them.

Ty: Okay.

Dr. Russell Blaylock: Virtually all of your flavonoids that I've discussed: curcumin, quercetin, ellagic acid, resveratrol, anthocyanins, they all reduce glutamate receptor activity. And that's their advantage and they do it safely. So the brain can function normally but the cancer can't use it.

Ty: Fascinating information from Dr. Blaylock, that the glutamate actually acts as a fertilizer for cancer cells. I thought it was really interesting what he said. It's not the monosodium—most people have heard of MSG, monosodium glutamate. It's not the monosodium part that's the problem. It's the glutamate and there's many different types of glutamate. Let's listen to some more from Dr. Blaylock as he shares.

Dr. Russell Blaylock: Cancer cells use two major fuels, they use glucose and they use glutamine. Of the two, glutamine is the more powerful stimulant for cancer cell growth.

Ty: Okay. We hear that "watch out for sugar and glucose" because cancer cells do feed on it, but you're saying glutamine is worse.

Dr. Russell Blaylock: Yeah, because the Warburg effect is the fact that normal cells use both anaerobic and aerobic system, the Krebs cycle. The cancer cells only use the anaerobic system, it was thought. Glutamine can work the aerobic system and product a lot more energy. So if you're eating a lot of sugar and you're eating a lot of glutamine, you're really stimulating your cancer powerfully. So the idea is you want to cut down your glutamine intake. A lot of people are promoting glutamine as a way to heal the gut—the leaky gut syndrome. So, they're saying, take five, six, ten grams of glutamine. That is a powerful stimulant for degenerative brain disorders, a powerful stimulant for cancer growth. You don't want to do that. There's a lot better ways to repair the GI tract—they work better and safer and actually inhibit cancer.

Ty: But not glutamine.

Dr. Russell Blaylock: But not glutamine. The other thing is foods, for instance, beans, like black beans are high in glutamine, mushrooms are high in glutamine. So these foods that are high in glutamine, you don't want to eat either. You want to try to eat only low glutamine foods and a lot of those are your vegetables. Some cancer researchers think this maybe why people who are on vegetarian diets and juicing seem to have these spontaneous cures of cancer is because they have such a low glutamine intake and a low sugar intake.

Ty: So getting rid of the two fuels.

Dr. Russell Blaylock: Getting rid of the two fuels. Now, cancer cannot use fat for its fuel. So coconut oil is a good way to keep your energy up without having to resort to sugar and cancer can't use it.

Ty: MSG is one form of glutamate. What are some other sources of glutamate to avoid?

Dr. Russell Blaylock: Well, industry really got hammered when my book *Excitotoxins* came out and everybody was looking at glutamate. They started taking MSG off the label and they even put on the label, "Contains no MSG" and then they put sources of glutamate in it like hydrolyzed protein, soy protein isolate, soy protein concentrate, autolyzed yeast, caseinate, very common. All of those are extremely high in glutamate, but the law allows them to put those in the foods and still put on the label, "contains no MSG."

Ty: Because they're not monosodium glutamate.

Dr. Russell Blaylock: No monosodium glutamate, but they're just as dangerous and harmful as monosodium glutamate.

Ty: So you have to watch out for all of the forms glutamate.

Dr. Russell Blaylock: All the forms of glutamate, particularly soy. Soy is naturally high in glutamate and glutamine, as well as aluminum and fluoride and manganese.

Ty: Wow.

Dr. Russell Blaylock: It's got a lot of toxins in it. Soy is a very bad food and particularly a liquid food, if you get it in milk and soy and liquid products, it's very high in glutamate levels and your blood level will rise as much as 20 fold or 50 fold.

Ty: And that's even if it's organic soy, right?

Dr. Russell Blaylock: Doesn't make any difference, it's natural to the plant. In my estimation, people shouldn't be consuming soy products.

Ty: Dr. Blaylock mentioned that glutamate is not only a fuel, but it's also a fertilizer for cancer cells. Now when you hear Fuel for Cancer, most people who have been paying attention thus far in the series are going to say sugar and sugar is something that we must address. Sugar is one of the primary fuels for cancer.

In this next clip, we listen to a scientist describe what we need to really look out for when it comes to sugar. Are all sugars bad? Or are there certain things we need to look for as far as sugar is concerned, potentially the spikes of sugar, the glycemic index? What is it that we need to look out for in order to avoid sugar fueling cancer cells?

Dr. Subrata Chakravarty: The question then becomes from practical perspective, what is a cancer patient to do? Should they not eat sugar? Should they eat sugar? The good thing here is that the source of sugar matters. You know how you're eating when sugar makes a difference. But if you look at the patterns of sugar eating back in the 1960s, most of our sugar came from sugar cane, and that sugar cane, if you look at what it's made of, it's mostly sucrose. It is 50 percent glucose, 50 percent fructose.

Over time, what has happened is the high fructose corn syrup has caught up with it. There a lot of indications to show that high fructose corn syrup has brought several negative health effects. Inside cancer, there is a processing center for glucose and inside any cell is there is always a processing center for glucose. They're what we call the hexokinase receptors—XK2—so to speak in cancer cells and in normal cells as well. The only difference is that there are way more XK2s in cancer cells than there are in regular cells.

The problem that happens is now you've got a hungry dog out here and you've got a dog that is not so hungry that could get satiated easily. When you have a sudden spike of sugar, guess what? The hungry dog is going to overfeed on that sugar. What we are really looking to do is to stop the spikes of sugar. That's what we're looking to give people diets that have got a lot of low glycemic index.

A lot of people think, okay, fruits and vegetables. That is something that we recommend for cancer, a cancer patient should eat fruits and vegetables. A lot of people think, oh my god, fruits and vegetables are so high in sugar. How is that going to affect our cancer cells? The answer lies really in not so much the composition of the sugar itself, but in how it is delivered.

In the case of sugars, if you look at the balance of what content most fruits have, it's different. Some fruits have got a higher level of fructose, some fruits have got a higher level of glucose—some of them have sucrose, so you have various varieties. Apples, pears, they're pretty good to eat because they've got a relatively higher fraction of fructose to glucose, but they have both. They have sucrose as well. They also have a lot of fiber with them. When you're eating them, what the fiber does is it slows down the absorption of the sugars into the body and that makes sure that you aren't going through those incredible spikes that are causing the absorption of the sugar into the cancer cells, which then feeds into their mechanism of growth because the more sugar they get, the more they can grow and they can replicate themselves.

Ty: So just to reiterate, what we have to watch out are the sugar spikes and what might cause those sugar spikes? It's the man-made processed sugars, the candies, the sweets. We also have to watch out for sugar's effect on the immune system.

Dr. David Jockers: Sugar really impairs the immune system. In fact, in 1970s, a scientist named John Ely—and what John did—Dr. Ely, he actually looked in detail at what happens...how do white blood cells run? What's different about white blood cells and normal cells? What we found was that white blood cells actually need 20 times more Vitamin C than normal cells.

Now, he also looked at, what's the pathway for white blood cells to get the Vitamin C that they need. We know Vitamin C is an antioxidant, protects the white blood cells from oxidated stress and of course, most of your listeners—most of your people should know, white blood cells are kind of like your military. They're going out and they're fighting wars every single day and so they need a lot of protection.

How does the Vitamin C actually get into the white blood cells? That's the question. What he found was that it goes through the same pathway that sugar or glucose gets into the cell – through insulin – and so what that means is when blood sugar elevates, our body naturally produces this hormone called insulin. Insulin takes the sugar, puts it into the cell where it belongs. What we know is that cells, including white blood cells, they have a greater affinity for glucose—the insulin receptor itself has a greater affinity for glucose than it does Vitamin C. So what that actually means is that when blood sugar is elevated, we are unable to get the Vitamin C into the cell and so there is something that Dr. Ely came up with, it was called the phagocytic index, and it was just this measurement of how good a white blood cell is at destroying either abnormal cells like cancer or bacteria, virus something along those lines.

Ty: How many bad guys can it kill?

Dr. David Jockers: Exactly. That's exactly what he was looking at. Here is what he found was that a blood sugar of 120 actually reduces your phagocytic index by 75 percent. So, we look at our blood sugar of 120, we know that if you have a fasting blood sugar of 120, you are considered pre-Diabetic, 125/126 is diabetic. Most people say, I don't have a fasting blood sugar of that, however, most people in society – let's say we eat cereal in the morning – just eating the bowl of cereal in the morning for the next three to four hours, you're going to have a blood sugar above 120.

Ty: Just from cereal?

Dr. David Jockers: Just from cereal.

Ty: Not even sugared cereal just because of the grains?

Dr. David Jockers: Exactly. Just eating Cheerios. Having a glass of orange juice with that. Your blood sugar is going to be pumped up and what's happening there is, you are actually reducing your white blood cells' ability to break down cancer cells. Then if you go and at lunch and you have a sandwich, have these high carb meals all throughout the day, you're actually reducing your phagocytic index. Most people are spending 16 hours a day with reduced immune function.

Ty: As we just heard from Dr. Jockers, sugar actually burdens and impairs the immune system. It fuels cancer cells, but that's not the only reason to stay away from processed man-made sugars like candies and sweets. Another reason we need to stay away from it, is it's been recently shown through studies that have been published in peer-reviewed journals, that sugar actually *creates* cancer cells. This is called oncogenesis.

Sayer Ji: A new study came out that showed for the first time that cancer doesn't only just feed off of sugar, but that sugar can induce a cancerous phenotype in cells. Which means it basically changed from a cell that just likes glucose to one that exhibits invasive activity where it's basically now becoming an independent cell that wants to go out and invade other tissue. So it was the first time we saw that sugar is a cancer risk, much like smoking is. It's not just that it feeds cancer is that it can actually *cause* cancer.

Ty: So in light of this information that Sayer just shared with us that sugar is oncogenic. It actually causes cancer. Does it make any sense to have bowls of candies and sweets in the office of oncologists that are treating cancer patients?

Suzanne Somers: In oncologists' office I've seen it where you go into their office and they have candy bowls with candy there because cancer patients on chemotherapy are so weak and they need a little pick me up and I have looked at that at different times in Oncologists' office going…

Ty: What are they thinking?

Suzanne Somers: What are you thinking?

Burton Goldberg: When you finish your chemo in a conventional setting, they give you cookies and ice cream or candy. That is tantamount to putting gasoline on a fire. That means these oncologists are guilty of crimes against humanity. They are killing their patients.

Dr. Roby Mitchell: One of the tests we use to diagnose cancer is a PET scan. So with a PET scan, we take radiated sugar, and we inject it in you because cancer cells take up sugar so much more efficiently than normal cells, they will take up that radiated sugar and then we're able to see on the CAT scan where the sugar is, which that tells us where the cancer is, right? So, yes, we're very aware of the dependence on cancer cells for prodigious amount of sugar and that's why cancer patients die of starvation is because the cancer cells will suck up all of the sugar from normal cells.

Jenny Hrbacek, R.N.: We're going to pretend these are both cells. The little pins I stuck – and I have ten pins in this ball – these represent insulin receptors. We know that when we eat a piece of whole wheat bread, that has as much glycemic rise as a little Snickers bar, but we don't think about the bread as being sugar. That's a lot of the—me included got in the situation. But you eat that, your blood sugar rises and the pancreas puts out some insulin and comes and opens these little doors so the sugar can get in a cell for energy.

Ty: Okay.

Jenny Hrbacek, R.N.: So the doctors use—what happens is, we run high blood sugar systemically as Americans, standard American diet.

Ty: Because we eat a bad diet.

Jenny Hrbacek, R.N.: Yes and so the body—the body doesn't like that. It doesn't like that high blood sugar because it burns your neurons, it messes with your vision, people get numb feet, their wounds won't heal. So the body is going to put more and more of these little receptors in to try and get the sugar out of the blood into the cell. So eventually you end up with this and this is what a cancer cell looks like. A cancer cell, from what my research is of 15 to 16 times the number of insulin receptors as a regular cell.

So when you go for your PET scan, which in the United States right now in 2015, the way that they diagnose cancer is with a positive PET scan or a biopsy. It takes years for the tumor to get to be at least a half a centimeter so it will show up. So you go in for the test, they start an IV, and they inject you with radioactive glucose.

Ty: Sugar.

Jenny Hrbacek, R.N.: Yes. It goes around the body, you wait for about an hour, in a little room by yourself because nobody else wants to be around you because you're radioactive. And the radioactive glucose—the glucose will go to these insulin receptors and it goes into a cell. When they take your picture, these cells light up, so you have to wait long enough for enough of these cells to grow to absorb enough of that radioactive glucose to light up on the screen.

Ty: I know, you're kind of sad right now. Don't want to give up the sugar because you have a sweet tooth and I do too. So does my wife, Charlene. I think everybody that's watching probably has a bit of a sweet tooth. The good news is you don't have to give up sugar. You don't have to give up good tasting food to be able to live a healthy lifestyle. You do have to give up man-made processed sugars if you're going to be healthy, but nature produces all kinds of natural sugars that are really good for us. The reason they're good for us is because they contain a whole spectrum of nutrients. They contain the fiber and so when we eat nature's candies, when we eat these fruits, especially the fruits and the vegetables that nature produces, we're going to be able to satisfy that sweet tooth. While, at the same time, keeping our bodies healthy through nature's pharmacy.

Dr. Patrick Quillin: Welcome to my pharmacy. This is where we start talking about—people think that modern medicine has to be controlling, invasive, disabling, expensive, and dangerous. And that's what most modern medicine is. In fact, real medicine is phytonutrients that nourish the body. They're antioxidants, they regulate abnormal growth, they stimulate apoptosis or programmed cell death.

We're going to start with one of my 60 fruit trees, black raspberries. What we have here, Ty, is arguably one of the most impressive medicines that you can find: anthocyanins, antioxidants, ORAC (oxygen radical absorbent capacity) off the charts, add ellagic acid which stimulates cancer cells to commit suicide and what you have is this feeds the brain, the lens of the eye, prevents cancer—this is real medicine.

We move on—you can see these figs and we'll see if we can find something that is ripe because it's the early part of the harvest. Here we go—Ty, you get to taste that. Longueverde means green, but inside they're purple. If you'd show the camera what we have inside there.

Ty: Okay.

Dr. Patrick Quillin: Ficin is one of the more important phytochemicals in figs and again, proven to stimulate apoptosis or programmed cell death in cancer cells. Delicious and if you think of all of the ingredients—one of the things you're looking for here is prebiotics, plant food, fruits, vegetables, greens, legumes contain substances that we cannot digest, but our hundred trillion cells in the gut are using it for food and if we feed our gut properly—it's called the microbiota, we end up making vitamin biotin, Vitamin K. We're also stimulating the immune system. What they find now is two thirds of the immune system surrounds the gut and by things that we cannot digest—that prebiotics—are going to improve our immune system. This is—

Ty: Incredible.

Dr. Patrick Quillin: This is Black Mission figs. This one is not quite ripe, but you can see we're going to have a great harvest here and people will think, you're some rich doctor in California, I can't afford that. Sixty-two percent of Americans own their own home. You don't need much land. About 20 years ago, Sierra Club put out a book called *Edible*

Landscaping, in which they talked about. If you're going to spend time on it, if you're going to water it, make it something you can eat. Two-thirds of Americans could do the same thing and if you don't have land, there's a lot of cities where they're taking land that's unused—downtown Detroit and other places, and they say this is a community garden, put some fruit trees in. It might be a couple of years before you get a harvest, but a garden you're going to get in a couple of months.

Ty: Grow gardens, not grass, right?

Dr. Patrick Quillin: Exactly. I live in a desert, southern California is a desert. We're in the worst drought in history; why would you water something unless you can eat it? And here's an interesting point, we were good to mother earth and it nourishes us. So there's this symbiotic relationship. I feed the soil and then the plant feeds me and the same thing for you folks.

Ty: By the way, Patrick, that fig I just ate, that's the sweetest fig I ever tasted.

Dr. Patrick Quillin: Isn't that delicious?

Ty: That's incredible.

Dr. Patrick Quillin: I tell you what. One of the things that I do, I add Epsom salts to the soil. Epsom salt is magnesium sulfate. If you look at green plants—what you have here is green chlorophyll and chlorophyll takes the energy of the sun, combined with water and carbon dioxide and it makes sugar. And then from that it makes proteins and all of these exotic phytochemicals that protect us from disease. Well the beauty of this whole business that the middle of that chlorophyll molecule is magnesium. If the plant doesn't get enough magnesium it doesn't make enough chlorophyll, doesn't get enough chlorophyll it doesn't make enough sugar, it's not going to get sweet enough and all of the other chemicals that it makes. I put like a handful of Epsom salts in a gallon of water and dissolve it at the base of the tree, about three times a year—delicious fruit.

Ty: That's a great tip for people growing their own food.

Dr. Patrick Quillin: You see any bugs or anything on that?

Ty: No.

Dr. Patrick Quillin: It's all biodynamic, organic and I'm not fighting any bugs. Essentially, the plant has its own immune system, just like you and I do. Just like you people do. These are Surinam cherries. Fascinating. Surinam cherries, I've got three harvests a year out of this—

Ty: By the way you guys are missing out. You have to be behind the camera. I'm going to eat these. This is incredible.

Dr. Patrick Quillin: The hard part is to eat and talk at the same time. I find I salivate so much and I can't talk well which is…

Ty: I'll let you do most of the talking and I'll do most of the eating.

Dr. Patrick Quillin: Perfect.

Ty: Happy here.

Dr. Patrick Quillin: Think about this. What you have is these beautiful dark cherries and they're sweet, aren't they? Delicious. And what nature is saying, is, all right, what I've got is some sugar here and the fungus living around us in the trillions wants to eat this. The plant has to create its own protection. It creates a substance called phytoalexins and that is one of those is resveratrol. People have heard about it in red grapes. Red grapes are another thing. So the sweet thing in the grape has to protect itself. So if a fungus lands on this and it eats that phytoalexin, it dies, it's sort of its own—it's a pre-drug essentially. The drug companies can't duplicate this stuff and that's the beauty of what we've got here is you cannot patent a natural substance and that's why the $280 billion dollar a year drug industry can't come up with something as effective as this. Phytoalexins in red and green fruits and vegetables have been shown to be anti-cancer, the same way that they protect the plant against fungus. Mulberries. These are Oscar mulberry.

Ty: Now this one wasn't ripe last year.

Dr. Patrick Quillin: You're right. Right, it came at a different time of the year. Dark purple is going to have this rich mixture of phytochemicals, bioflavonoids, carotenoids, the medicinal value is beyond argument.

Ty: That's ridiculously sweet.

Dr. Patrick Quillin: Delicious. We're not denying ourself people. People think if I can't have my Twinkies and Coke every day—no this stuff is delicious and once you develop an appetite for it, what's fascinating is the human tongue has got four sensors: sour, sweet, salt, and bitter. That sweet is for fruit. The earliest food of humans was fruit, eggs, and insects. I'm not telling you you have to eat insects, but eggs and fruit are good, and the sweetness is to make fruit taste good and feel good in our body.

What the food manufacturers have done is said, we're going to create all of these substitute sugars, which are not good for you and now we're eating 140 pounds per year of refined white sugar, which is killing us. Obesity, diabetes, depression heart disease, cancer among other diseases that come with refined sugar. This is a different sugar. What you find is, if you take the fructose and other natural sugars that are in the matrix— matrix means mother in Latin and literally here is this sugar sitting in the middle of this cell membrane and it's got all of these phytochemicals around it and fiber and it works. And if you take a different sugar and take all of the matrix away—which is white sugar, corn syrup, now it's killing people instead of healing people.

Dr. Ben Johnson: There are so many good non-toxic ways to treat cancer that it's laughable what standard medicine is doing, but they all work in different ways. For instance, the salvestrol works on an enzyme system. CYP1B1 is the enzyme system that it works on. This is a natural product found in fruits and vegetables that CYP1B1 enzyme converts into a toxic product so this fruit extract—vegetable extract acts as a pro-drug. It's not a drug, your normal cells don't have that enzyme system so it can't convert it, so it doesn't hurt normal cells. But the cancer cells have the CYP1B1 so it converts it into a toxic substance killing the cancer cells. So that's just an instance of how a particular natural therapy might work.

It was found because—and why don't we have salvestrol today in our body? Well, natural fruits and vegetables produce it just in the last day or two right as they become ripe because that was when they were higher in sugars and that's when fungi tend to attack the fruits and vegetables. So that's when they make salvestrol. Who eats vine ripened fruit today?

Ty: Unless you have your own garden, you don't.

Dr. Ben Johnson: That's it. Nobody because it's all picked green—I don't care if you're eating it a natural food store or organic food store, it's still picked green to ship to you. Because that's the only way they can get it there and not lose half their produce to spoilage. So we are eating all of this food that's salvestrol-depleted and one of the very agents that mother nature uses to kill cancer cells, which ma and pa got back on the farm. In the city, buying it from the store we don't get.

Laura Bond: Things like celery—we know that celery stimulates the parasympathetic nervous system which is that calming part of the nervous system. So you know, a perfect snack is celery, some peanut butter, or nut butter might make it a little more tasty. The reason it does that is because it contains the plant hormone called apigenin. And apigenin is powerfully anti-cancer and anyone can Google "apigenin" and they'll come up with a lot of scientific references.

The other thing which I often recommend food-wise for people with stress is foods with B-6. Sweet potato, pumpkin seeds, seafood, B-6 stimulates serotonin in the body, which is that feel-good neurotransmitter. That's all of these studies recently showing a high blood levels of B-6, are powerfully anti-cancer, so you can reduce your risk of cancer of about 49 percent by eating a Vitamin B-6 rich diet.

Dr. Joseph Mercola: One of the best strategies I learned at Hippocrates Health Institute here in Florida is growing sprouts and there is a number of different sprouts. There's dozens and dozens you could use, but the most efficient and effective one that I found that seems to provide the best value is sunflower seed sprouts. You can purchase them at many health food stores, or even Whole Foods, but you'll pay $30.00 a pound, but you can grow them yourself for about $.10 or $.20 cents a pound, which is really a simple strategy, you grow them from seed to harvest in about a week, maybe 10 days.

Ty: Really?

Dr. Joseph Mercola: That's all it takes and you'd say why would I do that? It's easy, simple, it's fun, your kids love to see that—you know, it kind of catalyzes or piques an interest in gardening. But also they are 30 times more nutrient dense than the organic vegetables you grow in your backyard. So it's a really powerhouse of nutrition. It's all condensed and concentrated in those sprouts.

Ty: You can grow it at your own house.

Dr. Joseph Mercola: Yeah. Easy to do—simple to do. That's actually the biggest component in my salad are the sunflower seed sprouts.

Dr. Bradford Weeks: The thing which I'd paid a lot of attention to recently is eating seeds. Now, I'm going to use that term generally—seeds would include nuts, it would include beans, anything which you can put in the ground and it'll grow—a pea would be a seed in that regard. Eggs, something like that. Caviar in particular, fabulous. Seeds are tremendously valuable because the seed is such a wise little packet of concentrates, nutrients, about 20 fold and 30 fold more than the rest of the fruit, so it's this fabulous packet of concentrated nutrition and what we know is that it's got all sorts of genetic spare parts if it's not going to be a seed that grows into a plant that's available for you and I to repair our DNA and our RNA with. It also has tremendous stem cell precursors, especially in the husk of seeds.

Gosia Kuszewski: The day my mom was diagnosed with cancer, on the same day my daughter was born, so I had two big news in the same day. So one beautiful news and the other one pretty sad. It was very sad, but at the same time, I was determined and I believed that I can do something about it, that we can beat the cancer. I believed that I could save my mom. Although, everybody around me was panicking and really scared that mom was diagnosed. By the way, they told her there was nothing she can do and it's only that she has six months to live. I was determined that something positive will come out of this, that we will save her with natural treatments. However, when I was talking to my mom, I understood that she didn't want to try natural methods that she was ready to go the conventional path and go through chemotherapy and I knew what that meant. I knew that once she had the conventional treatment that was bad news. I knew the consequences of that. So that was devastating.

I had a baby and at the same time, I was watching my mom just getting worse and worse every day. Injecting chemicals into someone's bloodstream, even if you're the healthiest person, fit, healthy person – if someone would inject chemicals into your body that would make them sick. Cancer patients are already unwell and on top of it, they inject—they are given the chemicals. So I can't find any sense in it unfortunately.

I feel that both experiences were taken away: experience of my mom bonding with her granddaughter and for my daughter to just remember, just a little bit of her grandma. That was taken away. Because I couldn't save my mom's life, I felt with every patient after I did everything I possibly could in order to save their life. Because of that you had countless cases of people recovering from cancer and that means everything to me. The experiences that I didn't have with my mom – I thought that I lost them – that I will never get them back. However, helping other people regain their life and watching grandmothers with their grandchildren, and husbands and wives, and the families being together is just beautiful and I'm really grateful that I can experience that moment looking at the families being together and lives saved. So I'm very grateful for the experience. So the very thing which I thought I lost forever, now I found in experiences of other people. Watching them going through life, happy lives, with the families loving each other and experiencing life together.

Ty: Wow. That's so encouraging that Gosia was able to able to regain what she thought she had lost in the death of her mother. Through helping others experience abundant life, by helping them detoxify and nourish their bodies with nature's medicine.

Another amazing remedy from nature's medicine chest is the chaga mushroom, or as Dr. Boris Grinblat from Russia refers to, the Russian curcumin.

Dr. Boris Grinblat: Another very famous thing in Russia is chaga.

Ty: Chaga mushroom.

Dr. Boris Grinblat: Chaga mushroom. It has so many benefits, it's almost like curcumin. So, you can say it's like Russian curcumin because it basically does everything. It's anti-cancer, it's anti-inflammatory, it's got lots of minerals and 15 percent of chaga is ash. And ash has lots of manganese and manganese is a very important factor in enzymes, activating enzymes.

Ty: Manganese.

Dr. Boris Grinblat: Yes. So it's unique, but it's taken from a birch tree so in those places where there are birch trees, I think chaga is very good.

Ty: So you have medicine growing on the tree in Russia.

Dr. Boris Grinblat: Absolutely, absolutely.

Laura Bond: There's a study from Liverpool University here showing that a serving of broccoli everyday reduces the risk of colon cancer 50 percent. Imagine if you're having broccoli sprouts which contain up to 100 times more sulforaphane than normal broccoli. People are always a bit like, what do I do with the broccoli sprouts. They've got kind of mustardy flavor and they are quite strong, but I find if you put them in your juicer, with beetroot, and celery, and carrot—if you're not mad about the flavor it does mask them a bit—sprinkle a few on salads. They are so potent you only need a little bit of them.

Ty: Nature's medicine chest is truly phenomenal. The sulforaphanes in broccoli, the sprouts with all of their amazing nutrient profile, chaga mushrooms – Russian curcumin as Dr. Boris Grinblat called it. Now, let's learn a little bit about the citrus fruits, grapefruit and oranges.

Laura Bond: From the National Institutes of Health In America, I think it was Mark Levine, studies in 2008 showing that over 50,000 milligrams, Vitamin C can take on cancer and leave healthy cells intact.

Ty: So like a detoxing.

Laura Bond: Exactly. My mom did that. There's also studies from Japan showing that women with uterine cancer live 15 times longer when they had Vitamin C.

Dr. Patrick Quillin: I find grapefruit a fascinating subject Ty, because every pharmacist, every medical doctor tells all their patients, don't touch grapefruit. What happens is, grapefruit accelerates a detoxification enzyme in the liver, which changes the pharmacokinetics of drugs. So if you take a drug it will have different activity if you're on grapefruit than if you're not.

Ty: Okay.

Dr. Patrick Quillin: So they tell you don't eat grapefruit if you're on drugs, and I agree, I'm not against that. I have another idea. Get healthy and starting eating the grapefruit, because it improves the function of your liver and detoxification pathways. So, while everybody says don't eat grapefruit, get healthy and then start eating grapefruit. Blood orange. Here we go Ty. Blood Orange.

Ty: Okay.

Dr. Patrick Quillin: What we have is—you want to use your strong Texas hands just to rip the thing open—basically oranges are good for you. Citrus has got everything from bioflavonoids, rutin, hesperidin, Vitamin C, fiber – all of those things that I mentioned, but blood orange goes a step further and it develops these red pigments that we were talking about. Not unlike the mulberry and the deep inside of the fig. So, this is going to look a little bit like a beet inside.

Ty: Yeah it is darker.

Dr. Patrick Quillin: And so the ORAC score, once again, oxygen radical absorbent capacity, is just phenomenal.

Ty: Pop this thing open.

Dr. Patrick Quillin: There you go.

Ty: So you can see.

Dr. Patrick Quillin: Pop it open.

Ty: Don't want it to get too close to this white shirt because it is dark as you can see. Wow, I've never seen an orange juice that way, look at that.

Dr. Patrick Quillin: So blood orange is another one of these things—if you live in a reasonably warm climate, you can eat this thing and it's...

Ty: It's really sweet.

Dr. Patrick Quillin: Off the charts for all of the phytochemicals that are going to protect you against heart disease, cancer, aging, inflammation. It's phenomenal. I have a few silent partners that work with me – the birds. I give them my tithe to them, 10 percent, they eat the insects and everybody is happy.

This is a peach tree and there was a study that came out of Harvard which they showed that people who ate peaches twice a week lowered their risk for breast cancer by 40 percent. How simple can it get? If that was a drug it would have been headlines in USA today, CNN, everywhere and the drug company's stock would have doubled.

There's at least 8,000 different carotenoids at least 20,000 bioflavonoids in fruits and vegetables. They find that these things are extraordinary as anti-aging, anti-oxidant, anti-inflammatory. There are 12 million Americans who are on the Viox/Celebrax drugs. They have chronic inflammation, chronic pain. Eat more fruits and vegetables. And here's the sound bite I hope our viewers can take home...

A healthy human body is self-regulating and self-repairing. It will protect itself from infections, it will slow down the aging process. If it finds any cancer, it will eliminate them. It will keep the blood vessels open. Why don't you and I have a headache right now? Some people have a headache. Why don't you and I? Because the body is self-regulating and self-preparing. It takes in these various minerals, it regulates blood pressure, and this miraculous process occurs because we feed the body properly. And much of that comes from fruits and vegetables.

Ty: I feel even better than I did when I got here because of all the fruits I've just eaten.

Dr. Patrick Quillin: Well, you're looking good.

Ty: Fantastic.

Ty: In that last clip, when Dr. Quillin gave me a taste of that incredibly sweet mulberry— remember that it was incredible, it tasted like just pure sugar, but it was nature's medicine. One of the things he mentioned, was that the food industry is creating all of these substitute sugars. What was he talking about? That leads us to excitotoxin number two tonight – aspartame.

Dr. Russell Blaylock: Aspartame has been studied for a long time and what a researcher did, he said, I'm going to look at the research that's been done, those that are sponsored by the makers of aspartame versus independent studies. What he found, virtually all of the independent studies found harmful problems. None of the ones sponsored by the maker found any problems.

Ty: So you've got to look at who does the studies.

Dr. Russell Blaylock: So what the maker does is he goes out and he pays scientists to come up with articles or ghost written articles that says it's safe and fills the literature with it. And then when it goes before a camera, he says, look, these are the piles of studies that shows it's safe. And so the news commentator looks at this and says, well gee, there's hundreds and hundreds of studies that shows it's safe. They don't even show the real studies that were done, the carefully done studies that shows it's not. Now the carefully done studies show that it's a carcinogenic agent and that if combined with other carcinogens like nitrites, from your food, to become even more carcinogenic. They found in the original studies to get approval for using NutraSweet and the research said they found increased brain tumors, about a six fold increase in brain tumors, they found increased lung tumors, breast cancers, breast tumors, all sort of tumors and thyroid cancers were found. What the investigation did after the approval, because they approved it over these findings, they find out that they taking out the tumor from the experimental animal and throwing it away and writing down that it was normal.

Ty: Really?

Dr. Russell Blaylock: All of this was discovered. It's under oath in Congressional hearings. A lot of these amoral shenanigans were done to get it approved in the first place. The guy that's head of the committee that approved it – after he approved it, within months – he went to work for the company that was a promoter of aspartame. It's sort of this revolving door we talk about between industry and government.

Dr. John Consemulder: What I found out, through the example of aspartame being the best example of how bad the situation actually is, the medical deception. That's its neurotoxic, it's cancer promoting, it's ruining your immune system, your endocrine system. It's a very dangerous substance we should not be drinking or eating in what way whatsoever. I didn't believe this when I first heard this. Research was now this is the best example of how bad this industry is doing its job; how good it's actually doing to ruin our health and I found out more. I found out there is not just conflict of interest, but there is actually a revolving door policy between the authorities that are supposed to be guarding the hen house, but the fox is guarding the hen house, so to speak.

Dr. Russell Blaylock: The Italian study was a study—I think his name was Rossini, but he is one of the most respected researchers on carcinogenic agents. What he does is he tests these agents to see if they cause cancer. So they gave him this project and said, look at this aspartame and see if it will cause cancer in animals. He did the largest animal study ever done. Now his research is considered impeccable, almost unquestionable, because he's so careful in doing it. So respected. He did it and he found, there seemed to be an increase in lymphoma and leukemia and probably breast cancer and maybe brain tumors.

And so they wouldn't accept it. He re-did it with a lifetime study of the animal as you would in humans—because humans would be drinking this stuff for a lifetime. He found a definite increase in leukemia and lymphoma, most likely increase in breast cancer and brain tumors.

So then it went to the United States. The CDC said we'll look at his study and give a final determination for the American audience and everybody knew how it was going to turn out and it's exactly what they said. We've had some criticism of how this study was done. You know what the criticism was? You did a lifetime study. We cut it off at two years and he said, "of course you do, that's when the tumor start appearing." They cut off the study before the tumor starts showing up.

Ty: It's the same thing that Monsanto did with the GMO studies.

Dr. Russell Blaylock: Exactly. They knew at which point you would see the problems of GMO, so they cut the study off before that appeared. And they said, "We didn't find anything."

Ty: And they did the same thing with aspartame.

Dr. Russell Blaylock: It's prestidigitation. It's a magic act.

Ty: What about weight gain? Do you, or do you know someone that drinks diet soda because they think it will help them to lose weight? This is an area that we've all been lied to in addition to the other areas that we've been lied to that we're learning about in this series. Let's listen to Dr. Blaylock describe the effect of aspartame on leptin and the way that affects obesity.

Dr. Russell Blaylock: What they found is, in the hypothalamus is where leptin operates to curb your appetite. And there's receptors there in this particular nucleus – arcuate nucleus. Unless that leptin can react with that receptor it doesn't work. Glutamate is a transmitter for that receptor and aspartame has aspartic acid, which is also an excitotoxin just like glutamate. So it burns out that nucleus so now the leptin won't work. Leptin levels start rising, which is inflammatory and you start gaining weight. So actually what they found is aspartame is not good for weight loss; it actually stimulates gaining of weight. The other thing that the tauricine in it, the phenylalanine, stimulates hypoglycemia, which makes you hungry.

Ty: So you're going to eat more.

Dr. Russell Blaylock: You're going to eat more.

Ty: That's really amazing isn't it? Diet sodas actually make you hungrier after you drink them because of the effect of aspartame on leptin. It's truly amazing. Something we need to pay attention to if we're diet soda drinkers. I'm not personally, but I used to drink them before I knew this information. One of the things that we need to remember is that once we have this information, now we're responsible for it.

Pepsi recently removed aspartame from their diet sodas but they replaced it with Splenda or sucralose. Is this really a step in the right direction?

Dr. Robert Scott Bell: They didn't choose stevia. They didn't choose organic whole cane sugar. They went to a form of sugar that's engineered in a lab and basically they take sucrose and they turned it into what they call it as sucralose and they've added chlorine atoms. Three extra chlorine atoms to this and it still has some level of sweetness and they say, okay, zero or less calories, fewer calories, so we're good. We're not aspartame anymore because they couldn't beat back the bad press on aspartame.

So I've joked. I said listen, if you want sucralose, pour it in your pool out back instead of buying chlorine because you got it, it's going to sanitize your pool. You think about what is chlorine designed to do? It's designed to kill microbes. What about your gut flora? You put this stuff in your gut flora, you're going to wipe it out. It elevates the PH of your colon, which also causes all kinds of aberrant issues. Headaches have been commonly linked to this, sometimes seizure disorders, damage to DNA. Mouse studies are showing damage to DNA from sucralose. So no, not a good substitute. Maybe you can say marginally better, but that's not saying much.

Ty: Stevia would have been a better choice...

Dr. Robert Scott Bell: Much better.

Ty: Or even organic cane sugar would have been better.

Dr. Robert Scott Bell: And if you get the chromium with it you're good.

Ty: So, as we just learned from Robert Scott Bell, one of the main reasons to avoid sucralose or Splenda is because of the fact that it devastates the gut and the gut is where we generate our immune system so it can't be good for us. Maybe it hasn't been proved to create brain tumors like aspartame has yet, or it's not quite as devastating, but it's still not going to be good for us. But, don't be discouraged. As we mentioned earlier, nature's pharmacy is very tasty and there are certain herbs that nature produces that are very sweet. One of them being Stevia. One option for you is if you like soda (and don't drink them very often because they're very acidic), but if you like sodas, and you want to have a diet soda, there are sodas now that are sweetened with Stevia so you don't have any of these toxic additives like aspartame or Splenda being added to the drink. It's a good option.

Dr. Robert Scott Bell: From a nutrient perspective, the three basics that are so simple and selenium is number one on the list. Because there is nothing as far as trace mineral, one humble trace mineral, that has been identified as the most powerful preventive mineral in terms of preventing cancer, but remediating it—talking about reversing cancer as well. This is where a good friend, Jonathan Emord, has sued the FDA seven or eight times now on the issue of actually being able to label as a preventive, much less a reversal for cancer, the science—the journals are replete with selenium preventing cancer. Selenium reversing cancer.

So I argue that we must do a food form, not a synthetic isolate, because in food, it comes in many forms in combination of all the cofactors and I utilize 200 micrograms a day as a preventive. When I talk to someone with breast cancer I'm saying going up to 1,000 micrograms and sometimes 1,200 micrograms, but I bet you'll hear people object and say that's dangerous, that's toxic, selenium will kill you.

Ty: Not if it's food.

Dr. Robert Scott Bell: Not if it's food form and the studies that the FDA used to say that selenium was dangerous was based on synthetic isolates. Wrong form. They can bioaccumulate and of course the toxicity associated with too much selenium is brittle nails, skin issues, hair falling out and if you stop the selenium intake within a few days to a couple of weeks, that's reversed. So you're not going to die of it. The whole food form is not going to cause you that. Then the chromium.

This is interesting because the GTF chromium is something that's been robbed from the soils, it's been robbed from the foods that contain it like whole grains. Even the sugar cane that has the highest content of chromium, and this chromium is critical because it robs the cancer cells of their ability to grab the sugar. If you eat anything with sugar, anything with sugar and you don't have adequate chromium stores, you can't lock it away before the cancer cells get it. If you took 100 micrograms, three a days of a GTF (Glucose Tolerance Factor) of a whole food chromium, you have a transformation ability to starve the cancer cells. Even if you get a little bit—I'm not arguing that we should eat refined carbs, that's not the point, but there's always going to be some level of carbohydrate and you have to be able to bind it with minerals. That chromium is like the dock workers that helps to off load the sugars into the cells and also relinquish from the cells that have it, that is stored as fat or some other solid form to bring it back out for your healthy cells to utilize as energy.

Ty: Wow that's a huge—

Dr. Robert Scott Bell: Keeping it away from the cancer cells.

Ty: Chromium then and so what's the third?

Dr. Robert Scott Bell: The third is preventing metastasis. How do we do that? Strength and integrity of connective tissue. Chromium we've talked about, we've talked about selenium. Silicon, or silica is another mineral that has been so robbed from the soils, so ripped from the food because it's all processed. Without silica we don't have integrity of our structure, our very connective tissue and that's everything: skin, nail, hair. A lot of people know the entire matrix of cellular matrix that holds us together. The skeletal system, the visceral system, the nervous system. You name the system and it's dependent upon silica for integrity of connective tissues so if you don't have adequate silica in the system, the metastasis, the chewing through, the enzyme breakdown of these cancer cells, chewing through it, spreading, metastasizing.

Ty: And that's what kills people.

Dr. Robert Scott Bell: Right. And so we can prevent that by ramping up silicon intake and of course, you can take the horsetail extract, you can drink some of the tea, but you can't get enough. So, we concentrate that tea into a food form that you can take in a tablet form and you've got it. Three basics, man, awesome.

Ty: Three great supplements to prevent cancer.

Ty: Over the summer, we traveled to Tijuana, Mexico, to the "Hope for Cancer" clinic and we were able to get a tour of the clinic and see the different innovative therapies that they are using. Joining us now is Dr. Tony Jimenez, the Medical Director for the clinic, takes us on a tour.

Dr. Antonio Jimenez: The first room we're going to go into is the Sono Photo Dynamic Therapy Room.

Ty: Sono Photo Dynamic Therapy. Say that six times fast. Okay, so what do we have here?

Dr. Antonio Jimenez: At the core of "Hope for Cancer" is energy medicine and we know we use energy medicine for diagnosis, PET scan, positive emission tomography, that's energy. We use MRI, CT scan, ultrasound. For heart, we check EKG, those are all energy diagnostic tools. But, when we're using energy to help patients with cancer, then that's not conventionally accepted.

We know that in 1954, Michael Gerber, MD, wrote a book called *Vibrational Medicine*, which at that time he was far ahead of his time. Now, here at "Hope for Cancer" we have the Sono Photo Dynamic therapy and this therapy is available at "Hope for Cancer." We've been doing this for nine years now. We're using sound to affect cancer cells. So we provide what's called a sensitizer and the patient takes this under the tongue based on their body weight. This is absorbed by cancer cells 70 to 1. For every 70 cancer cells, 1 normal cell absorbs this molecule.

Ty: What is the sensitizer?

Dr. Antonio Jimenez: The sensitizer is a derivative of chlorophyll or seaweed, so it's a naturally occurring product, has no toxicity and it's absorbed by cancer cells 70 to 1. We wait 24 to

36 hours after administration. This way most of the cancer cells if not all will absorb it and normal cells release it. We don't know the mechanism why normal cells release it. I think it's a God thing, but that's another story…

Ty: But it works.

Dr. Antonio Jimenez: But it works. Cancer cells retain it, but this substance by itself does nothing until we wake it up or activate it and that is done using sound therapy, a specific frequency amplitude intensive. This is something that patients can do not only while they're at "Hope for Cancer," but for an extended period of time at home at a home program because it's totally non-toxic.

Ty: Then we have the photo part.

Dr. Antonio Jimenez: Then we have the photo therapy and this is—as you see it has red lights, blue lights and a row of lights that are not on, but guess what they are on—it's just invisible like an infrared spectrum. So photo dynamic therapy will also wake up the sensitizer and allow it to activate itself within cancer cells and that forms oxygen radicals, O-minus. O-minus, as you know are toxic to cancer cells and they set off the apoptosis or programmed cell death. In addition to that, it provides local inflammatory response, so thereby, the immune system can come and target that area.

Now we're going to the Hyperbaric Oxygen chamber room and here we have hyperbaric oxygen. What this does is the patient comes in here, it's lying down very comfortable. We're increasing the pressure of oxygen to about 4.0 to 4.5 pounds per square inch. So we know that oxygen and cancer don't combine and so the one hour that the patient is in here, you're saturating the cells with oxygen.

Ty: What's the normal pressure? You said 4.5 pounds per square—what's the normal pressure?

Dr. Antonio Jimenez: About 1.3.

Ty: So it's like four times as strong.

Dr. Antonio Jimenez: Exactly. Yes.

Ty: So that pressure is then forcing oxygen into the cells.

Dr. Antonio Jimenez: Patients love this therapy because you feel that oxygen load and some patients say, "Can I stay in here two hours or three hours?" Literally you can because you can't get too much oxygen in this sense, but one hour is the duration of the treatment. This is one of the preferred treatments at "Hope for Cancer" and not only for its efficacy, but because it allows the patient to relax there for an hour. You are in kind of a bubble and you forget what the fears and the conflicts you have, and it's just a good therapy in that sense as well.

Charles Daniel: In January of 2007, I was diagnosed with invasive bladder cancer. The recommendation and the mainstream medical treatment for invasive bladder cancer is to remove the bladder, prostate, and surrounding lymph nodes. This treatment had a cure rate of about 90 percent and would not require chemo or radiation.

Ty: So that's what you went with.

Charles Daniel: Yes, my daughter was 11 years old at the time of surgery and I wanted—with a 90 percent shot of cure—that's pretty good odds. So, I went with the surgery, however, when they did the surgery, they found that the cancer was also in my lymph nodes. This was previously undetected on my initial test.

So, suddenly I went from a possible cure rate of about 90 percent down to about 40 percent and I was going to have to have chemo. The initial procedure when they thought it was just confined to my bladder, I was only going to have to have surgery and no chemo and no radiation. My surgeon set me up with an oncologist – one of the best around.

Ty: Okay.

Charles Daniel: When I met with the oncologist, he requested another scan. So the scan results came back. I had three tumors in my liver that were previously undetected on the initial scan. At that time, I asked my oncologist, was there a chance of a cure? He said not really. He added that with bladder cancer metastasized to the liver that the average life expectancy was 9 months, some people die in four months, and he had never seen anyone last longer than 12 months.

My brother, his wife, my wife and I really started researching alternative cancer treatments, clinics, and so forth. May of 2008, I came to "Hope for Cancer."

I completed an inpatient program and continued with their home program and I'm proud to say that since then, all of my tests and scans have indicated I am cancer free.

Ty: Wow. That's awesome.

Charles Daniel: It is awesome. It's a great day to be alive.

Ty: It is. Wow, seven years.

Charles Daniel: Seven years and counting. I count every day, every minute.

Ty: I tell you what. And that's from a pretty bleak prognosis, less than a year, you're alive eight years later.

Charles Daniel: My urologist who did the initial surgery says that I'm a miracle. My oncologist says that he's never seen anyone with bladder cancer metastasized to the liver live this long.

Ty: I'm glad you're the first.

Charles Daniel: Hey, it's good to be in that group of one.

Ty: It is isn't it? And now your 11 year old girl is 19?

Charles Daniel: At the time of that initial prognosis of maximum 12 months to live, I didn't think that I would see her even through middle school. Now she's graduated from high school and just completed her first year of college.

Ty: That's so awesome.

Charles Daniel: It is awesome.

Dr. Antonio Jimenez: This is pulsating electromagnetic field therapy. Again, to affect the cell, we could pulsate water, we could pulsate the cells, we can help reduce the tumor size by energy. And can I try that on you, Ty?

Ty: Absolutely. Sure.

Dr. Antonio Jimenez: Okay.

Ty: You want me to sit down here?

Dr. Antonio Jimenez: Have a seat please. Make yourself comfortable. I know you've had a long day. Put this around your neck.

Ty: You're not tying this to a truck or anything are you?

Dr. Antonio Jimenez: No. We'll start with a three minute session. I'm going to increase the intensity. You're going to feel maybe your muscles jumping a little bit and here we're affecting—do you begin to feel that?

Ty: Yeah. I feel it twitching.

Dr. Antonio Jimenez: Yeah. Feel it twitching. So, now we're sending electromagnetic fields.

Ty: That's interesting.

Dr. Antonio Jimenez: This goes back to the papimi in Greece when this was developed. Many years ago, it was like a washing machine. Now technology has consolidated it and we have this…

Ty: Wow it's very interesting.

Dr. Antonio Jimenez: It's very good for pain, very good for inflammation.

Ty: I've been having pain in the back of my neck. Should this help?

Dr. Antonio Jimenez: This should help. We're waiting for the three minute cycle to finish.

Ty: I like this, though, it actually feels good.

Dr. Antonio Jimenez: Yeah it does. It does.

Ty: Yeah, at the very first—at first it was kind of odd.

Dr. Antonio Jimenez: Uh-huh.

Ty: But now it feels good.

Dr. Antonio Jimenez: So Ty, is it done?

Ty: Yeah.

Dr. Antonio Jimenez: You wanna see what kind of energy we gave you?

Ty: Yeah.

Dr. Antonio Jimenez: All right can you stand up for a second please?

Ty: Sure.

Dr. Antonio Jimenez: And hold this like this. This is a chain, as you see.

Ty: Wow.

Dr. Antonio Jimenez: So I take it—it closes—and closes…

Ty: Some serious energy.

Dr. Antonio Jimenez: Serious energy. If I crank it up, more maybe we could take it this way so we can see it. Hold the bottom.

Ty: Okay.

Dr. Antonio Jimenez: It forms a loop, it stops.

Ty: Right.

Dr. Antonio Jimenez: I take it away—All right. And it's stabilizing the energy.

Ty: Wow. That's interesting.

Dr. Antonio Jimenez: Right?

Ty: Yeah. So this is the favorite treatment of many patients?

Dr. Antonio Jimenez: Yes. For sure. Very simple to use, very effective, and one of the staple treatments at "Hope For Cancer."

Ty: Very cool. Thanks for showing us.

Dr. Antonio Jimenez: Glad you enjoyed it.

Ty: You let me be a guinea pig. It was enjoyable, actually.

Dr. Antonio Jimenez: Okay, excellent. This is a *near* infrared sauna, as opposed to a *far* infrared sauna.

Ty: So, Dr. Tony, what's the difference between a far infrared and a near infrared? I've got a little personal far infrared at the house, but I think it was one of your patients today that I talked to—he said no, it's not far infrared, it's near infrared. What's the difference?

Dr. Antonio Jimenez: Near infrared light has a greater depth of penetration than far infrared. Near infrared light is more detoxing—you that saunas and infrared light pulls out toxic and heavy metals. Also most far infrared saunas in the market, have too much EMF, Electromagnetic Fields that are toxic, like a cell phone. There's a book called *Sauna and Detoxification* by Dr. Lawrence Wilson, MD, out of Arizona. There, he's considered the guru of sauna therapy and he talks about what I just mentioned to you – the importance of using near infrared as opposed to far infrared.

Ty: So near infrared is less EMF and it penetrates further.

Dr. Antonio Jimenez: Further. Here we have local, direct, hypothermia. What is hypothermia? High heat. We know, science knows, that cancer cells are heat sensitive. Normal human cells are heat resistant. That's why when we have a flu, a virus, an infection, we get a fever to kill the bugs, but it doesn't kill our healthy cells. So now even in the US they're using hypothermia with radiation and they're saying, wow, the results are better. Well, of course, because most of the damage selectively to the cancer cells are being done by the local hypothermia.

Ty: So that's what this is, it's a local hypothermia machine.

Dr. Antonio Jimenez: Yes and it's a very easy, non-invasive therapy. This is the one. Of course, let's say the patient has a tumor in the breast, right? We put a conductive gel, natural non-toxic, we crank up the device and then the treatment is done externally.

Ty: Okay.

Dr. Antonio Jimenez: And this is using both capacitance and resistant different types of energy to get to superficial, as well as to deep tumors. This is another favorite, Ty. I know I told you several of them are favorites, but this is not only a feel good therapy, but a very effective therapy. With the combination of Sono Photo Dynamic Therapy, and local hypothermia, we're getting at least a 52 percent decrease in blood supply to the cancer tumors or masses during the stay of the patient here. We know that angiogenesis right is one of the characteristic hallmarks of cancer. We could decrease the blood flow to the tumor we're well on our way to having an effective therapy. And maybe you saw some patients today who had an 80 or 90 percent.

Ty: We did as a matter of fact. Now, as opposed to what we've already seen with the near infrared sauna, that's also hypothermia, isn't it?

Dr. Antonio Jimenez: Correct.

Ty: This is just a different machine, it does the same thing?

Dr. Antonio Jimenez: Not exactly. It doesn't do the same thing because that's more for pulling out toxins, that's more for superficial opening up of the pores for cleansing, detoxing. This local hypothermia and we also have full body hypothermia here is a therapeutic treatment for cancer, meaning it's going after the cancer cells, it's going after the bugs.

Ty: Got it.

Dr. Antonio Jimenez: The viruses, the bacteria, the fungus.

Ty: So it's good doing both.

Dr. Antonio Jimenez: It's good doing both. Yes.

Ty: Great.

Just to summarize Dr. Tony's protocol there at "Hope for Cancer" clinic in Tijuana, he's using sono photo dynamic therapy, hyperbaric oxygen chambers, far infrared and near infrared saunas, a drastic change to the diet, restricting sugar almost completely. And my favorite, as you saw was the PEMF, which is Pulse Electromagnetic Frequencies. If you saw him put that little thing around my neck, if he turned up the voltage it would have taken me like this [*indicates getting a shock*]. But at the low voltage that they use of that, it actually is a selectively toxic treatment for cancer cells.

Trina Hammack: The initial feeling was absolute terror and disbelief and sure death. I watched my mother die at 48 of breast cancer and my grandmother at 36, she died of ovarian cancer. Here I was, 46, and was it my time because that's what happened to my family. I was absolutely terrified, but I also knew inside of me that I really—there was no way you could have dragged me down the conventional path for chemo or radiation or anything like that. I knew that every part of my being, not to do that. I knew to have the surgery to have this mass removed. I knew that, but there was no way I was going to do chemo. You'd have to straightjacket me and drag me in to do it because I knew not to do that.

Dr. Tony was my hope because I knew him and I've known him for years and I'd seen the success that I'd send my clients—I'm in the holistic world too and I would send my people down there when they needed cancer help and they always said, "I wish I would have come here first." And so I remembered that and that was my hope and so I called him up and I said, "Hey, this is what's going on," and so he gave me my hope. They gave me my hope. But it's hard to have hope when you're indoctrinated into this world and your belief system is cancer equals death, or cancer equals chemo and radiation. So there's a lot of fear out there and you have to really look inside yourself and not be afraid. It's terrifying. It's absolutely terrifying to get that diagnosis where your whole world implodes in on you.

You know, my son was nine and he was my big reason why I had to do something different because I watched my mother die, my grandmother died, both from these cancers and I knew that I wasn't going to leave my son without a mom. So I just looked death in the eye and I said, "No." My will was so strong because I was not leaving him without a mother.

There's another piece to this story in that, five years before, I didn't have a diagnosis, but I became really ill and it turned out I had Lyme disease in my brain and that set me up for cancer down the road. This weak immune system. And back then when you have a little guy running around, you have to do whatever it takes to get well to be there. I had to do that twice and he was my saving grace twice. I had to figure out the Lyme and the doctor said there's nothing wrong with you, it's all in your head. It really was, it was actually in my brain. So I had to heal myself. I did and he was my motivation.

So for anybody out there that is faced with these kinds of things. You look to your why? Why do I need to get well? Is it my kids, is it my grandkids, is it my husband or my wife? What is it? Why do you need to get well and you focus on that because that's what's going to get you through it. It has to be a really strong reason why you'll do whatever it takes—whatever it takes to get well. I did whatever it takes and that's why I'm here. I still to this day have not looked at the statistics for ovarian cancer, but according to other people, I shouldn't be here.

Ty: While creating this series has been fun and exciting, it's really a very serious responsibility because every topic we cover, every fine detail, has a purpose. And no, it's not to make money. It's to give you what you need to save and protect your life. We did not receive any financial kickbacks from any expert, doctor, clinic, supplement, or product of any kind. Every piece of information was solely for the purpose of giving you vital information you and your loved ones deserve to know, and it's the greatest honor for us to give you that as a gift simply because we believe that your life is precious. You deserve to be healthy and happy, free from toxicity, free from every negative influence on your body. And through this episode you've seen clearly how to avoid toxins, and how to eat foods that foster life and vigor.

Today you've seen that excitotoxins are to be avoided at all cost if you truly desire to live a life free from the fear of cancer. You've seen how these excitotoxins not only excite and kill healthy cells, but as the documented evidence proves, these excitotoxins actually cause cancer to originate in the body which is called, as you know from tonight, oncogenesis. I know you'll never look at a product containing aspartame, Splenda, sucralose, or any of its other evil artificial relatives the same again.

I know for some of you, watching this episode may result in a trashcan full of junk food that you remove from your fridge or your pantry. Now, that's a quick way to say "no" to cancer. Seriously, coupled with healthy living, that's the single best way to eradicate cancer from your body – right now. And what a better way to restock your home and body than with Nature's Pharmacy? You've seen how nature can heal your body, and promote health. And that the garden should actually be better understood as a pharmacy. With plants containing actual medicines that are lethal to cancer while exponentially strengthening immunity and vitality.

You've also seen how sound and light therapy are in fact advanced scientific discoveries that have been proven to dramatically aid the body in the fight against cancer as countless cancer survivors have confirmed. You've seen with Trina, with a Stage 4 ovarian cancer diagnosis, who beat cancer with the aid of sound and light therapy, and a combination of non-toxic therapies. Once again proving that cancer is not, in fact, a death sentence.

Ty: Wow, it's really amazing the amount of material we covered in just a short time tonight. I hope you learned a lot. And I hope you're ready for tomorrow's episode because we're going to cover more ground. It's vital in your fight against cancer or to prevent cancer. Tomorrow night we're going to hit some of the blind spots, some of the things you may not be aware of that could have a direct impact on a cancer diagnosis. Whether it be your mouth, root canals, metals in your mouth, the spine. Did you know if your spine is not properly aligned that it could result in cancer? Emotions – the emotional aspect of cancer. Recent studies have shown a direct link between emotions like fear and stress and a cancer diagnosis. And heavy metals, not just in your mouth, but in vaccines.

Yes, tomorrow night we are going to talk about vaccines, a very controversial, very contested topic today. A lot of people are very opinionated on it. We're going to try to keep the opinion out and stick straight to the science.

Tomorrow night's episode is going to be extremely valuable in your journey, in your quest to learn all that you can to prevent and/or treat cancer. You don't want to miss it.

In the meantime, have a great evening. God bless you and we'll see you tomorrow.

[credits roll]

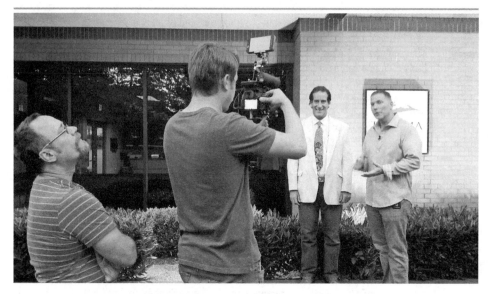

Above - with Dr. Gaston Cornu-Labat in Seattle, Washington
Below – The TTAC Team in Tijuana, Mexico

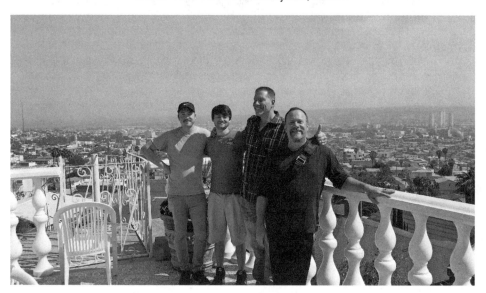

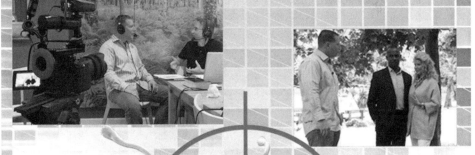

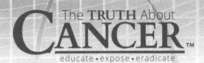

Ty: Welcome back to *The Truth About Cancer: A Global Quest.* I'm so glad that you joined us tonight. I'm really looking forward to an episode that's going to help empower you with knowledge in your fight to stay healthy and prevent cancer. But just in case you missed last night's episode, here's a brief recap for you.

[Video plays: Summary of Episode Four]

In tonight's episode, we are going to cover some of, what we called last night, the blind spots regarding cancer. Things that you wouldn't think about that might have an impact on a cancer diagnosis—things like your mouth. Not your words that you say, but the things that are in your mouth: fillings, mercury fillings. People call them silver fillings but they're actually half mercury. Root canals. Do they have any kind of impact on cancer? We'll learn that tonight.

Did you know that your mind plays a big part in the cancer equation? Your emotions have a drastic effect on a cancer diagnosis, and we'll learn more about that later. But to begin the episode, we're going to learn about what is potentially the *biggest* blind spot in the cancer equation, and that's your spine. Did you know that your spine has a direct bearing on a cancer diagnosis? Let's listen to doctor, Terry Harmon as he explains.

So I appreciate you being here and really looking forward to getting your input on the importance of the spine in overall health, which was a little bit of the piece of the puzzle that we missed in the last documentary. Why is the spine so important?

Dr. Terry Harmon: That's a big thing because, oftentimes, even when patients come to see me, they're thinking nutrition if they're coming with a cancer diagnosis. But when we start to study the body and you're looking at the quest for cures and other things out there, we look at what system is the most important system for fending off cancer, and most people will say the immune system, right? Most people say absolutely the immune system. I would agree with them. But then we look at the immune system is comprised of a series of glands and organs that make this immune response and those glands and organs are controlled by the nerve system.

Ty: First of all, what are the glands and the organs of the immune system?

Dr. Terry Harmon: We're going to look at the thymus, we're going to look at the spleen, we're going to look at the bone marrow, and then the gut. When we look at the gut, a majority of our immune response comes from the gut tissue, and yet all of that hinders upon, or rests upon the vitality of the nerve system. When we look at the spine, the spine is the tissue that surrounds and protects the spinal cord. The brain communicates to the body via the spinal cord. And so when we look at it, oftentimes, as we work with patients, a lot of people don't understand that our spine is designed to have a certain structure; a very specific structure. And any deviation off that structure directly interferes with the nerve system's ability to adapt and respond to stress. And what are we doing more of now than ever before?

Ty: Stressing about everything.

Dr. Terry Harmon: Stressing about everything. We're sitting more now than ever. We're looking at our technology more than ever. And even if we go to the gym, we're kind of thinking fitness, we're not thinking structure. When we look at all the research, some of the most amazing research on the planet's coming out nowadays, and it says that the nerve system controls the immune system. And then I tell people, "What impacts your nerve system?" And they say, "Everything." Everything we do impacts the nerve system. The only question is, are we doing the things that make it healthier or are we doing the things that break it down. Thomas Edison said, *"The doctor of the future, will give no medicine but will interest his patients in the cause and prevention of disease and the care of the human frame."* Hopefully, that's where we're at now.

Dr. Steve Klayman: Keeping your spine healthy and not having nerve impingement is really important because it's recently been found that having pinched nerves in your spine is actually mimicking a chronic fight or flight state. Fight or flight is really good if you have to run away from the dragon or fight the bear or whatever. That's what fight or flight is designed for.

Ty: That's interesting. Nerve impingement causes you to be in constant fight or flight.

Dr. Steve Klayman: Correct. Correct. It sets up this adrenal gland secretion in your body, and your adrenal glands are the glands that are your stress glands. You need the adrenal glands for energy. Without adrenaline, you don't survive. When you wear those out, then you go into exhaustion. So it's important that there be some reversal of the stress process every day. Meditation is a great way to do it. Exercise is a great way to do it. Yoga's a great way to do it. Going to a bar is not a great way to do it.

Ty: Unless it's a juice bar, right?

Dr. Steve Klayman: Unless it's a juice bar. There you go.

Dr. Terry Harmon: Hippocrates said, *"Let thy food be thy medicine and let thy medicine be thy food."* He also said this. You ready? "Look well to the spine for the cause of disease."

Ty: Hippocrates. He knew what he was talking about.

Dr. Terry Harmon: He did know what he was talking about.

Bill Spalding: I was diagnosed in October 2011 with renal cell carcinoma. I had a large tumor on my right kidney. I had kidney cancer that had also progressed into the vena cava vein. After a diagnosis in late November of 2011, I had surgically removed my right kidney and the tumor, and then also had got the cancer out of my vena cava vein. So they sent me home, they said I was cancer free, but there was a big percentage likelihood that my cancer would return. So they suggested to do CT scans every three months to see that if there was any cancer that had returned. In August of 2013, they done a CT scan and noticed a spot on my left adrenal gland. It turned out I got a biopsy and my cancer had been back. It metastasized to my adrenal gland. I was now considered Stage 4.

Ty: So it's Stage 4. What was the prognosis at that point with Stage 4 renal cell carcinoma?

Bill Spalding: They said there was a zero percent chance of survival five years, but if I took the treatments that they were suggesting that there would be possible I could have a few months to live and even possibly maybe a year or two to live max. And the oncologist said, "Me nor no one else can cure you."

Ty: So basically, there was no hope.

Bill Spalding: There was no hope, none whatsoever. The only hope you had was to try to get a few more months to live, and to go home and get your affairs in order. We went home. Me and my wife had made the decision that we were not going to do cancer treatments, so I hit the Internet and tried to do all of the possible research I could on what I could do to help myself naturally. And then through that research is whenever I came across a Quest For The Cures with yourself, and then listened to the doctors, and the documents, and the scientists, and different survivors.

And then I started getting hope that there could possibly be a future for me and maybe I wasn't dying. The more research and the more things I was hearing. All the survivors I was finding in the cancer world were surviving naturally with natural products and protocols. So then I started taking the Protocel, and my oncologist told me before, after I had metastasized, that renal cell carcinoma, it will go to your lungs, your bones, your liver, and your brain. That's why you're not going to be here very long. It will metastasize. So using the product Protocel, I used it for about 13 months and I really believe that it kept it from going other places. But different than a lot of people, it didn't really not cure me because I couldn't get rid of the tumor on my adrenal gland.

And then that's whenever I came to listen to you speak, and there was a Dr. Terry Harmon from Morganfield, Kentucky there speaking. Me and my wife were so impressed with what he was saying that we decided to make an appointment and just sit with him and let him talk to us. And to this day, I still see Dr. Harmon, and he told me the value of my structure and my spine. He had said there was like six inches of my spine that he called "dead." He said there's no energy coming out of it. And he showed me on a graph. He says, "Now, see, this six inches is dead. That controls your adrenals." And he said, if you get the spine adjusted through traction or whatever, to move the spine, and then also if you go on a what's called a cellular healing diet where I could get my body in ketosis, where I would get ketones in my blood that would help burn and get hot. He said that would burn the tumor. And also, with the spinal adjustment, it would help get rid of the tumor.

I believe Protocel really got me to the point where I had time to do that. And then with diet change, supplements, you done lab work, I was low on vitamin D, magnesium. I took seven or eight different supplements to get my numbers where they needed to be. Dr. Harmon told me if I create an environment in my body where he would say, where it's supposed to be, that cancer would not be able to survive. Fired my oncologist and quit doing CT scans because I just hated that feeling of the chemicals going through my veins and me going through that. I never did like that.

Finally, I found out through Dr. Terry, found out about thermograms, thermography. I started doing thermography, which is non-invasive. It's just a picture image. The last thermography I'd done, which was a couple months ago, shows no cancer activity at all in my entire body. Since the day at the oncologist, whenever the news was I had no chance, I have not been sick one day. I was told by Dr. Terry that I wasn't sick because I had cancer. I had cancer because I was sick. And the thing that I like to tell people is they took out my right kidney and my tumor. The tumor was larger than a football, so I had to have the surgery. But what they did is they removed the symptom, a cancer symptom. The symptom was the tumor that was on my right kidney. If they would have removed the *cause* of cancer in August of 2013, I wouldn't have cancer again. So they removed the symptom, left the cancer cells in there, which was so tiny it's undetectable by a conventional X-ray or CT. And it took a year and two months for the cancer cells that's remaining in my body to start forming another tumor on the left side of my body on the adrenal gland.

The one thing I would really want to say is try to get people to educate themselves that, you know what? The tumor in your body is not your cancer. That's hard for people to fathom. And if you get to the cause that caused the tumor, cancer don't have to be a death sentence.

Ty: What an encouraging testimonial from Bill Spalding, sharing with us how he used spine adjustments, chiropractic, and other natural remedies to cure his late stage and supposedly terminal renal cell carcinoma, kidney cancer. It was really humbling for me to be able to talk to Bill because one of the things that Bill shared with me, and he just shared with us on the interview, was that he learned about these natural remedies through us, through *The Quest For The Cures*. It's really a blessing for us to be able to share these life-saving truths with the world. Now, another one of the blind spots that many people don't realize has a direct impact on their health and cancer is the mouth. Let's learn more.

Bill Henderson: I've been very fortunate the last 15 years or so to be educated by some dentists, particularly wonderfully educated dentists about health and how it relates to our mouths. These dentists are quite rare. I refer people to them every day around the United States and in other countries. But they're so rare. It's like 2/10th of one percent of dentists that really know this. They've taught me a lot about it and of course I've read a lot of different books and so on. But what it boils down to is that every one of the 32 spots in our jaw are directly connected to organs in our body, whether you have a tooth there or not. This connection is quite intimate and if you've had some dental work done that is toxic – and this is really every root canal filling that has ever been done.

Most of the removal of teeth, including wisdom teeth and other infected teeth, is done in a way that there are toxins left in the jawbone. Where the tooth comes out of is not always cleaned up correctly. It's called a socket and it has a ligament in it that holds the tooth into the jaw. It has a bone surrounding it that is always infected. If the tooth was infected, the bone and the ligament are infected. And they are not removed correctly by the dentist. And this is true for root canal-filled teeth as well. If the person recognizes how toxic they are and tries to get them removed by a normal dentist, they may remove the tooth but they don't clean up the socket correctly. The effects of it simply don't go away.

Dr. Leigh Erin Connealy: Breast cancer, 97 percent they say are related to a root canal because your teeth drain into your body. But it's also a burden just like viruses are a burden to the body and increase the patient's risk of getting cancer.

Ty: That's interesting that there's a direct correlation between breast cancer and root canals. That's not something your oncologist is going to tell you, is it? Dr. Thomas Lokensgard is a biological dentist and he has a practice in Nashville, Tennessee. He's actually my dentist and the dentist for the rest of my family. In this upcoming clip, he further elaborates on the direct correlation between root canals and cancer.

Dr. Thomas Lokensgard: There's been a lot of information and concerns about root canals. Root canals, they fail quite often. They fail most of the time. It has been said that dentists are the only doctors that leave dead tissue in the body. When you do a root canal, there's the pulp tissue that you have to seal off. And when you do that, you leave the dead tooth in the mouth because if you want to keep your tooth in your head, you have to pretty much do a root canal. Otherwise, you have to extract it. But the problem is there's these dental tubules called canaliculi that, once you fill the root canal, they become dead space, and so then they fill up with anaerobic bacteria.

Here's basically essentially what happens. You have a tooth that goes bad, and then the voltage drops in that tooth. And when the voltages drops, then the pH drops. When the pH drops, then the oxidation goes out of the tooth and out of the area. When the oxidation drops, then the bugs come in, and the bugs come in and they set up housekeeping. Well, bugs don't have teeth, but they need to eat. They wake up and they're hungry, they want to eat. So what they do is they begin to produce all kinds of enzymes. They begin to liquify you and they start having us for lunch.

That begets an infection and an infective process that you cannot leave in your body because then it crosses the gingival sulcus barrier, goes right into the cardiovascular system, goes right to the liver, produces highly specific C-reactive protein and some other—that's a general inflammatory marker. And it says to your body, "Hey, we're chronically inflamed. We have all this inflammation," so then all of these pathways get turned on. So then what you have to do is what we've started to do is bio-oxidative therapies for root canals that are failed because sometimes root canals in the anterior segment would be okay because they're single rooted. But you leave all these dentinal tubules and all these canaliculi that are open to bacterial infection and you can't have bacterial infection which becomes systemic. It's a real problem.

Bill Henderson: For the last 100 years it has been well known that there is no safe way to do a root canal filling. And they're still done the same way they were back in 1923 when the study was completed.

Ty: That's interesting to me that Bill Henderson just cited a study that was a 1923 study that showed that these dental toxins, these, basically, poisons in the mouth are one of the primary causes for degenerative diseases, including cancer. And it is odd, as Bill mentioned, that 100 years later, we're still doing root canals the same way. It looks like dentistry really has not progressed that much in the last century. And one of the ways that these biological dentists, like Dr. Lokensgard, they have progressed is they're using what's called bio-oxidative therapies to treat disease. Now, bio-oxidative therapies is introducing molecules like ozone or hydrogen peroxide into the system in order to kill pathogens. Let's learn more from Dr. Tom.

Dr. Thomas Lokensgard: This is very commonly done in Europe and in England, Switzerland. They've been doing this for years. They're curing all kinds of diseases with bio-oxidative therapies. Our Food and Death Administration, bless their hearts (in a Tennessee way), they don't really get into therapies that really cure a lot of things because that interrupts the monetary flow, and I'll stop right there [chuckles]. But you know what I'm talking about. I try to leave the politics out of this, but we know that there's a political component when it comes to cancer.

Chronic inflammation affects most all chronic degenerative disease. And we call it oral inflammation, we say it starts here. Essentially, there's a switch called nuclear factor kappa beta, NF-KB, and I go around and I talk to dentists, I talk to physicians, and I say, "How many of you guys out there understand and know what nuclear factor kappa beta is?" And I usually get these blank stares. What it is, it's a genetic transcription cytoplasmic switch that turns on inflammation. It's a genetic switch. The body is so intricately and amazingly designed to just—I don't know how anybody can look at the human body and not see a miracle, especially a little baby. But what happens is inflammation, in its nascent state, it's good for us because an inflammation is what causes the voltage drop and it causes healing to occur.

But when we're constantly chronically inflamed and we've got this saber-toothed tiger behind our back, it ramps up the sympathetic nervous system, decreases the parasympathetic nervous system, it turns on the nuclear factor kappa beta, and it turns on all of these pathways, all these inflammatory pathways that affect hypertension. It affects stress levels, which stress is a killer. We all know this. It affects every organ system in your body so you have to control inflammation. As I said, inflammation starts here. It starts in the mouth.

Ty: All the more reason to make sure that your mouth is not inflamed because the research shows that chronic inflammation leads to cancer. We've heard that thus far in this documentary mini-series and we'll hear more about it in the next few episodes. But there's no doubt, the research is conclusive: chronic inflammation leads to cancer. So we've got to deal with chronic inflammation. And one of the ways that you can deal with chronic inflammation in your mouth is through the bio-oxidative therapies. They help to reduce chronic inflammation.

One of the other things that you can do for your mouth, if you want to lessen your chances of cancer, is to get rid of the toxic metals. And who thinks they have metal in their mouth? I'm not talking about braces. I'm talking about those metal fillings. We may call them silver fillings, but in actuality, they're about 50 percent mercury. This is toxic to your mouth. Let's learn more about this vitally important subject.

Dr. Thomas Lokensgard: The silver fillings, you're right, they're about 40 percent silver, the rest is copper-tin and mercury. Forty-three to 55 percent is the mercury in a silver filling. It's a huge problem. The question is, do they outgas? The ADA's position (the American Dental Association's position) is that they do not outgas, is that they are inert. Well, I have news for the ADA. This is not true. They do outgas, and they outgas from the time they're put in to the time they're taken out. When they outgas, what happens? Mercury is a known toxin, not a dental toxin; it's just a known toxin. It's very toxic to the neurological system. It's very toxic to the gastrointestinal system. It ties with candida. Candida some people call it. So if you have candidiasis or candida infection or you have gut dysfunction, it's going to mess with that. It's going to be very difficult to fix your gut.

It has an affinity for fat tissues. Since we're all fat heads, it goes to your brain. It has a great affinity to cross the blood-brain barrier, to cross the placental barrier. That's really bad news because that's supposed to be a sterile environment. It causes memory loss. It causes fatigue. It causes brain fog. I can tell you story after story after story of patients that have had their mercury fills removed the proper way, we've put all the garb on them, we make sure that there's no vapor escaping and crossing the blood-brain barrier, the placental barrier. And they come back months later and we say, "How are you feeling?" They go, "I feel a whole lot better."

Dr. Robert Scott Bell: If you look in a Homeopathic Materia Medica, there are pages and pages and pages, almost more than any other, let's say, substance listed in that Materia Medica, of potential effects and actual effects at even minute doses, minute exposure to mercury. And this affects every system of the body: the endocrine, the neurological system, you name it, the digestive system, the epithelial tissue. Mercury is the biggest baddie of them all and, ultimately, I believe facilitates cancer.

Ty: We're going to learn more about the toxicity of mercury and its relation to cancer later on when we address the topic of vaccines. But before we get there, let's listen to what Dr. Tom, a dentist, has to say about fluoride.

Dr. Thomas Lokensgard: I used to argue with my wife about this. When I first got into dentistry, she came in and said, "Tom, I don't want the kids to have fluoride." I go, "What? What do you mean you don't want the kids to have fluoride." To a dentist, this is heresy. It is. You're telling me I'm not supposed to give my kids fluoride. Well, it turns out she was right. I'll just say this. The journal of *The Lancet* – the very prestigious medical journal, The Lancet – has just labeled fluoride as an excito-neurotoxin. It causes cancer. It causes osteosarcoma. Kids have died from this stuff. Eating tubes of toothpaste. It says right on there. I mean, you can—

Ty: Call poison control.

Dr. Thomas Lokensgard: Exactly.

Dr. Edward Group III: Fluoride calcifies the pineal gland. They knew that back in Nazi Germany when they put fluoride in there for one reason: to reduce our consciousness, to make us non-aggressive, to make us controllable, to make us like zombies – literally.

Dr. Daniel Nuzum: In 2011, there was a *Time magazine* article. This is mainstream. This isn't coming from us researchers in the national medicine world. This is *Time magazine*. They listed fluorine or fluoride as one of the top ten most toxic household chemicals. Fluoride disrupts the metabolism of other key elements that we need for bone growth. It activates the osteosarcoma genes. It activates other things like leukemia, and things like that too, that are bone-based cancers. Those genes get activated by elevated fluoride levels in our bodies. Why it's in our system, our food chain, and our water system, there's no good reason for it.

Dr. Edward Group III: Iodine is one thing that I would highly recommend every single person look at – a detoxified iodine – because we found that it's crucial in the oxidation. Like I was talking to you about glucose oxidase, a new project we're kind of secretly working on, what we're finding is that every single person—and Dr. Brownstein has also verified this with testing of over 9,000 patients. Every single person is deficient in iodine. And when you're deficient in iodine, cancer can be one of the consequences, but also every single cancer patient should be on probably a minimum of 10,000 to 20,000 micrograms of the detoxified iodine a day.

Dr. David Brownstein: Every cell in the body needs and requires iodine to function optimally. We can't function optimally in an iodine-deficient environment. I've tested – along with my partners – over 6,000 patients. Over 96 percent were low in iodine; the vast majority, significantly low in iodine. When I talk to clinicians around the country who are looking at this, they find the same numbers that I'm finding. Iodine has a lot of jobs in the body. The immune system can't function without it. You can't fight infections without it. But one of its main jobs is in the endocrine glands.

The endocrine glands include the thyroid, the breast, the ovaries, uterus, and the prostate. What are we having problems with out there? The thyroid, the ovaries, uterus, breast, and prostate. I've mentioned the prostate. I've mentioned the breast. The fastest growing cancer in the United States is thyroid cancer. We have uterine, ovarian cancer growing at epidemic rates. All these tissues are—we're having epidemic rates of problems with them. Iodine's main job is to maintain a normal architecture of those tissues. In iodine deficiency, the first thing that happens is you get cystic formation in the breast, the ovaries, uterus, thyroid, prostate, and let's throw in the pancreas in here as well, which is also increasing in epidemic rates—pancreatic cancer.

Cysts start to form when iodine deficiency is there. If it goes on longer, they become nodular and hard. If it goes on longer, they become hyperplasia – hyperplastic tissue, which is the precursor to cancer. And I say that's the iodine deficiency continuum. The good thing about iodine is iodine has apoptotic properties, meaning it can stop a cancer cell from just continually dividing, dividing, dividing until it kills somebody.

Dr. Daniel Nuzum: Virtually everyone in our nation is iodine deficient. There's a few things: one, you can't have thyroid issues without being iodine deficient. You can't be Type 2 diabetic without being iodine deficient. Woman can't get PCOS (polycystic ovarian syndrome) without being iodine deficient. That covers a huge portion of our society. So correcting this is something—we have to find a way to correct this.

Ty: And just to throw this in, last year, with *The Quest For The Cure's* Dr. David Brownstein mentioned the fact that he believes—he's done more research on iodine than a lot of people that I know. I mean more doctors. And he says that iodine deficiency is directly linked with cancer.

Dr. Daniel Nuzum: Absolutely. Iodine is necessary for the thyroid to produce the hormones that activate the mitochondria in our cells. If the mitochondria in our cells aren't activated, we go from a oxygen respiring metabolism to a sugar fermenting metabolism, which is what produces cancer.

Ty: As we just heard, iodine is vitally important, and that's why myself and my family, we take an iodine supplement every day. Now, iodine used to be in the bread. They replaced it with bromine, and so now we're not getting something that prevents cancer. And then we heard about fluoride, that we are getting something that *causes* cancer without our consent. It's being dripped into the water. If you're drinking municipal water, you're getting fluoride whether or not you like it. This issue of freedom is near and dear to our hearts with The Truth About Cancer. The freedom to choose what you do put in your body and what you don't put in your body.

You got a choice in your food that you eat. You got a choice in who you marry. You got a choice in where you live. You should have a choice in these other areas too. But as we learned in Episode One, with the forced chemotherapy issue, many people, including a lot of children, don't have a choice in whether they are force medicated with chemotherapy. But it gets even worse than that. What if you didn't have a choice whether someone injected you with a vaccine that contained known cancer-causing agents; toxic chemicals that can create autism, or brain swelling, or even immediate death? That would be an issue, wouldn't it?

And that's actually happening right now in the United States with Senate Bill 277 in California, which recently passed, which is the Forced Vaccine Bill. That's right. In other countries, I'm not aware of this happening yet, but it's happening in the United States. And what happens in California usually follows in other states, and eventually around the globe, so this is going to be a global issue down the road, I firmly believe. And it's an issue primarily of health freedom. Let's listen to Dr. Steve Klayman address this issue of forced vaccines.

Dr. Steve Klayman: This SB 277, the mandatory vaccination rule that now passed and is supposed to go into effect July 1, 2016 in California. Of course, they'll fight on a lot of grounds, including its constitutionality and its violation of Nuremberg Codes of forced medical procedures without informed consent. Of course, Dr. Pan, who led the charge was given $95,000 by the pharmaceutical industry to his coffers.

Mike Adams: It's a dangerous precedent because it strips away medical choice from parents and citizens, and it establishes a precedent where the state believes that it owns your body or the bodies of your children. And that it can then mandate that you must be injected with any substance that the state says is in the interest of public health. And yet that same state *never* talks about what is in those vaccines. They never talk about the ingredients: the mercury, the formaldehyde, the MSG, the antibiotics, the aborted fetal cells that are used in them, and in the past, the hidden cancer viruses like SV40, which was found in the polio vaccine injected into as many as 98 million Americans. They never talk about that.

If you really start digging and get to the truth, the vaccine mandate is linked to cancer because of the ingredients, and it is something where the state is now denying you personal freedom and the power of your own choice to decide what interventions you want to undergo.

Ty: Very similar with the vaccines, we're seeing these forced chemotherapy incidents. They're linked, aren't they?

Mike Adams: Yes.

Ty: It's an overarching tyrannical government that comes in and says, "You don't have any choice. We're going to tell you what's best."

Mike Adams: It was best called by John Rappaport – scientific totalitarianism. I think it's a great term for it. Some people call it medical fascism. It means that the so-called science, which is really just corporate driven fraudulent science, but the so-called science driven medicine is being forced upon you now in absolute violation of the American Medical Association's Code of Medical Ethics. Which says that the patient must be given the choice. The patient must be informed. They talk about informed consent. This is supposed to be a pillar of the ethical practice of medicine in the United States of America, and really all around the world.

That is now being stripped away. Parents are being told, "You *must* submit your children to these interventions, whether you like it or not." That's a violation at every level – of human rights, of human dignity, of parental rights, of children's health, of even the genetics of some children who are especially susceptible to these vaccine ingredients. It's a kind of genocide, if you really get down to it.

Ty: Wow. Mike Adams just used some pretty pungent terms, right? Totalitarianism, fascism, genocide. These are all phrases that you might associate with Nazi Germany, not the United States of America today. Why do we bring in Nazi Germany, the Nuremberg trials, into this discussion? The reason is that the same thing that was happening then is happening now. The forced vaccines that are currently being implemented in certain states in the United States of America are equivalent to the medical experimentation that went on in Nazi Germany. Believe it or not, many of the convicted war criminals at the Nuremberg trials were then shipped over to the United States and took positions on the boards of directors of major pharmaceutical companies in the United States. That's Operation Paper Clip.

Fritz ter Meer, who was found guilty of slavery and mass murder in Auschwitz, he served only seven years in prison, and then he became the chairman of the board at Bayer in 1956. Carl Krauch, executive member of IG Farben and the head of military economics for Hitler was found guilty of mass murder. He served just six years in prison, and then he became the chairman of the board for BASF. This is the same vaccine industry today which protected and employed Nazi war criminals. The very industry that produced the Nazi gas chambers was purchased by Bayer. Do you still want those vaccines? Exactly who are you trusting for your health and for your children's health?

Mike Adams just mentioned SV40, which is the monkey virus that was added to the polio vaccine that has resulted in thousands of cases of cancer. Previously in *The Quest*, we learned from vaccine expert Sherri Tenpenny as she addressed the SV40 virus in the polio vaccine.

Dr. Sherri Tenpenny: The polio vaccine has been known for many, many years to have a virus in it called SV40, which stands for Simian Virus 40 because those polio vaccines are made from monkey kidney cells, and so simian virus is a monkey virus. In 2002, *The Lancet* published a paper that said it was suspected that more than half of the 55,000 cases of non-Hodgkin's lymphoma that were out there, with a very high probability, could be associated with the SV40 virus from the polio vaccine. That's something in the published literature that came—that was in *The Lancet*. That came out in 2002.

There's two other stray viruses that end up, and they're from avian cells, which are all the vaccines that are made from eggs because they're passed down through the chickens and they get into their eggs. There are two different viruses that are known to be associated with breast cancer. I've written a couple of articles about that.

Ty: That's really amazing. Over half the cases of non-Hodgkin's lymphoma were actually *caused* by the polio vaccine. That's published in *The Lancet*, one of the most prestigious British medical journals. Investigative reporter John Rappaport has been doing research for over 30 years and has written for many prestigious periodicals and newspapers. He's also a vaccine expert. Let's listen to his perspective on this vitally important issue of vaccines.

John Rappaport: I think that people have to look at vaccines from the ground up. Let's take away all of the propaganda and so forth. You've got a needle, you're injecting it into babies, into adults even, into children of all ages. What's in the syringe? You've got many different chemicals, some of which are obviously carcinogenic, like formaldehyde, for example. You've got aluminum, which is extremely toxic. You've got other heavy metals. You've got unknown elements in vaccines, germs that were not intended to be there that are there, partial genetic sequences of things that were either put there on purpose or not. And it's all right there in the syringe, and these toxic chemicals, and these germs, and the whole soup. You're basically saying to a mother, "Look, this is what we want to do to your baby, okay? I'm going to take this needle with a syringe full of this stuff that I just explained, I'm going to shoot it into your baby, who doesn't really have any immune system at all, except derived from you, the mother, and this will be a good thing."

Desiree Rover: What I often do when I speak to parents, I say, "See this beautiful green apple I have here? Now, I'm going to inject into that formaldehyde, aluminum hydroxide, polysorbate 80, phenoxyethanol, this, that, and the other." Are you going to feed your kid this apple?

Dr. Sherri Tenpenny: It's just amazing to me how we think we can inject something that's never been tested for carcinogenity, never been tested to see if it's mutagenic, which means changes your DNA, never know whether or not it can cause any autoimmune diseases, but we can perfectly say that it's safe and effective and causes no harm. If somebody died and made me health czar tomorrow, what I would do is I would round up all the medical doctors, all of them, and I would put them in a big football stadium and have them read all of the package inserts, particularly the pediatricians. Read the VAERS report from the vaccine adverse event reporting system, and then take an entire test, a written test on immunology to prove that they know something about the human body. And then have them, with good conscience, say that what we are injecting into human beings is harmless.

Dr. Robert Scott Bell: They sacrifice children on the altar of this church of pharmaceutical mysticism with the needles of big pharma, as I call it. They argue that the only way we can survive childhood is to somehow elicit an artificial antibody response by injecting toxic poisons that you wouldn't put in the bottle of that same baby to make them drink. In fact, if you did, you might be charged with a crime – attempted murder.

Ty: Robert Scott Bell is accurate. If you were to take a bottle and fill it with aluminum, and formaldehyde, and mercury, and aborted fetal tissue, and other ingredients that are in most vaccines and give it to a baby, you could be charged with attempted murder. But vaccines are even worse than that because when you inject something directly into the muscle tissue, it goes directly into the bloodstream from there. It bypasses many of the protective mechanisms that have been placed in your digestive tract to keep us from dying of poisoning.

John Rappaport: When you're injecting anything into the body, you're intentionally bypassing a lot of portals of immune defense that would normally be active and working because you want this to penetrate deep into the body. Well, that's the idea of vaccination. Beginning from there, I say fundamentally, yes, vaccines can cause cancer. No question about it. Vaccines are not safe. They're not effective. They don't do what they're supposed to be doing. They're not responsible for the major declines in infectious or contagious diseases in the West. That was done by revolutionizing society – better sanitation, better nutrition, less overcrowding, development of the middle class, et cetera, et cetera. The fundamental environmental things that you would do in order to improve life for people. That's why those diseases basically went away. And when they return, it's basically because those factors have diminished again, which we are now seeing, especially when it comes to nutrition because it's gotten a lot worse over the last few decades. The whole thing to me is a gigantic hoax.

Ty: John Rappaport said the whole thing's a gigantic hoax. What hoax? What's he talking about? Let's learn a little bit more about the history of vaccines from vaccine expert Desiree Rover in Amsterdam, Netherlands.

First question being about vaccines. I know you're an expert. You've been looking at vaccines for 25 years. We hear they're safe and effective. We hear they don't cause cancer. We hear that they prevented all these diseases. What's the truth?

Desiree Rover: The opposite. That's a short answer.

Ty: The opposite.

Desiree Rover: Totally opposite, yeah. I wrote a book in 2009 on the HPV vaccines – Cervarix and Gardasil – and then for the book, I delved even deeper into the history of vaccination. To my big, big surprise, I found out that vaccines or vaccination—the foundation for vaccination is a folk myth that Edward Jenner followed, that cowpox—if you had had cowpox, you were supposedly protected against smallpox. But these are two viral entities, so it's a nonsense story.

What he did, he was the first guy who introduced proteins and DNA and RNA from animals – from other species – into humans. It was called inoculation or variolation. They made a scratch and then they put in the smallpox pus. That's how it originally started. And Jenner did a variation on that and he put in the cowpox pus, or the goatpox, or the pigpox, or whatever. All sorts of crap. He did that with his son and the son of his gardener, and both boys never got older than their 20, 21 years old because they died of tuberculosis, which is an illness related to cows. The studies that have been done with vaccines, that's being paid by the manufacturers. But the FDA in America, and the [FDA equivalent] here in Holland, for adding it to their program, they go with these studies. So it's the foxes guarding the henhouse.

Ty: Well, look at the HPV vaccine. On the package insert, it says it may cause other kinds of cancers.

Dr. Sherri Tenpenny: Yes, and we've already known that it has with the various report that there have been many girls who've been fully vaccinated with the HPV vaccine. That was in three months to about two years that are diagnosed with cervical cancer, massive cases of venereal warts. We know that less than four percent of the women in the United States have actually ever been exposed to the two viruses that are in the vaccine. So if the vaccine did anything, which it doesn't, and it can cause a lot of harm, there are at least eight strains of HPV (human papilloma virus) that are supposed to be associated with or are known to be associated with cancer. But the vaccine only covers two of them, so it gives this false sense of security to moms who think they're protecting their girls to think they won't get cancer. And that will say to the girls, I don't need to get a pap test because I've been protected. But there are other strains that can cause the cancer.

Jefferey Jaxen: Vaccines are not tested. On the insert, it says, "Not tested for carcinogenic and mutagenic properties." It also says it's not safe for pregnant women, and it's not tested in children for those same properties. What that is is that's your consent form that the doctor doesn't give to you. When a doctor is pushing or a nurse is pushing a vaccine, this is uninformed consent at the highest level. This goes against the Nuremberg principles. Nuremberg principle number four, actually, five, that were in 1940s after World War II. They did this so there was no more human experimentation on people. And this is medical experimentation because we are the last phase of the experimenting process.

As they're manufacturing these, we are—it depends on the lawsuits that come back to the company to tell the company if this product is actually safe. There have not been studies for the vaccines, but now there's not been studies for two, and three, and four vaccines stacked on each other, and up to 60, 70, however many they're going to push. There's no studies for all of those on top of it. You're looking at uninformed consent at the highest level.

Ty: Jefferey Jaxen mentioned that this is uninformed consent at the highest level. Uninformed consent means that you're not being informed of the potential dangers from a medical treatment or intervention like vaccines. You're supposed to be informed of the possible negative side effects. This is uninformed consent because people are not being told this. But you would think that if vaccines are actually harming people it would have a lot of lawsuits and the people would actually be getting money from these big pharma companies that are manufacturing the vaccines.

Sayer Ji: The government has paid out since 1986, through the National Vaccine Injury Compensation Fund, over $3 billion—

Ty: Billion?

Sayer Ji: $3 billion for literally thousands and thousands of cases of children that received the vaccines and they were injured, and their families have suffered profoundly. They are just a fraction of those who were compensated. It's been declared by the government that vaccines are unavoidably unsafe, and yet they claim that they are safe and they claim they're effective. If you look at the research on effectiveness, Cochrane Database Reviews, which is the most authoritative source, you will find no evidence, unequivocally, that the vaccines in the schedule today are safe. It doesn't exist. It's completely a lie.

Mike Adams: Many vaccines, if you just read the inserts, will say things like, the HPV vaccine, for example, says that "upon receiving this injection, you may lose consciousness and pass out, or fall down and hurt yourself." And that's just considered normal. Or you may have seizures, you may have fever, you may have to go to the emergency room. These are all listed on the vaccine inserts. And somehow, the American public has been brainwashed into thinking that this is normal healthy medicine. It isn't! If someone gives you a shot of something and you pass out, how is that not causing a neurological side effect that could damage your brain? I mean, think about it if you still can. Some people can't because they've been injected with these things.

Across Europe, $90 million in damages was just paid out by the UK government to cover children who were provably brain damaged by the swine flu vaccine. Do you think they would pay $90 million if it wasn't conclusively proven that that caused it? Of course not. They know what caused it. That's why they're paying the money. Yet the vaccine industry has complete immunity, even though it's causing all of this damage, and cancer as well. There was a town in Mexico recently where 75 percent of the children who were vaccinated wound up either in the hospital or dead – 75 percent.

Ty: Are the vaccines affecting our mental cognition?

Mike Adams: Yeah, the vaccines are brain damaging the population. Think about it. The vaccines still contain mercury, like in flu shots. They still contain aluminum another known neurotoxin. They still contain formaldehyde and MSG. Almost every one of these preservatives or adjuvants is a neurological poison. How can they not cause brain damage?

The medical establishment today says you shouldn't smoke cigarettes because the chemicals in the cigarettes go into your body and cause damage, right? They probably say you shouldn't sniff glue, or you shouldn't snort crack, or whatever. Why? Because those chemicals go in and cause damage. But then they're injecting you with a vaccine that contains chemicals that they know causes damage. How is that allowable? By the way, I'm not against the theory of vaccination. Let's be clear here. Why can't they manufacture *clean* vaccines without the chemicals that are single dose vaccines that could be given with a margin of safety that doesn't exist today?

Dr. Rashid Buttar: I'm not against the principle of vaccination at all. Stupidity is what I'm against. And to give the body a live virus at a time when the body can't even build an immune response – meaning the first six months of life, because the immune system isn't developed yet – along with certain substances that are acting as preservatives that suppress the immune system, under the false pretense of building up the immune system. That's just hogwash. There's no validity to it.

Dr. John Consemulder: We have the same position here like in FDA in America because the [NEVM], like I mentioned, is also not open to discuss, even just go into a dialogue about the non-safe and non-effective vaccines. I mean, if we are crazy, show us. Give us the evidence. Give us the independent evidence that vaccines are actually safe and effective. But if we show them the independent evidence that they're actually not safe and effective at all, they do not even want to discuss these matters. I'm like, "Science is science, right?" It shouldn't be a double standard, but it is.

Mike Adams: Chemotherapy destroys the immune system. Vaccines weaken the immune system. If you combine them, that's how you get a lot of fatalities. You get people who are just being injected and poisoned from multiple angles, all of it under the auspices of public health. But it's really profiteering on the part of the drug companies using human bodies as the vessels of profit generation. It's like *The Matrix*. You're like the Neo character in *The Matrix*. You're in this vessel and the tubes are plugged into you, and they're generating profits off of you, and that's your only role in society according to these corporations. They just want you lined up, stacked up, towers of human bodies that they can make money off of. It's a medical Matrix.

There's such a scientific dictatorship out there that you're not allowed to ask any reasonable question at all. Someone who says, "Well, what if we spaced out the timing of the vaccines so that a child can recover more before they get hit with another insult to their immune system?" Space them out. It's a reasonable thing, right? You can't ask that question in the vaccine industry. Suddenly you're anti-science, you're condemned, you're a heretic.

What if you ask the question, what if we took the mercury out of the vaccines? They've done it in Europe. They have mercury-free medicine is a pillar of the United Nations, the future of medicine. Get the mercury out of everything because it's toxic. Why do we still have mercury in flu shots that we're injecting into pregnant women and children? But if you ask that question, you are attacked and you are condemned.

It's really a kind of insanity in the vaccine industry, just like in the cancer industry. Many people who are pushing these poisons are themselves clinically insane, or they're tied to the profits in such a way that they are unable to discover the personal ethics required to tell the truth. And it's sad because children are being harmed and killed every single day because of these greed-driven people or these insane people who parade as scientists, but they're not. They're the kind of scientists maybe that the Nazi regime would have loved to hire, willing to carry out experiments on Jewish prisoners. That's their ethics. But they're not the kind of scientists that we should have practicing medicine in America today.

Ty: I know that vaccines are a very emotional topic, they're hotly debated, they're very controversial. But we felt like it was important to bring you the truth about vaccines, especially their impact on cancer because you can't make an educated decision if you don't know about this. How are you feeling now that you've learned this about vaccines? That you learned about these potentially carcinogenic ingredients in vaccines? Does it make you angry? Are you upset? Are you in disbelief? It's okay to be temporarily angry or upset, but we don't want chronic anger, or chronic stress, or chronic fight or flight with the adrenaline rushing through our bodies, because that's what can lead to a compromised immune state and can lead to cancer.

As a matter of fact, the emotional aspect of cancer is one of the blind spots that we're going to deal with tonight. It's one of the most overlooked blind spot for cancer. Many oncologists – most oncologists – don't even know that there's an emotional aspect to most cancer diagnoses. We were privileged to travel to the Hope 4 Cancer Clinic in Tijuana, Mexico, and we interviewed Dr. Xavier Curiel, who is an emotional expert. He's a medical doctor but he understands the impact of emotions in cancer. He discussed with us a revolutionary scientific technique for dealing with emotional baggage, which is called recall healing.

Dr. Xavier Curiel: Recall healing is basically a system that has put together different knowledges to the benefit of the patient in emotional healing. The importance of emotion in cancer, to my opinion, is fundamental, is crucial. Especially in the last four to five years, I started to pay a lot of attention to that. Before that, I will consider it important—be stress-free, whatever—but I did not really have understood the deepness of the importance that that is because I believe today, I'm convinced that probably that's the main trigger, the main factor that can actually codify, program certain information at a genetic and cellular level. There's a lot of research that demonstrates the impact of psychological, social stress, and emotional. In the University of Berkeley, I like an article they have by the Department of Psychology. It's called *The Emotional Expression in the Onset and Progression of Cancer*. There's a certain group of conflicts—

Ty: There's specific conflicts and trauma that trigger different types of cancers.

Dr. Xavier Curiel: Exactly.

Dr. Francisco Contreras: The reason why we're failing in oncology so much is that we become mechanics of the human body and we're not paying attention to the emotional and spiritual needs of our patients.

Dr. Henk Fransen: When the body starts to heal itself, you can see that old emotional wounds and spiritual pain comes to the surface to be released also. But like we have to assist the body in this detoxification process, most cancer patients also need help in this process. We have many techniques like EFT, emotional trauma therapy, and others, to help assist people to let go of their emotional pain.

Ty: What is EFT?

Dr. Henk Fransen: EFT is a way of using affirmations while we tap certain acupuncture points to release all the pain and to substitute them for new ideas and a new mindset. This detoxification of the emotional and spiritual level with this physical level should go hand in hand.

Ty: There are many devices that have been invented over the years that deal with the emotional aspect of cancer. One such device is called the EVOX machine.

Liliana Partida: I compare the EVOX to what I would consider emotional acupuncture. It's pretty amazing because it's done with biofeedback, and so what it's doing is picking up voice recognition. We use a cradle, it works on galvanic response. A patient will have a microphone on, and then I just ask them to speak their name so that I can just pick up the patterning. Then it'll come up with a little mandala. It'll have what we call PIs (perception indexes) from 1 to 12. Each area is associated with an organ and also with an emotion. Oftentimes, the patient doesn't know what's really running their life, and potentially been running their health in regards to their crises that they're experiencing.

What's really fascinating about it is the patient doesn't even really have to tell me about it. The feedback actually comes up with the areas of stagnation, or what we call extreme energy, or let's say even if you were thinking in terms of acupuncture, where there would be extreme excess in a specific organ. Through that determination, the program is equipped to sense specific frequencies to unlock those emotional stagnations. It's pretty amazing. Each time we do a recording (we do about five recordings) we can actually see the unlocking of those emotions, and that is kind of like an onion. Each voice recording you go deeper and deeper in regards to what potentially is the underlying of even that emotional stagnation.

Ty: So kind of peeling off the layers off the onion.

Liliana Partida: Exactly.

Ty: And then eventually you get to the real root cause.

Liliana Partida: Eventually, we get to the root cause, which is really pretty amazing for the patient because, oftentimes, they'll have an a-ha moment. They'll be potentially experiencing a lot of depression, and really, what we're looking at as we go deeper and deeper, the depression is based potentially on unworthiness or repetitive thinking. I always ask them, "How does that show up for you in your life?" We've tried to get some feedback, and they'd say, "Actually, you know, I just churn things until they just really turn into butter. I can't let go of things when they happen to me." When a patient's able to really identify what they actually do, they can begin to actually recognize, "Oh, I'm doing it again. This is a stuck pattern." And just even that begins to unravel those energies that are stuck.

Ty: So this can be really beneficial for cancer patients because of the emotional link that we've seen to cancer. We have so many cancer patients that have this emotional trauma, these things that have happened in the past that they can't let go of, this baggage, whatever you want to call it. This allows them to help release that, doesn't it?

Liliana Partida: Absolutely. We're definitely a believer in Hammer's work in regards to every disease has an emotional component, whether it's a sore throat or cancer. It's pretty exciting that we have this information so that we can really look at potentially, is it the emotion that's causing the problem or is it the actual organ function that's causing the emotion?

Ty: One emotion that's very detrimental to a cancer patient is fear. But let me ask you a question. What emotion is it that an oncologist will elicit in the cancer patient when they look them in the eye and they say "you've got three months to live?" And then they rush them into chemotherapy.

Dr. Bita Badakhshan: In Kaiser, they would get the diagnosis of cancer, they didn't even have time to research. Within a few days, they had to do chemo. Otherwise, the doctors would tell them they're going to die or it's going to spread everywhere. They would come—one patient I had, she had urinary infection, and next day she had to do chemo. I said, "No, hon, you have to take care of your kidneys first, or urinary infection, get rid of the bacteria, and then do your research." It's no rush. You didn't get cancer overnight. Cancer is a process of 10 years, 12 years. I mean, within eight years, you get the tumor. Sometimes people don't get diagnosis until 10, 12 years. They kind of tend to scare the patients and they get worried. They don't have time to research, then they start the chemo.

Mike Adams: Oncologists and ISIS use many of the same tactics of fear to manipulate your behavior. Yes, I'm comparing oncologists to a known terrorist organization because they use the same tactics to try to control people. In fact, terrorism is the use of fear. The definition is the use of widespread fear or the threat of fear, the threat of violence, in order to achieve a desired behavior or decision-making outcome among people.

By definition, what many oncologists do today is a cousin of terrorism. That's why it's unacceptable. That's why some of them are going to jail. That's why they're criminals. That's why more of them should be arrested. And that's why you as a patient should be extremely skeptical of anything that an oncologist tells you because it is in their interest that you say yes to what they are pushing.

Ty: Mike Adams just compared fear tactics that oncologists use to the fear tactics that terrorists might use. Is this over the top? You can decide that. I did recently see an HBO special where the oncologist told a lady that she had six months to live, and if she did not do chemotherapy that she would eventually die within six months, and that she would feel like she was drowning as she died. In my opinion, it should be criminal for an oncologist to treat a cancer patient that way.

Peter Starr: I was diagnosed with prostate cancer ten years ago. I had the fear of death put into me by the urologist. He had a bedside manner of a Neanderthal, as far as I was concerned, and it prompted me to study natural medicine. When the doctor tells you you've got cancer and he says it just like that—there's two things you know about cancer. One is, you're going to die, and you're going to die soon. That's the average person's view of having somebody say that you've got cancer. It's the most irresponsible thing that a doctor can do.

Dr. Francisco Contreras: The power of life and death is in the tongue. So if you pronounce somebody dead, they see the doctor as an authority. They buy it. I'm dead, no matter what.

Dr. Darrell Wolfe: What the medical system has is very archaic. The only reason why people use the medical system, whether it be chemotherapy, radiation, or surgery—sometimes surgery is needed—is because of fear and panic.

Dr. Leigh Erin Connealy: Once you enter into the system and you need a surgery or you need a chemo or radiation, you are losing your life because even surgery—just say you had a little lump, one centimeter. Surgery is a major assault and attack on the body. It affects the nervous system, it affects your physiology, and it's outrageously stressful.

Ty: Talk about stress and the immune system and cancer.

Valerie Warwick, R.N.: Stress really diminishes the immune system because it increases your cortisol, which suppresses your immune system, which depletes your melatonin, your vitamin C, your niacin. So there's this big cascade actually where chronic continual stress will deplete your micronutrients.

Ty: Stress, mental anguish, negative thoughts and emotions. These are all detrimental to our health. Previously in *The Quest*, Dr. Tony Jimenez has shared with us the impact of negative thoughts.

Dr. Antonio Jimenez: A negative thought can kill you faster than a bad germ. One of the main things to detoxify is here. *[pointing to head]*

Ty: The mind.

Dr. Antonio Jimenez: The mind.

Dr. Irina Kossovskaia: Think about yourself. When you come home all stressed out and tired in the end of the day, and your dog runs to you and puts its head on your lap and looks at you. You're getting this energy of love, unconditional love,from them. That's the most coherent energy that charges you up, and your headache disappears at that time. There are studies done that actually show blood pressure going down 10, 20 millimeters just from petting your cat.

Dr. Edward Group III: We know the body can heal itself just with thought. There's been proof of that to where people have manifested with and visualized their cancer going away, and their cancer went away with no other type of medicine, internally or externally.

Ty: Curing cancer simply by thinking about it sounds too good to be true, but it's reality. Dr. Group knows many people that that has happened for. Early in this episode, we heard from a chiropractor, Dr. Terry Harmon. Chiropractors are oftentimes thought of as quacks, but the reason is not because they're practicing inferior medicine. It's because of the Flexner Report of 1910 and its effect on the perception of medicine in the United States and actually worldwide.

Another area of medicine that's oftentimes referred to as quackery is homeopathy. Let's listen to Dr. Suzanne Kim, who's a medical doctor, describe to us her first experience with the practice of homeopathy.

Dr. Suzanne Kim: When I started learning a little bit about nutritional medicine, that was really very, very helpful. That's the foundation, I believe, for all health. That then led me into homeopathy. As I learned about homeopathy, it kind of expanded my thinking and challenged me because it really was very far off from what you learn in medical school. After that, I just said I will try it and it just worked amazing.

Dr. Keith Scott Mumby: This is homeopathy in two or three sentences, okay? You pick a substance that copies the illness; not one that opposes it, but one that copies it. For example, if someone has scarlet fever, you choose belladonna because if you take belladonna, your face goes all bright red, you throat's sore, hectic temperature, you feel ghastly. Taking belladonna is like having scarlet fever, so it's a good remedy for scarlet fever. It's called "like cures like," so you're looking for a mimic of the disease.

A commercial doctor would take an antagonist. You take aspirin to lower the temperature. Different kinds of opposing ideas. This is, first of all, identify something that copies your illness, then you dilute it. This is the weird part that doctors and scientists can't get hold of. It's called *potentization*. You can dilute it one in ten, one in ten, one in ten, one in ten, one in ten, and after twelve dilutions, you've passed the Avogadro number so we know there is no belladonna left. Interestingly, if you hitch it up to a spectographic transmitter, you find that the more you dilute it, the more it starts transmitting energies.

You can't argue with a spectograph. It's the most exquisitely sensitive scientific instrument we have. That's what tells you there's manganese on a star that's a thousand, billion light years away. You can't argue with a spectograph. And yet the homeopathic remedies actually start to broadcast the more you dilute them.

Dr. Robert Scott Bell: What is homeopathy? The million, zillion dollar question. Well, we take substances from the three kingdoms: mineral, plant, animal kingdom. And in their mother state, they would cause certain symptoms to occur if you ingest them, or are exposed to them topically, or whatever. Catalog these symptoms that are associated with the mother substance if you will, like the venom of a bee, it stings, right? You take the venom of the bee (Apis) and you use it homeopathically to reverse the stings like that or exactly that. And we can use that for many different things including we can use a lot of toxic substances that you would never use, although modern medicine would like mercury, and we can convert that into a homeopathic form that is non-toxic that can actually facilitate the detoxification of mercury, for instance. So that's the shortest version.

It's a worldwide system of medicine. In the United States it's regulated as a drug because of the passage of the Food, Drug and Cosmetic Act of 1938, passed in 1939. Thanks to Senator Copeland who was a physician and a homeopath. He made sure that the HPUS, the Homeopathic Pharmacopeia of the United States, was grandfathered in at that point. And so that allowed a legally-recognized drug system. Even though it was non-toxic, no side effects, that it has equal standing in the sense that it can be labelled and sold as a medicine in America.

Gemma Hoefkins: Since 1996, I was sent home to die, really. Previous to that, when I was 23 years old, I had hydrocephalus and they said that was a very successful operation. Hydrocephalus is water on the brain, which is a tube going from your head going down to your abdomen, draining fluid. Everybody's got cerebral fluid that goes down. A couple of years later on, I was getting problems: memory problems, dizziness, headaches. They kept doing scans. I was worried about the shunt coming down, whether that was damaged or not working properly. They're giving me MRI scans and checking and checking. Nothing wrong. Then they finally found there was a tumor in my pineal gland, which is right in the middle of your head.

On the first radiology session, they leapt into the room and said stop it because they'd found another tumor. This was on my pituitary gland. It then went down my spine. They did some more radiology down my spine, and then I got the results and they look into it, and they said, actually, it's quite good because the ones in my back had actually gone. I think that's great. But then they said it's not an improvement enough. We need chemotherapy.

Which is kind of confusing. I'm thinking, well, why don't they carry on with what's working? But the doctors said no. I thought, okay, good news, but I was a bit confused because it was going on to chemotherapy. I had the chemotherapy. I was supposed to have three sessions of it. I think I had two. I said I didn't have the third one, and they said to me, basically, the treatment is making it worse. All my hair fell out with the radiology in two weeks, and I was nauseous and vomiting.

After my chemotherapy, they came in and basically they said, "Would you like to stay in the hospital? Would you like to go home? Or would you like to go to a hospice?" Actually, my sister ran after them after they said about did I want to go to a hospice, et cetera. She ran after them and said, "Look, the family needs to know how long have we got. What's the prognosis?" Basically, he said to me at the time, "Have a good Christmas." This was only October, and I was thinking, oh—I realized that he was probably saying "because this is going to be your last one." He basically gave me about three months to live.

Ty: Gemma, I want to read a letter here. This is a letter that I've got, you gave me. It's on hospital letterhead from a hospital here in London. I'm not going to read the doctor's name or anything, but this is the actual doctor's letter dated November 19, 1996, so almost 19 years ago. Doctor says, "I have discussed the findings. I've explained that the chemotherapy has not helped her since her disease has progressed during treatment. I have also stressed that there are no other viable options for treating the disease."

Gemma Hoefkins: I thought, I don't want to go into a hospice. As far as I was concerned, you go into a hospice because you die. And I thought, I don't want to stay in this hospital. Everybody's dying around me. I was in the oncology ward and I could hear people having their last rites in the middle of the night, and things like that. I couldn't wait to get out of there. I thought, I'll go home to my mom's because there's nothing like your mom to look after you—mom and dad. I went back to their place. That was the point where I could barely get out of bed. I couldn't get out of bed on my own. I used to have help. I couldn't even open up my eyelid. I'd have to lift it up with my finger. And then I had to have a stick to walk with, and to go to the toilet. I'd have a hand on there, stick on there. My balance was really, really bad.

Ty: And you were late 20s.

Gemma Hoefkins: I was 26, 27. My sister-in-law phoned me up and she said, "I've heard about this woman. She's helped me with my daughter's eczema. It's gone completely away. Do you want to speak to her? She's a homeopath." I go, "What's that? I don't know what that is."

Ty: You didn't know what homeopathy was at that point.

Gemma Hoefkins: No idea what homeopathy was, I didn't know. But I thought, I'm really, really poorly. I might as well give it a go. I'm not getting anywhere. So I started having some treatment from her, and so I had a bit of faith in her. I didn't have a lot of faith in her. I was very skeptical about anything alternative, to be honest. I thought, all these things are happening to me, they were coincidence. But they kept happening again and again and again, so I'm like, "Okay." So I kept on with that. And then when I was sent home to die, I've just kept it going with homeopathy ever since then. And now, this is 18 years later on, and I've never needed to go to a doctor again.

Ty: Eighteen years since you began the homeopathic treatments, have you had any contact with the doctors that told you there was nothing that they could do, that their treatments were making you worse?

Gemma Hoefkins: Oh, yeah, I went back. I called back two years later, I think. I went back two years later. I'm very proud about doing this because I could walk down the road on my own, get on a bus, and get to the hospital on my own. I told them to put it down to homeopathy. It's in my notes. He puts it down to homeopathy. But he said it was a remarkable recovery and he couldn't understand it. And then he turned around and he went to shuffle some papers, and he said, "Well, maybe it's the delayed effect from the chemotherapy."

Ty: Really?

Ty: So what do you think? Was Gemma's cancer cured because of a delayed effect of chemotherapy? I'll let you be the judge on that one. Due to her positive experience from homeopathy and it actually healing her brain cancer, in 2000, Gemma became a homeopath and actually treats cancer patients in England. But homeopathy, in many areas, is not tolerated.

Mike Adams: We talk about tolerance in this country. Well, there is no group that is more intolerant than the pharmaceutical industry, and the cancer doctors, and the vaccine pushers. They are completely intolerant of any other opinion. They do not welcome freedom of thought. They do not even believe in the scientific method, which involves questioning and seeking answers to those questions by letting the evidence tell you what is true. They *hate* that process. They want to dictate science to you, and that's a contradiction. We cannot stay stuck in the compartmentalization of chemicals that is based on the 1940s and 1950s understanding of science and nutrition medicine. But that's what we're stuck in today with the cancer industry. We've got to move past that if we hope to actually heal.

Dr. Bita Badakhshan: We need to educate people. We need to tell them there's other ways to go. Going with the conventional surgery, radiation, chemo is not the way to go.

Dr. Howard Fisher: If it doesn't make sense, then it's non-sense. Don't listen to nonsense.

Dr. Sunil Pai: And now we see commercials on television, right? I always tell people, you can watch television this week, and one commercial will be going to a beach in Bahamas, and swim with the dolphins, and the next exact commercial will be, "Come to this cancer center for your treatment." It's becoming very, very common. The problem is making it so common, not due to its prevalence that more people are getting it, but just makes it that as common that we expect to get it. It should be alarming that why are they advertising me to go and check in at this place. And they're competing, so every hospital is competing. The one in Texas, it could be the one in Arizona, in Florida, and the one in Chicago. And they're really spending a lot of marketing dollar to get your admission. I call it the healthcare amusement parks or the Disneyland, for example, of—they want you to come and spend your vacation, but instead of taking a vacation, you're actually being treated.

Ty: But you sit in a nice, comfortable lounge chair with a view of the golf course while you're getting chemotherapy dripped into you.

Dr. Sunil Pai: That's not the ride I want to be on.

Ty: Wow, what a liberating feeling it is to discover the blind spots that could potentially trigger cancer. And to become empowered to understand and address the issue before it becomes life threatening. Even if you're in a dire situation, isn't is amazing that by correcting these root causes, that are hidden in these cancer blind spots – whether it's in the spine, the mouth, or another area – that we can enable the body to eliminate cancer. As you saw in the story of Bill Spalding who beat cancer simply through correcting a root cause.

It wasn't a subject we wanted to cover necessarily, but we knew that we had to. We knew that the topic of vaccines must be addressed. I hope that you've seriously considered this information as it relates to important decisions in your life. And that you can take the steps that you know are the safest and most reliable in avoiding toxic substances that detrimentally affect your health, cause disease, and promote cancer growth. I'm glad we could help equip you with this essential information.

We've learned the science behind homeopathy, and the valuable contribution it's made to health and wellbeing. We're so glad to help reinforce the true science and evidence which supports this important area of natural medicine, and it's invaluable contribution to preventing and beating cancer.

Finally, we've learned that what you think and feel *does* matter. As you've listened to this information, I hope you thought about your own life. And what thoughts and feelings may be seriously injuring your health and happiness as we've shared important action steps you can take, as well as avenues to pursue. We hope that now, in this moment, you resolve to forgive and to forget. As the old saying goes, "Don't worry. Be happy." And remember that laughter is the best medicine. Smile, laugh, tell someone you love them, breathe, relax, let someone know that you're grateful for them. Take time to fill your life with the things that bring you joy and happiness.

Ty: Wow. We really covered a lot of ground in tonight's episode. I hope that you've learned a lot and I hope that you're pumped for tomorrow night, because tomorrow night's episode is going to get even better. We're going to travel all the way to Cologne, Germany, and visit a German cancer clinic. As you know, the German cancer clinics are renowned in the world for their natural treatments for cancer and for their medical devices that are only available there. We're going to get a tour of one of the best cancer clinics in the whole country of Germany.

Tomorrow night's episode will also focus heavily on detoxification. If we're going to be healthy, we've got to get the toxins out of our body. Tomorrow night, we are going to hear from two of the most renowned experts in the world on detoxification.

If you've learned thus from *The Truth About Cancer: A Global Quest*, please tell your friends and family to join us for tomorrow's episode. You'll be glad that you did because we're going to share more lifesaving information that could save your life or the life of a loved one from that cancer diagnosis. In the meantime, have a great rest of your day. Join us tomorrow night. God bless all of you.

[*credits roll*]

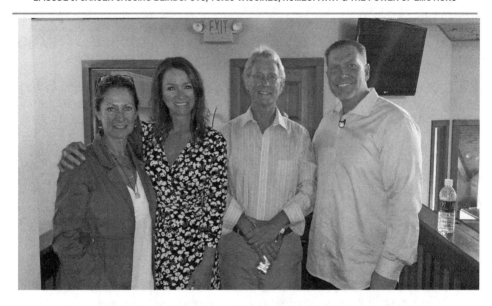

Above - with Charlene at the office of Dr. Thomas Lokensgard in Nashville, TN
Below – with the BetterWay Health crew along with Dr. Jockers and AJ Lanigan in Atlanta, GA

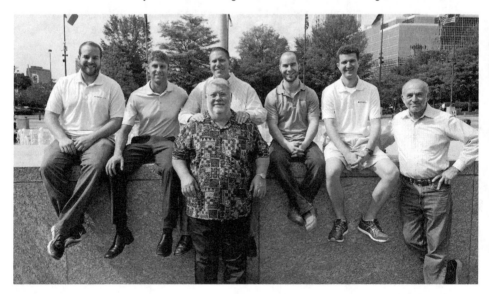

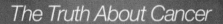

The Truth About Cancer

A GLOBAL QUEST

Episode 6

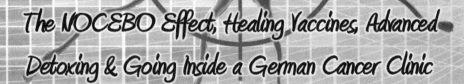

The NOCEBO Effect, Healing Vaccines, Advanced Detoxing & Going Inside a German Cancer Clinic

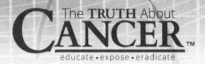

The TRUTH About
CANCER™
educate • expose • eradicate

Ty: Welcome back to *The Truth about Cancer: A Global Quest*. I'm so happy that you joined us tonight. I hope you were with us last night. We had an episode that was chock full of lifesaving information. But just in case you missed it, here's a recap.

[*Video plays: Summary of Episode Five*]

Now in last night's episode, we learned a lot about vaccines and the toxicity that most of these vaccines contain. In contrast with tonight, we're going to learn more about vaccines, but we're going to actually learn about vaccines that are helpful – not harmful. I know that may sound weird, but when we get into tonight's episode I think you'll understand it a little bit more.

But before we get to that, we're going to deal a little bit with detoxification, because detoxification is a huge part of the cancer puzzle. We've heard from detoxification experts in the past, but some of the experts that we're going to hear from tonight have never shared the information that they have shared with us until these interviews.

We're going to travel to Cologne, Germany. We're also going to travel to London as we learn more about this vitally important process of detoxification.

Dr. Raymond Hilu: These cells on the body are interconnected by interstitial tissue, or by matrix. This area in between the cells is where things happen. This is where the nutrients are and where they enter into the cell. The dirt inside the cell goes out into this area and the lymphatic system drains it away.

This interstitial tissue, this matrix, has to be clean. If it is contaminated, then oxygen won't be able to go through and the cell can become cancerous. The proper nutrients cannot go through and the cell can become cancerous. Potassium and magnesium cannot go through so the cell becomes *acidic*, in this case, and it can turn cancerous. That's why detoxification is very, very, very important.

Dr. Leigh Erin Connealy: Then you talk about all the environmental pollutants, everything from phthalates to benzenes to fire retardants—I mean chlorine, chlorine! It's the pharmaceuticals now that are in our body that you are not even taking!

Ty: They're in the water.

Dr. Leigh Erin Connealy: They are in the water so we're getting them in another way.

Dr. Edward Group III: We are living in a world where—we're all living in a toxic world. The world is sick. The world has cancer right now. Trees are dying. The chem trails. The soil is sick. The water is contaminated. The air in the world is contaminated.

The only thing that we can do is to keep our self-healing mechanisms strong. In order to keep our self-healing mechanisms strong we have to keep our bodies clean. It all comes back to simplicity. After years of looking out here for the answer, I finally realized that the answer was right here and realized that no disease can exist inside of a clean body.

Ty: No disease can exist inside of a clean body, but how do we get our bodies clean? Through detoxification. When I was in San Diego, I was able to do an interview with Dr. Daniel Nuzum. We sat down and he discussed the one, two, three of how we can detoxify our body.

Dr. Daniel Nuzum: Okay, first off, the garbage shoot. We've got to take the garbage out, clean the colon.

Ty: Clean the colon. And how do we do it?

Dr. Daniel Nuzum: Coffee enemas. We can use colon hydrotherapy. My preference is usually with herbal supplements, using herbal cleanses like…

Ty: Psyllium

Dr. Daniel Nuzum: Psyllium, cascara sagrada.

Ty: Cascara sagrada.

Dr. Daniel Nuzum: Bentonite, slippery elm bark. Buckthorn is very very good. Very good. Those are good, good, good herbs. Humic acid, excellent for the entire digestive tract. You've got to clear one exit to clear the next. Your colon would be number one.

Dr. Edward Group III: When we opened our cancer clinic in 1998, our main focus was how can we keep the intestines clean on a regular basis. We found prescription drugs, over 900 prescription drugs, 90 percent of them cause constipation. They also kill the intestinal flora. Chemotherapy ruins the intestinal lining.

Dr. Darrell Wolfe: The most important step to care for the human body is daily, gentle detoxification. Natural health practitioners still don't have it today. They don't understand it today. They still look at trying to do a cleanse on somebody every few months. They still teach people to pile their crap up, create a manure pile, start to feel sick and then do a deep cleanse. Let's dump all those toxins out real fast, overload the body that's already overloaded.

It is like everything in life. If you exercise a little bit each day, you show that you love your family a little bit each day, and you show you love your body a little bit each day. Then we wouldn't get into this mess would we?

Ty: So it's daily gentle detox. There's a tea that you've developed that we drink in our family, great for daily detoxification.

Dr. Darrell Wolfe: It's called the daily cleansing tea.

Ty: Daily cleansing tea. Okay.

Dr. Darrell Wolfe: You know what? It's like this. Your large intestine is the mother of all organs. It houses almost 60 percent of your immune system and whenever you're in trouble, what's the first thing that sticks out?

Ty: Belly.

Dr. Darrell Wolfe: Yeah, if it sticks out it is full of gas. If it sticks out and hangs down, that's your immune system falling down, that's your guts falling out. Meanwhile you can walk down the street and you see three guys talking together on the corner and they're all rubbing it and seeing which one gets the wish first.

Ty: Like little Buddhas.

Dr. Darrell Wolfe: Yeah, it's an epidemic.

Ty: Dr. Wolfe is accurate. It is an epidemic. Step one, we must cleanse our colon. So now let's go to step two in the detoxification process for the entire body.

Dr. Daniel Nuzum: The next best exit to go to would be the urinary tract, the kidneys, bladder. Clear that urinary tract system.

Ty: How would we do that?

Dr. Daniel Nuzum: Parsley, asparagus.

Ty: Parsley, asparagus.

Dr. Daniel Nuzum: Your marshmallow root and those types of things are very good.

Ty: Lots of water.

Dr. Daniel Nuzum: Lots of water.

Ty: Which you'd want to go back to your colon if you're taking psyllium husk. You need to drink a lot of water.

Dr. Daniel Nuzum: Right. That's going to swell up and take up space and so if you don't want to bloat you've got to keep it moist so it moves easy.

Dr. Nicholas Gonzalez: The liver and the kidney are the body's main detoxification organs. That's for environmental chemicals, our own metabolic waste, the dead cancer process – metabolize and prepare for excretion.

He opens up the *Merck Manual* and low and behold there are coffee enemas. The interesting thing, the sad thing is, the ironic thing, Kelley was brutalized in the media for his use of coffee enemas. We get attacked about it today too, but they come right out of the conventional medical literature. He didn't learn about it from alien space beams being injected into his brain through some mystic psychic experience.

He didn't learn about it through some alternative throw-away journals and stuff. He learned about it from conventional medical textbooks. The *Merck Manual* was a compendium of conventional therapies, and they were in the *Merck Manual.* Coffee enemas were in the *Merck Manual* right up until the 1970s.

Dr. Daniel Nuzum: Once the urinary tract was cleared, your best bet would be the liver. Follow that with the liver, clean the liver, clear the liver.

Ty: And coffee enemas, as Dr. Nick Gonzalez shared with us the last time, one of the best ways to clean the liver—

Dr. Daniel Nuzum: The best ways. Your turmeric, milk thistle, virtually all of your root vegetables – beets, ginger, burdock – all of those things are very, very good at cleaning the liver.

Ty: Are you recommending that people eat those or that they take extracts?

Dr. Daniel Nuzum: If you want to clean it quick, extracts. You need the concentration. They need to be concentrated.

Dr. Group III: And this goes back years and years and years in research is actually drinking oils because oils are the only thing that are going to actually push the congestion out of the liver. So we developed a program based on ancient philosophies and techniques combined with modern philosophies and techniques and experimented with different products and different herbs.

We developed an herbal formula that uses borututu bark and chanca piedra, which are rare rainforest Brazilian herbs that will actually loosen and dissolve stones in the liver. Then we have them do that for four days.

On day five they drink an extra virgin olive oil with some Epsom salts and they push so it causes contractions of the liver. It actually pushes all of that congestion out. What we found with evaluating over 100,000 liver cleanses is liver cleansing is probably one of the most effective ways of boosting your self-healing mechanism.

Each liver cleanse is going to boost the liver production and efficiency by 10 to 15 percent, which means another thing we found in research is that most cancer and degenerative disease patients need multiple liver cleanses.

The beauty of cleansing is you can do it in conjunction with any doctor who you are seeing or any cancer doctor. As a matter of fact, we've had fourth stage cancer patients who have just done intestinal cleansing and balancing and multiple liver and gallbladder cleansing without taking any other supplement. Fourth stage with two weeks left to live who have been sent home to die, that have continued liver cleansing and intestinal biosis, fixing their intestines and just doing liver cleanse, liver cleanse, liver cleanse.

Ty: That's very good information from Dr. Nuzum and Dr. Group about how to keep your liver clean and the importance of detoxifying the liver. In this next clip we hear from Cherie Calbom, the Juice Lady, about her gentle liver detoxification recipe.

Cherie Calbom: My morning shake is lemon – the juice of one lemon and one lime, and you can add orange too if you want to. For me that's too much sugar. My body just does not like sugar at all, even orange juice. But you can put orange juice in there for sure.

Then you add about a cup of water, a bunch of ice cubes, as many as you want to make it the temperature you want, a tablespoon of olive oil, one garlic clove, and a little chunk of ginger and that's day one.

Day 2 it's two cloves of garlic and two tablespoons of olive oil, and then day 3, three [cloves of garlic] and three [tablespoons of olive oil]. [Day] 4 and four [of each]. Day 5, five garlic cloves, five tablespoons of olive oil and the rest is the same. Don't breathe on anyone that day!

Ty: Oh, because of the garlic.

Cherie Calbom: I'm teasing you.

Ty: Right. Well, make sure that your husband or wife is drinking it with you, right?

Cherie Calbom: Or chew on parsley. That takes away the garlic breath. That is, along with a carrot salad, a beets salad, and potassium broth soup, and a beet juice drink, and a green juice drink. That is your liver cleanse, gentle liver cleanse program. Then you can add salads and soups and stir fries but it should be an all-vegetable week.

It's a wonderful, gentle, very gentle liver cleanse. There are many others that are more heavy duty with herbs and different tinctures that you can add in. But if you want to do a gentle one, that is a great way to start working into it.

Beets are wonderful for the liver. They are known as a liver food, a liver cleanse food along with many others: the dark leafy greens and carrot, olive oil, lemon juice. All of that is just wonderful for liver cleansing.

With my carrot salad and beet salad, I make them with the pulp. I juice a beet first and pull out the pulp, and then I juice all my carrots to get a cup of pulp and then add lemon juice and olive oil dressing to each of them. They are separate. I put cinnamon in there, in my dressing, because it just sparks up the flavor a whole lot. I love cinnamon.

Then you eat your beets salad a couple tablespoons at a time throughout the day. Your carrot salad you can eat all at once, but it is done for you so fast. It's all done for you.

Ty: And it really cleanses the liver, all these steps together.

Cherie Calbom: Yes, and if anyone has had chemo and radiation it's extremely important that you cleanse your liver. I say to everyone who has cancer, who has had cancer and has been through chemo and/or radiation, "You must, must, must cleanse your liver, cleanse your whole body because those things are so toxic. If you don't it's going to stay in your body, and it *could* contribute to cancer coming back along with all the other toxicity that was there and contributed to cancer in the first place."

But before you cleanse your liver – and we talked about it earlier – always cleanse your colon because we want that channel of elimination very open and as clean as possible so that when the liver starts dumping the toxins they can get on out and get through your body.

I do want to say, for everyone who does a cleanse, if you don't feel well, don't worry. This too shall pass. It's going to come on through your system. You want it out. So if you end up with a headache or you feel tired or a little flu-ish or achy all over, it's not going to hang around like the flu or a cold. It's going to move on through your body. As those toxic things move out you're going to feel a whole lot better, and you're going to be preventing disease from coming back or coming to you down the line.

Ty: So step one, cleansing your body, total detoxification, the colon. Steps two and three are the kidneys and the liver.

Dr. Daniel Nuzum: You have two kidneys, one liver. You have 100 lymph nodes. If you don't clean out those lymph nodes there is no way to then drain the tissues. So if we clean the colon, clean the kidneys, clean the liver, lymph nodes would be the last thing to focus on.

Ty: Okay and how do you do that?

Dr. Daniel Nuzum: That? You need things like cat's claw, pau d'arco, burdock root, the Essiac formula.

Excellent for cleaning out lymph nodes and draining those lymph nodes. Even the lymph fluid drained out.

Ty: And would you use that in conjunction with a daily rebounding?

Dr. Daniel Nuzum: Rebounding, excellent. Yes. That would be excellent, especially if you're trying to drain it. The lymphatic fluid is what's called a thixotropic fluid. A thixotropic fluid is like butter. The warmer it gets the softer it gets, the more fluid it gets. The colder it gets the harder it gets.

Ty: So as you heat your body up you heat your—

Dr. Daniel Nuzum: Exactly. So you heat your body up and get it moving, bounce on the trampoline, do those types of things, you will get it moving, raise the temperature a little bit. That liquefies that lymphatic fluid. It flows easier. You can do that while you are doing things to clean the lymph nodes that are going to clean much faster, more efficiently and probably with fewer hiccups with, you know, the detox effect.

Ty: And so that would be last?

Dr. Daniel Nuzum: That would be last.

Dr. Rashid Buttar: You've got two types of circulation in the body. You've got the blood that everybody recognizes as circulation, but then you've got the little-known cousin that a lot of people don't recognize, the lymphatics. The lymphatics are the lymph nodes and the drainage system in the body that is there to remove waste product.

When people get lymph nodes that are enlarged, and the doctor said, "Oh my God, lymph nodes. We've got to take them out." You're just taking out the oil filters. Don't ever have your lymph nodes taken out. If a lymph node gets hard when you've got cancer, it means it's doing its job. it is filtering the cancer. It is holding onto that stuff and keeping it from disseminating out.

You take that filter out, that's like your car. You've got a filter that's blocked and what do you do? You take out the blocked filter and say, "Okay now I don't have a problem. Nothing is blocking it." But now you've got all that sludge that was going into the filter before now going right into the engine. You don't want that to happen! The lymph nodes are part of the lymphatics drainage system.

Dr. Robert Scott Bell: Well, if you understand anything about a lymphatic system, a critical drainage canal of the body, any restriction of that could put you at risk, particularly women who wear bras, the underwires, anything that restricts that area because there is a lot of lymphatic tissue associated with the fat cells as well. That's part of the detox processes.

In fact Sydney Singer, who we interviewed on our show together some years ago, wrote a book, *Dressed to Kill*, talking about the risk of wearing a bra 24/7.

Your risk is what, three out of every four women are definitely going to develop cancer, whereas if you wear it only 12 hours a day, the likelihood of cancer drops to one in seven. If you don't wear a bra at all, or it's a very loose-fitting scenario where there is no restriction of lymphatic tissue, your risk is no greater than anybody. In a sense you're not likely to suffer from the breast cancer.

Erin Elizabeth: We don't want to cut off that lymph, the system when we're wearing those tight bras. I think it's another thing in society where women feel that's what they're supposed to do. Buy more bras, get more underwire, more support, more you know. But yeah, the fewer hours a woman can wear a bra, the better.

Dr. Robert Scott Bell: And that doesn't even get into the issue of underarm deodorants and antiperspirants that have a lot of issues blocking the normal detox processes through the pores by sweating. If you stop that sweating you will actually bio-accumulate even more. The lymphatic system will be under additional burden because of the toxic things like aluminum that are put in these things to stop you from perspiring or sweating.

Erin Elizabeth: We're meant to sweat. I quit probably 20 years ago or more wearing antiperspirant. I still wear a natural organic deodorant. Even for men it's kind of a taboo subject as this is, I definitely don't recommend antiperspirant for men or women. We're meant to sweat.

Ty: So detox step number four is to clean the lymphatic system. And as you're about to hear from Dr. Edward Group, step number five is a parasite cleanse.

Dr. Edward Group III: And then we do a parasite cleanse after the first liver cleanse because we know that then the intestines will be ready to expel them. Then the liver would be able to deal with the toxins produced by the parasites once we start killing them off inside the body.

Ty: Great. What were the ingredients in the parasite cleanse?

Dr. Edward Group III: We looked at a lot of different ingredients, and we decided that we would use the black walnut hull from the green hull. We would use American wormseed, epazote. We would use wormwood. We would use clove, kamala, and that combination with a couple of other ones with bromelain. We would be able to also, using diatomaceous earth as a flow agent, be able to get rid of and purge the majority of the parasites inside the body.

Ty: And how long does the parasite cleanse portion take, how many days?

Dr. Edward Group III: Parasite cleanse takes six weeks because that's the cycle of most parasites from the time that they lay eggs until the time they are an adult. If you do a parasite cleanse for a shorter period than six weeks, there might be eggs still left in there that might hatch.

The good news is this can all be done in conjunction with whatever doctors, supplements that you're currently taking, whether you are doing ozone or anything. There are not any contraindications of doing an oxygen intestinal cleansing, doing liver and gallbladder cleansing, doing parasite cleansing. The last thing we would do would be chemical and heavy metal cleansing, which is also another factor that needs to be considered in conjunction with your cancer care.

Ty: Dr. Group just mentioned heavy metal detoxification. One physician whose entire practice is built around detoxification, specifically heavy metals, is Dr. Rashid Buttar out of North Carolina. Dr. Buttar's entire medical practice is built around a five-step program, the first of which is detoxification.

Dr. Rashid Buttar: We have a five-step program that has been evolving since 1997. The five steps I always outline. The first is systemic detoxification. You have to clean up the body. If you don't detoxify the body then there are too many things in the way for the body to function correctly. Most of these toxicities that cause a detrimental effect in the body, they increase oxidated stress, etc.

What we know as poisons, different mechanisms of how these poisons affect the body you are probably familiar with. I know you are familiar with the seven toxicities, my whole philosophy that I have all the different toxicities and it goes from heavy metals, persistent organic glutens, the opportunistics (the bacterias and viruses, plasma, yeast).

The fourth one is energetics, like electromagnetic radiation, microwave energies, this, that and the other. Cell phone radiation is a big one.

The fifth one is the most important in my opinion and that is emotional/psychological toxicity.

The sixth one is foods, what we *do* to the foods which I know is near and dear to your heart – the irradiation, the homogenization, the pasteurization, the genetic modification of foods – all these things that we do to food and change the basic molecular structure of the things that we're taking into our body just to sustain ourselves. These are severely detrimental to the body.

And then the seventh toxicity is spiritual. These toxicities that I'm talking about, that's the first step. We deal with all those things.

Trina Baird: I was diagnosed with Stage 2A breast cancer December of 2010. I was 45. Then in 2011 I ended up doing chemo first, six rounds of chemo, starting the first of February 2011. Then after that, I had surgery, a double mastectomy in July of 2011 and then radiation in October/November 2011. So I had the full gamut of treatment.

I remember thinking, "I just want to close my eyes, and I just don't want to wake up." I was so mad at the world and the doctors. I just thought this isn't working and how can you feel so bad? My tongue was swollen, but I didn't know it was swollen. I had all kinds of issues, was hardly eating and just sick. I thought I just want to close my eyes and not wake up the next day and do this again.

Then when I woke up the next day I thought, "Well, darn it. I've got to go through this, I've got to go through another treatment." I wanted to quit but felt like it was a sign of weakness. And me being type A, we've got to go through it and just get to the finish line.

I thought, "this is not really a way of living. This is being poisoned." I felt it and just didn't have the courage to stop it.

Dr. Rashid Buttar: The second step is physiological optimization. What I mean by that, is this: If you have two people and one has shortness of breath when he walks up the steps and the other one runs three miles every day, the one who is running three miles every day is more physiologically optimized. I want to optimize a person so their bodies are functioning at the highest level.

When you're dealing with cancer, the way you deal with that—I'm not saying the people have to run, although I have cancer patients and one of them if you want to talk to does run three miles every other day and she's Stage 4 with multiple metastatic disease.

The proudest thing that I see in my patients, none of them look like they have cancer. That's the thing that—you know.

Ty: That's a big thing.

Dr. Rashid Buttar: Yeah, that's the best way of being able to look at—

Ty: That means that they are not in cachexia cycle.

Dr. Rashid Buttar: Absolutely, yeah. So it's an old saying, when growth stops, decay sets in. So to me this is not a static process. Either you are getting worse or you are getting better. There is no such thing as staying right there in the middle.

So physiological optimization where you're dealing with a cancer patient would be, for example, the use of oxygen. The use of oxygen is highly detrimental to cancer because cancer is an obligate anaerobic metabolizer. It likes an oxygen-free environment. If you can give oxygen, it is detrimental to the cancer.

Cancer is an obligate glucose metabolizer so it needs sugar to sustain itself. The brain needs sugar, the body needs sugar, but we reduce the amount of glucose that's coming into the body so that there is less fuel for the cancer. These are the types of techniques, and there are many different ways of doing this.

Betsy: I was diagnosed with cancer the first time in 2014 by an oncologist here in Charlotte, NC. It was Stage 2 ovarian cancer. Then five-and-a-half months later, unfortunately for myself, my family and also for Dr. Buttar, I was diagnosed with this secondary primary breast cancer that was also developing at the same time, unaware to my oncologist.

The conventional treatments in my case, the only conventional treatment I did was surgery. I was one of the fortunate few that had a cancer, primary cancer, and organs that were not necessary for life. I had a full hysterectomy. It did work in that it did remove the cancer, a primary portion of the cancer, and it had not spread and it was not in my lymph system yet.

However it was the treatment that the oncologist wanted to do – the chemotherapy – and it was not just plain "use one port and put chemotherapy" – administer it up here. They also wanted to put a second port on my rib cage, and they wanted to do something called intraperitoneal chemo where they would have been giving me chemo, blowing out my abdomen like I'm pregnant every Monday and blowing out my veins with a second chemo.

It was the over the top, aggressive chemotherapy they wanted to do that made me cringe. I lost 20 pounds after the surgery just thinking about the chemotherapy. I dropped to 106 pounds and was in menopause and was just a mess. My oncologist was ready to put poison in my body. I was like, "I can't do this."

Dr. Rashid Buttar: It's amazing when you look at the standard oncology practices when a person is becoming cachectic. They recommend Ensure®. Are you familiar with Ensure?

Ty: Sugar.

Dr. Rashid Buttar: Yeah.

Ty: Sugar and cream.

Dr. Rashid Buttar: That's exactly right. During my surgical residencies I can tell you that Ensure was a precious commodity. The surgical residents, we'd go through the different wards and open up the refrigerator and find the Ensure and drink it because it is very tasty – I'm not going to deny that. But for a cancer patient, it's poison. It's literally poison. It is like pouring gasoline on a fire. It is feeding that fire of cancer.

The third step is immune modulation. Now immune modulation is an important component. You notice I didn't say increasing the immune system or decreasing the immune system. I said *modulating* the immune system. Each patient is going to be different.

Generally speaking, a person who has cancer has a suppressed immune system. If the immune system has been damaged and it is lower, we want to repair that immune system. We want to get it back up.

They're just recognizing now that the immune system is important in cancer. I have had patients tell me that they have shown their doctors the natural killer cell profile that we do before and after the lymphocytes population to measure our results, to see where is the patient at. How much further improved have we been able to help their immune system get to.

She's had—I've had patients tell me, including this particular patient, that when they showed their oncologist this paperwork, these two lab tests, the response that they got from more than half the doctors was some of them said they didn't know what that meant or they didn't know how to interpret it.

But more than half of them said, "What relevance is this? What's the natural killer cells have to do with cancer?" For God's sake, that's why they call it *the natural killer cells* because they naturally kill things that are not supposed to be in the body like cancer!

It's a really severe disconnect that the conventional side has, and when I say conventional, there is only one medical science. It's just that you've got these different groups, and some are open to innovation and some are not. I consider myself as in the category that is open to innovation. The ones that are not, they are just too vested in the status quo, too ingrained in it the way it is right now.

The modulation of the immune system is key because you cannot have cancer if you have an adequate and functioning immune system. If you don't have a functioning immune system, now you can get cancer. But there is no such thing as "Oh, my cancer has nothing to do with my immune system because my immune system is fine." There is no such thing. If you have cancer, you don't have an immune system. Your immune system has been damaged. That's it. Our focus is to get that immune system back up.

Trina Baird: At the beginning of last year I was doing blood tests every six months. My blood tests came back elevated. So I went in for another bone scan, CT scan, PET scan this time and found it in sternum and a spot on my left hip.

I did one round of chemo and then at point that is where Ty Bollinger and Chris Wark and even Kelly Turner's book *Radical Remissions* had just come out and it was just released. I saw that the day I went in for my round and couldn't get the book in time so I had that first round of chemo and came home that day, got the book, started reading the book and then that's when I stopped the chemo.

In talking with Chris, I asked him who he recommended, if he knew of anybody here in the Charlotte area and he recommended Dr. Buttar. That's how I got to Dr. Buttar. I think it was God just saying, "There's another option for you." That's when I said "Okay, stop. I don't care what happens. I've got to look at something else. This is someone else speaking to me, someone else higher is speaking, and I need to listen." I just know I would not be here today, not at all. I wouldn't have made the 12 rounds, the 12 treatments.

Dr. Rashid Buttar: Our goal in this fourth step is target acquisition. We want to acquiesce the target. We want the body to identify the cancer has been formed because right now the cancer is mimicking a fetus and saying, "Hey, hey, I'm supposed to be here and that's why you see cancer secreting alpha theta protein in the human chorionic gonadotropin.

Even though it may be a male it doesn't matter because it's trying to show the body that "I'm okay. You don't have to be worried about me. I'm supposed to be here." So we *want* the body to identify the cancer as being foreign.

The way we do that is to through AAROSTA, and that stands for Autogenous Antigen Receptor Specific Oncogenic Target Acquisition. This fourth step is to acquiesce the target, meaning having the body identify the cancer and being able to do what it needs to do to follow the way that the Ultimate Engineer designed our bodies. Our bodies were designed that we identify cancer. The body's immune system identifies the cancer and starts doing what it's supposed to do.

But because the immune system is defunct and not functioning it can't do that, we fixed that with the third step, which is immune modulation. Then with the fourth step now the immune system may be strong and able and capable to fight, but it doesn't know what it's supposed to fight. It doesn't know who the enemy is.

That fourth step, AAROSTA, is designed to allow the individual's immune system to identify the cancers being formed. It's a fancy term for creating a vaccine specific to that individual's cancer. But it's not a vaccine. It's allowing the body to identify the cancers being formed. When we give those injections, then the person's body starts responding. We are basically getting the proteins from the cancer and creating a treatment that is specific to the patient because where does the cancer start from?

It starts from the DNA. That's what is unique about the cancer. It is specific to that individual's DNA. We give it back to them and the body now sees that as being foreign. As soon as it sees that thing is foreign, it sees anything with the same morphological characteristics as being foreign and all of a sudden the whole body lights up wherever the cancer is in the body.

It lights up because we just introduced it in a way the body can see it as being foreign, and boom, it snaps to it. That's why we call it the shift. That's when the person gets sick because their body is responding. All of a sudden, the treatment, the immune system, the way that God designed the system, now recognizes the substance, that cancer, that shouldn't be there and the body is fixing the individual, not me, not chemo, not radiation, not some other pill or vitamin. No. It's the body itself doing what the Ultimate Engineer created it to do to fight the cancer. Then the fifth step is arguably the most difficult: maintenance, meaning that once you've crossed that line you have to live your life a certain way.

Betsy: It was during a trip to Atlanta my husband and I took to Cancer Treatment Centers of America to get a second opinion from an oncologist there that we realized *The Truth About Cancer* series was playing free that weekend online and we didn't have any children with us that weekend.

I was very conflicted. I had been a pharmaceutical rep for 14 years and had known the medical industry. That had been my career. We were able to watch seven to eight episodes of Ty Bollinger's *The Truth About Cancer*. It was during these seminars online that we watched that gave us the courage and the confidence that many other individuals and survivors had gone through natural treatments and were living.

Dr. Buttar, I believe, hits cancer from many angles. You've heard or may have read his book about the seven toxicities that he mentions in his book, *The Nine Steps to Keep the Doctor Away*. I believe I had many of these toxicities. Not only was my body toxic with metals, it was also toxic with pollutants and, I also believe, emotionally and psychologically. I had gone through three miscarriages trying to conceive our second and third daughter. And during these times of grief, that really contributed, I believe, to the ovarian cancer and breast cancer diagnoses that I received that year.

His treatment hits all three of these toxicities. There is chelation and many different IVs that Dr. Buttar gives that help your body get rid of toxins. And I have seen my body get rid of so many toxins through the protocol at home, which is very aggressive, as well as through the chelation in the office.

Also the things that Dr. Buttar gives to build up your immune system are phenomenal. I can literally go to treatment and be in treatment all day, have six or seven bags of various great things that I believe God made to heal our bodies that my body even makes, just not in enough—I didn't have enough of those substances in my body to heal. I can go home and cook dinner and take care of my little ones.

The cancer that I had in my body is definitely going away. I hope to be cancer-free any day or any month now. We are doing some of those tests as we speak and all of my parameters, my blood work is of a healthy 30-something-year-old. This is really great news. My energy, my color, all of those things, my liver, my kidneys are all functioning at 100 percent and like a healthy individual would be.

So we are very grateful that the cancer markers are so very low and I may be cancer free today, but I hope to be cancer free soon if I'm not. Dr. Buttar has brought something to my family we thought we wouldn't have.

After the diagnosis last year, psychologically, mentally I just thought I was on my way out. I'm usually a positive person, but all I could see was myself laying in a bed after doing chemo treatments and being 85 pounds. Having my daughters, my little ones, not even know me, grow up without a mother as well as my eight-year-old just watch me die, not to mention my husband.

What *The Quest for the Cures* gave us and also Dr. Buttar, was hope that you can heal naturally, that there are so many things that I believe God has given us in the world that can build up your immune system, can remove toxicities, and can also just increase your vitality and your overall health. I believe that I've experienced all of those through the unconventional treatment that we chose and this path.

I have to be honest. We thought, because I was a drug rep as I mentioned for 14 years, we thought, "Okay, if this doesn't work, then we'll go back and we can always do chemo." That was kind of our fall-back scenario that we gave to friends and family because they were horrified that we were not going through with conventional treatment.

There is a lot of pressure after a diagnosis to start treatment immediately – start the chemo tomorrow. I think I've done so well with the therapy there is no reason to ever compromise my body and my GI tract with the only thing I had going for me at the time of diagnosis. That would have been wiped out after one chemo treatment. We are just so grateful and thankful that we had this option, and we hope that many others will also be brave enough to travel the road less traveled, so to speak.

Ty: Wow, those are some really encouraging testimonials from Trina and Betsy, two of Dr. Buttar's patients. We're going to hear the rest of their stories later on in the show. Dr. Buttar shared with us his five-step protocol for treating the disease.

The first step is detoxification. The next step, step number two, physiological optimization. Step number three is immune modulation. Step number four is target acquisition. Dr. Buttar uses a vaccine that is called AAEROSTA. It's a completely nontoxic vaccine.

And step number five, which he says is probably the most difficult, is maintenance. We're going to strap on our seatbelts now. We're going to fly across the Atlantic Ocean to Cologne, Germany, and we're going to meet another doctor who uses a completely nontoxic vaccine in his practice in Cologne.

Dr. Robert Gorter: What we do here is talk about fever range, total body hyperthermia, the local hyperthermia. We do ozone therapy. We do oxidases within the cells and all kinds of things for immune restoration including mistletoe, and also the preparations made from cannabis. So I'll give you the tour and we can start from this side. Here is the total body hyperthermia.

Ty: Total body hyperthermia. Okay.

Dr. Robert Gorter: We call this at fever range, total body hyperthermia, to emphasize we don't do extreme temperatures.

Ty: The heat?

Dr. Robert Gorter: The heat comes from these lamps. They send the infrared and it works principally so that the infrared doesn't go deep, maybe half a centimeter through the skin. The blood flow in the skin works like a central heating system where we have hot water running through the house so the blood is heated up, so to speak, and then it circulates through the body. Then the whole body is warmed up slowly but surely.

It's a very elegant way and so after about two hours the patient is at 38.5/39 Celsius. Then we switch off the lamps and leave the patient for half an hour and they have a steady state. Then we slowly cool them off and when they get cooled off they will have here a shower. They take a shower and then we give patients the vaccination with dendritic cells.

Ty: Dendritic cell vaccination.

Dr. Robert Gorter: Yes, a dendritic cell vaccination.

The Nobel Prize for Medicine in 2011 was awarded to three researchers who discovered the function of dendritic cells. And we right away jumped on their research and we further developed it how to make dendritic cells for the patient's own simple white blood cells. So that's what we do.

And you can sort of say that the dendritic cells be seen as the policemen of the immune system because these dendritic cells really migrate through your whole body. That's exactly why they can go to the tip of your nose, your liver, your prostate, and look for abnormal cells. When they find one then they quickly in a lymph node inform natural killer cells and they kill.

So dendritic cells can sort of see what is right or wrong, but then they inform cells which have as a function to kill, and that's what happens. And if it functions well, then within 24 hours a cancer cell which has been detected is also killed.

So and now when you get cancer, these policemen all need reading glasses. They can't see so well any more. Therefore cancer cells can get the chance. They are unnoticed and then they pass by and start to grow.

So what we do, we can make from a simple blood draw from monocytes or simple white blood cells we can make a whole new generation of policemen, dendritic cells, and they are given back and it is very safe because it's autonomous, our body's own tissue. There is no fear something from a donor comes from the AIDS epidemic. You are always afraid that he might transport something unknown through blood products. So it's perfectly safe. No side effects, no rejection and, that is what we do.

I say to patients let's say 20 million young, fit policemen, so from the police academy—

Ty: I really like that analogy, the policemen.

Dr. Robert Gorter: Yeah, the dendritics are the policemen. That image is really true because good policemen will recognize a rapist and a bank robber and a banker or other things. So they do so they don't only notice cancer cells, but also cells which are damaged by a virus infection or another way of mutation.

So the policemen are dendritic cells. Very important. The patient understands right away if you give them the image of the policemen that can see more than just one bad guy.

Ty: So you've got the dendritic cells that you are using here.

Dr. Robert Gorter: Yeah, and then we have the hyperthermia we like to do before we give the dendritic cells. The patients go through a moderate period of fever which we initiate by infrared lamps and also people have metastases or cancer in the lungs, or liver or elsewhere, then we treat that in addition with local hyperthermia.

And the principle is that we bring through a region with cancer – cancer tissue is electromagnetic fields – and then selectively only the cancer cells are quickly increased in the temperature. Then the cancer cells always make lactic acids. The production of lactic acid is almost tripled. Next, the pH goes down so it gets more and more acidity in the cell and the cell dies during the treatment.

Also no side effects, no toxicity except every once in awhile if people have a pacemaker. That's the only complication because a pacemaker can go astray when you're put a strong electromagnetic field on it. Often, even in medical school, it is often portrayed that fever is the *cost* of illness.

But it's the opposite. Your body, in the last attempt to activate your immune system, is to produce fever. When your body temperature goes up one degree your immune system is in an absolute state of alert. A normal core body temperature, your immune system is on automatic pilot.

It does its thing. But if there is any emergency the only way to activate the immune system is through fever. There is no other way. What do I say to a cancer patient who has end-stage disease and told there is nothing we can do. I say possibly we can still do something and give you hope, because we do things very differently.

Ty: I agree with Dr. Gorter, there is always hope and hope is often missing when it comes to cancer. Have you ever heard of the placebo effect? The placebo effect demonstrates the power of the mind in healing. The placebo effect is when somebody may be healed by taking nothing more than a sugar pill, but they *think* that they're going to be healed and so they are. Modern medicine tends to frown on the placebo effect, as if it's a bad thing. But is it really a bad thing?

Dr. Rashid Buttar: I will tell you this. I think that in modern medicine this demonization of placebo effect is the most ridiculous thing. We should be harnessing it! If we can actually elicit that type of response in an individual where we can get a benefit in that individual from just the power of belief, without changing the physiology, it's our ethical, fiduciary responsibility as healers, as doctors, to harness that power and get that result.

If we can do so with the least harm – that's the first part of being a doctor, right? Do no harm. And if you give somebody narcotics, but you are affecting them in a negative way you're affecting their liver, there is harm that's being done.

So if we can get the same result without giving them a narcotic, why shouldn't we and why is that poo-pooed? Why is that ridiculed that, "Oh, you got this result from a placebo." You should get a Nobel Prize if you can elicit a response from a placebo.

Sayer Ji: A placebo effect is the basis for evidence-based medicine. They have to control for it even to have this hierarchical power structure saying that they have the evidence and the truth, right? Double-blind, randomized placebo controlled trials. That's the absolute truth in their model.

Well, why are they controlling for the placebo? It's so powerful! It's even more powerful than most of the medications they're using, and the placebo is is this self-healing ability that I've now outsourced to you because you're the doctor. I believe in you. When you tell someone that their body is constantly self-healing, they can overcome cancer in the same way that they may from a scratch on their knee. They can watch it heal and they believe that, if they do the right things, then they will heal cancer. That is really the power that we have, that the medical profession really doesn't. They either don't know it or they don't want you to know about it.

Ty: Most of you probably have heard about the placebo effect. But have you heard about the "NOCEBO effect"? Let's listen to Sayer Ji.

Sayer Ji: This is one of the most powerful studies of our time published in the *New England Journal of Medicine* just three years ago which showed, based on a huge group of Swedes. We're talking about 500,000 in this study. When they were given the results for their cancer tests, looking at different types of cancers, and if they were told positive, what happened is that within one week of that diagnosis, they had up to 26.9-fold increased risk of death from heart-related events.

So what happens is it's like a shaman in an old culture pointing a bone at a member and saying, "You're going to die tomorrow." That person is so convinced that that authority is so valid that they go walk off into the woods and the next day they die, exactly proven by this new study.

The power of belief and what they call the "nocebo effect" which is if your physician who you trust more than your own self healing ability comes in and says "You're going to die; look at these results. You have six months." Guess what? You're probably going to end up dying.

But what this study showed was that the belief is so powerful your heart actually fails on you within one week. It just crashes. You die because of your belief, and it's not based on evidence. It's based on the belief that someone else knows your fate better than yourself. That is why we have to be extremely careful about conventional medicine and this type of diagnosis.

Ty: You mentioned "nocebo effect." What is the "nocebo effect?"

Sayer Ji: Yeah. The placebo effect is really "I will help," because if you believe your physician, like your mother, who is taking care of you is going to heal you...

Ty: Gives you your sugar pill and—

Sayer Ji: Exactly. The same thing is true that if you believe, or your doctor comes to you and you feel a negative vibe or you think they don't like you, or they think you're going to die, that means, "I will harm." It means you believe that. You incorporate it into your life, your belief system feeds into your physiology and then you end up having an adverse effect or dying.

Ty: "Nocebo effect." So it's like the flip side of that coin.

Sayer Ji: It's the exact opposite.

Ty: Placebo is positive; nocebo is negative.

Sayer Ji: It's true, and it also tells us that physicians have an ethical and medical responsibility to be aware of their effect, to be aware of their belief system and realize if they are quoting from some statistical data set of poor outcomes based on really outdated cancer therapies – let's say it's radiation and chemo which is just absurd ultimately – it's on them. They have to educate themselves and they should be inculcating into the patient a belief in the healing power that they have.

If they don't know, I understand. They weren't trained on this, but they should probably be doing something else than treating people with cancer if they don't know that.

It is no longer just about a bunch of people on the periphery like us saying you've got to do better. It's *New England Journal of Medicine*, one of the highest impact journals stating that this a lethal force. "Nocebo effect" is as real as the placebo. They are responsible for what they say, what they know and they should never pronounce someone dead based on statistics of an outdated way of treating people with cancer.

Ty: I have to agree that the big three treatments, chemo, radiation and surgery, they are outdated methods for treating cancer. But what about somebody who's already undergone those treatments or is currently undergoing chemo, radiation, or surgery, is there hope for them as well? You bet there is.

Jefferey Jaxen: But when it comes to people that have taken the chemotherapy or the toxic drugs associated with that, you're going to look at immune boosting. I like to say mushrooms: reishi, and cordyceps. They have to happen. In fact everybody, in my opinion, minus a toxicity or any contradictions which at this point there are none for the cordyceps, should be taking cordyceps in this environment.

What the cordyceps mushroom does is it ups your immunity and it ups available oxygen in your body. So a cancer, as you know, and everybody watching probably knows, thrives in a non-oxygen-based environment, or an anaerobic environment. When you take theses cordyceps, studies have shown that it ups your body's internal oxygen by 40 percent, ATP by 28 percent and then it also increases your natural killer cell activity by

400 percent and that was in people that had cancer for the last one with the natural killer cells.

The athletes in China – it's been in Chinese medicine for a long time. In 1993, it became right on the radar because the women's marathon team started shattering all these records. They were shattering them by not one or two seconds, but 30, 40 seconds, just huge amounts.

People were trying to figure out what was going one. They were taking cordyceps. They had supplemented with cordyceps.

Ty: More oxygen.

Jefferey Jaxen: More oxygen, exactly, more available oxygen for the muscles. So what happened at that point is the sports commissions and the sports regulation bodies said, "Look, we've got to regulate this stuff because it's very prominent in China and they know how to develop it and they have the best sources. It's not fair for other countries that don't have these sources. Now this is an unfair advantage.

Now it is disseminated everywhere. You can buy it everywhere. Cordyceps is the way to go.

Ty: Do you buy it at the health food store?

Jefferey Jaxen: Yep, health food store.

Ty: Do you take a supplement or the fresh mushrooms?

Jefferey Jaxen: That's a great question. You could take a tincture, which is the drops in the water, or you could take a pill; either way. Some companies are actually infusing it into coffee to go a step further.

Ty: I've seen that.

Jefferey Jaxen: So there you go. People that don't like to take supplements and they are coffee drinkers, you can do that. Now the other part of the mushroom I'm going to talk about is the reishi mushroom. The bio-defense and bio-shield departments of the United States did studies on the reishi mushroom for the big dogs for swine flu, bird flu, some of the really nasty viruses. At a one to 100 dilution it was showing huge virus-killing abilities with this stuff. It upped your microphages. It ups your immune system.

Ty: One of the substances in mushrooms that makes them so medicinal and so potent against cancer is called beta glucan. Here scientists and immunologist A.J. Lanigan who has developed one of the most potent forms, if not the most potent form, of beta glucan available on the market discussing that topic.

A.J. Lanigan: Just a couple of weeks ago, yet another study has been published, ironically, in the *Journal of Tumor.*

Ty: *Journal of Tumor*

A.J. Lanigan: *Journal of Tumor* demonstrating that even if people are going standard of care – chemo, radiation and so forth, which would typically drive white blood cell counts down – this material will actually mitigate and keep those white blood cell counts up.

Ty: So beta glucan is a substance you can use if you are currently undergoing chemo, radiation, to help your immune system stay strong and so that it won't be crippled by the treatment.

A.J. Lanigan: That is correct. One of the things that we do know [is] without that compound, the chemo and the radiation basically wipes out everything, and if it's not successful, we know that only the bad guys are left behind.

Ty: Right.

A.J. Lanigan: And the cancer is going to come back with a tear, and you have no defense at all. So keeping that immune system properly supported is really critical.

Ty: Again, the immune system is the key. There are foods and herbs that contain certain properties that can turn off or turn on switches in cancer cells. They can also prevent oxidative stress. People have heard of oxidative stress. What is it? How can you minimize it? What kind of a role does it play in cancer?

Dr. David Jockers: Absolutely. Well oxidative stress is kind of this chemical reaction. The best example for anybody to understand would be a metal when it rusts. It's got all these environmental factors coming against it, and it ends up rusting. We've all seen that happen.

Within our body, there is this war, this war against rusting ourselves versus our cells actually protecting themselves alone. God put this power within us to protect us from oxidation, from environmental stresses. Every single cell has a little signaling mechanism. It's called the KEAP1 pathway. Think about it.

Keep us healthy. Right? So that KEAP1 is this little receptor and he's got his hand out there and he's just checking the water. As the water gets hot, let's say as the water gets hotter, that's war of this environmental oxidative stress that is coming. Water gets hot; it sends a signal. It tags its partner, which is called NRF2 gene pathway. This NRF2 enzyme—

Ty: NRF2.

Dr. David Jockers: NRF2. You'll hear about that. NRF2. That then signals our antioxidant response element (ARE), the antioxidant response element. The antioxidant response element is a very powerful pathway. What it actually does is it amplifies our body's entire oxidative-stress defense system.

All the antioxidants are going. Instead of just like one antioxidant to quench one free radical, a one to one ratio, it sends out hundreds of thousands of signals to protect the whole cell, the whole genome, from oxidative stress. A very powerful pathway.

Ty: So it's like it opens the floodgates.

Dr. David Jockers: That's right, opens the floodgates. Full military defense. We're fully ready, stocked and on guard.

Ty: So how can you release – how can you open the floodgates? What substances might do this?

Dr. David Jockers: Yes, this is huge. Because if we want to prevent cancer, we've got to activate this response. We want it to be very sensitive. We want our system to be so good with this pathway.

There are four key compounds; many different lifestyle activities like exercise that help enhance that, but compounds that we can take in from nature that are really going to dramatically improve that antioxidant response is four things. Your listeners may have heard of some of these:

Resveratrol. We find that in berries. Consuming blueberries, consuming grape skins that's the number one source. We've heard about it in red wine, resveratrol, very powerful for ramping up that NRF2, KEAP1, ARE pathway.

You also have it in something called sulforaphane. Sulforaphane is found in cruciferous vegetables: broccoli, cabbage, collard greens, and brussel sprouts. Number one source from nature is going to be broccoli sprouts, which you can find at most health food stores. Most health food stores nowadays you find broccoli sprouts. Put them on your salad every single day; ramp up that pathway.

Also curcumin which is the active ingredient in turmeric. Curcuminoids help ramp up that pathway, especially if you combine them with a little bit of black pepper and also good oils. Making them fat-soluble ramps up that pathway.

And the last thing is going to be catechins which are like ECGC which is what we find in green tea, chocolate – most people like chocolate – dark chocolate, no sugar in it, loaded with catechins that ramp up this NRF2 antioxidant response element in our system to protect our genome.

Ty: Awesome information from Dr. Jockers. Now here's Dr. Nalini Chilkov discussing some of those same herbs that Dr. Jockers mentioned, but she'll be discussing the ways that they affect the immune system and also help in detoxification.

Dr. Nalini Chilkov: I really am a fan of some of the great traditional Chinese herbs. All of the medicinal mushrooms are extraordinary immune modulators, signal cancer cells to turn their apoptotic switch on and to die, and also manage inflammation really well. Also the medicinal mushrooms are really good for managing insulin and blood sugar.

So are the ones you put in your salad by the way. So that would be cordyceps mushroom. That would be reishi mushroom, ganoderma, shiitake mushroom, you can add to your food. Maitaki mushrooms. Coriolis is one of the most powerful, that's turkey tail mushroom. Those are very powerful. They can actually be used with chemo and radiation if a patient is actually having those therapies.

Ty: And they'll help.

Dr. Nalini Chilkov: Right.

Ty: It will help to mitigate the side effects?

Dr. Nalini Chilkov: Well, they'll help mitigate the side effects, but they also keep you stronger so that your immunity is not pressed down. All of the mushrooms have beta glucans and polysaccharides in them and that's what makes them medicine. They also have CLA which is conjugated linoleic acid. That is anti-inflammatory and it also turns on a gene that regulates blood sugar in insulin, ppar gamma.

In the same family is one of my favorite herbs – astragulus. Astragulus is huang chi in Chinese medicine. Also an enormous amount of research, also rich in polysaccharides and beta glucans and really ramps up your white blood cells and your natural killer cells. We're always looking for things that are going to increase natural killer cells.

These are the army of our immune system that go after cancer cells and also viral cells, and astragulus is also one of these things you can take safely for long periods of time. And for patients who've had their therapies like chemotherapy that depress their white blood cells and then they are vulnerable to infections, astragulus is one of the best things to increase white blood cells and natural killer cells, and acupuncture also does that. Very powerful. I'm also an acupuncturist.

A lot of the herbs that are good for detoxification are either rich in essential aromatic oils or they have alkaloids in them that stimulate us to excrete things. Or they are rich in sulphur so there's a lot of herbs and supplements that are rich in sulfur. So I actually very much like garlic. That's a simple, simple herb that anybody can use.

I try to put into these resources things that anybody can get no matter if you don't have a lot of money or you do have a lot of money. Everybody can do this. So garlic actually has some antitumor activity, but it actually stimulates the excretion of a lot of toxic chemicals.

So do the radish and cabbage family vegetables, which are rich in sulfur. So the garlic family and the cabbage family have all this sulfur in them. A traditional remedy actually used to be cabbage juice.

Ty: Yeah.

Dr. Nalini Chilkov: Before kale was so popular. It's the sulfur that turns on your liver enzymes to start producing chemicals that detoxify.

Ty: Sulfur does.

Dr. Nalini Chilkov: Yeah, sulfur does. Sulfur is one of the most detoxifying chemicals, so think that anascedial anticidal systane, lipoic acid, these are rich in sulfur. All the *sulfor*aphanes – are chemicals in the cabbage family that not only interrupt the development, progression, and metastasis traveling of cancer cells. The sulforaphanes interrupt every stage of cancer. They are very powerful, but they also promote detoxification. particularly of hormones.

So the hormone-driven cancers I always add the sulforaphanes in for that.

Ty: Why is sauerkraut the new super food?

Laura Bond: Sauerkraut's the new superfood because it's wonderful! A spoonful of sauerkraut delivers trillions of probiotics and enzymes which are just so powerfully anticancer. I've got health as the center of our immune system. Eighty percent of our immune cells are in our gut. Looking after the healthy bacteria there is so important for whatever you're doing – digestion, stress, any immune problem, which cancer, of course, is.

I came across an interesting article recently though from the University of Michigan. It was showing that healthy bacteria can help you get through chemo. The article was tied to gut reaction – "must survive lethal doses of chemotherapy," and they're talking about how important this healthy bacteria is. It's great for people going through chemotherapy, great for anyone.

Dr. Sunil Pai: We always want to recommend probiotics because the gut microbiome is one of the most important things to our health. What people don't realize is, that they understand that if I want to take an antibiotic, it lowers the good nitrate in my gut. But chemotherapy we would consider like 100 times stronger than an antibiotic, and that's why people lose weight. They have diarrhea and malabsorption. When we give chemotherapy it also knocks out the good bacteria in the gut. By doing that then they have malabsorption problems and then their nutrition is poor.

So no matter what they are eating, it goes right through them and they will lose weight. They don't have enough strength, their immune goes down and then sometimes they die from the therapy. Right? So we have to look at strengthening the GI tract. A lot of times when we work with patience looking at – how do we keep your immune system up? How do we decrease the swelling post-chemo or from the radiation? How do we decrease the burn, for example?

Or the tumor is dying off, rightfully so. There is still going to be swelling around that tissue. What natural agents like proteolytic enzyme formulas and what if you have a hormone-sensitive cancer? How can we help the excretion of the hormones? Through the liver, for example.

We have certain drugs that block it. We're mentioning here in the conference tamoxifen and all these other type of drugs. Okay, they block it, but it's still in the body circulating. How can we help the body augment that excretion? Even through diet. We can increase fiber, for example.

People eat a plant-based diet. They get about 40 grams a day. The study showed that women who had estrogen-positive breast cancer who had three bowel movements a day had the lowest recurrence rate because their bodies are able, once the hormones go to the liver, the gallbladder takes it out with the bile. It goes into the small intestine and fiber binds that and excretes it.

Dr. Eric Zielinski: When it comes to aromatherapy and using oils and internally and topically, these oils not only help with cancer, but the side effects. That's so critical because as you travel the world, Ty, and you talk to people that are cancer survivors and people struggling with cancer. It's really the side effects that get them. Often times it's not the cancer that kills them. It's a common cold or the flu or you name it. It compromises the immune system.

Ty: From a devastated body.

Dr. Eric Zielinski: And that's what the essential oils do when it comes to sleeplessness, nausea, and especially with myrrh. In the research on myrrh when it comes to the side effects inadvertently related to cancer are pretty encouraging for folks.

Ty: So Dr. Cass, tell us about what is chemo brain to start with, and how can you— what natural treatments can you use to remedy this condition?

Dr. Hyla Cass: Here we are at a cancer conference talking about natural therapies. What I have found many, many people who have undergone chemotherapy end up with this terrible condition called chemo brain. They can't think straight. They can't remember things. They can't remember where they put their keys, they can't remember—one woman she couldn't remember how to put dishes in the dishwasher. It's heartbreaking.

What they are told by their oncologist is a) be happy you're alive, and b) it will go away. It will get better. It doesn't! It doesn't! It may wear off, but usually not. There is a lot you can do to give the body what it needs, give the brain what it needs in terms of raw materials to make neurotransmitters.

Raw materials for building brain cell walls which help the circulation in the brain, things that are wonderful for helping chemo brain and people should know about this because their oncologist is not going to tell them.

Dr. Russell Blaylock: Now this is one of the things I wrote in my cancer book years ago. I said it's a good possibility that chemotherapy is damaging the brain. At that time the literature was denying it and they'd say, "No, it can't damage the brain because it can't get past the blood/brain barrier." I didn't believe that.

Well now it has been proven. They went back and they looked at cancer survivors and measured their cognitive ability – ability to think and remember and learn language – and in fact found that they were impaired, virtually all of them were impaired from the chemo.

And then when they did it in animals and they looked at their brains, yes, it was destroying parts of the brain that have to do with those functions. So now it is well recognized that it produced it. Well they have no way to protect the brain. These flavonoids like curcumin, quercetin, ellagic acid, resveratrol, naringenin, they powerfully protect the brain against damage by the chemotherapy.

Ty: Wow. They sound like miracle herbs.

Dr. Russell Blaylock: Well they are. I mean they are incredible. This is what you expect when God made something.

Ty: He didn't make any mistakes.

Dr. Russell Blaylock: And when you look at what these things are doing like curcumin for instance is one that's most researched, it does virtually everything that you want it to do. The difference between it and a chemotherapeutic agent is that chemotherapy attacked one thing in the cancer cell. The cancer cell finds a way to go around it very quickly and that's why it escapes treatment. Curcumin affects so many processes in the cancer cell it can't overcome it so it dies. So that is the advantage of these flavonoid things being used for cancer treatment versus chemotherapeutic agents.

Ty: It's very encouraging to see that there are a multitude of natural substances that can help to mitigate the side effects from chemotherapy, even chemo brain. But just in case you're still discouraged, maybe you are currently undergoing chemotherapy or you've undergone several rounds of chemotherapy and you're concerned about your immune system, we're going to share with you the rest of the story from Trina.

You heard about Trina earlier in the episode and you saw the fact that she underwent several rounds of chemotherapy. We're going to hear the rest of her story now, and it's going to really encourage you that there is always hope.

Trina: When you get that diagnosis, you're shell shocked and you just—it just takes all the breath out of you and… sorry. It just takes you right down to your knees. When I talk to other people, I tell them you have other options. I tell them about Ty and I tell them about Bill Henderson or Chris Wark or Dr. Buttar or a thousand other doctors out there that are actually trying to get the message out that you don't have to go the conventional way.

I feel better today than I have in probably 10 years. I have tons more energy. I started running again and I ran three to five miles until I broke my arm and now I'm back down to square one. But I feel better today than I have in probably 10 years. Thank you to Ty and Chris and Bill Henderson. I've watched all of Ty's documentaries, the whole entire thing several times. I continue to watch some of his excerpts on Facebook when he'll bring some of those out every once in a while.

Dr. Gonzalez. And a big thank you to each and every one of those doctors who participated because they truly saved my life and I think Dr. Buttar definitely is one of those—if I didn't have that I wouldn't think I would have had another option. So it's just a huge thank you. Thank you for doing what they're doing.

Ty: I'm so pleased that during this episode we've equipped you with knowledge about the most advanced ways to detoxify your body, removing harmful heavy metals, and other toxins from all your vital organs. I'm excited that we were able to share the amazing discoveries of healing vaccines and how this innovative cancer solution is saving lives through enabling the body to powerfully heal itself. I'm glad you were able to see the successful integrative therapies inside the German cancer clinic. I know it's been exhilarating for you to hear how the doctors and experts team up together with the patients to work with their unique needs and see them achieve total health and healing. Seeing lives restored is truly the most rewarding part of this mission. For me, what I experienced this day is such a blessing. I gained some important answers to my questions as I know you have also. And I found myself another step closer to discovering the truth about cancer. As have you, as we've joined arms and embarked together on this global quest.

Wow. We have really learned a lot in this episode, haven't we? And in the next episode we're going to learn even more. We're flying across the Pond to London where we're going to interview a doctor that uses what is called the Budwig Protocol.

This protocol is a very scientific protocol and it deals with the electricity in the cells. We're going to also visit a clinic in the United States that deals with using electricity to treat cancer and we're also going to visit Amsterdam, Netherlands as we talk about the effect that light has on the cells. We're going to be traveling all over the world tomorrow. I hope you join us.   [*credits roll*]

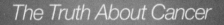

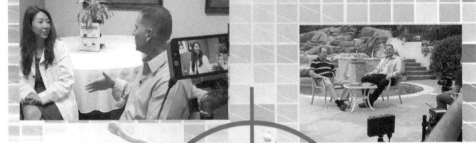

A GLOBAL QUEST

Episode 7

Heal Cancer with Clean Electricity, Unique Water, Natural Sunlight & Combining Superfoods

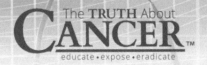

The TRUTH About CANCER™

educate • expose • eradicate

Ty: Welcome back to *The Truth About Cancer: A Global Quest*. We're so happy that you've joined us for this episode. If you missed the last episode, here's a little recap of what we learned.

[*Video plays: Summary of Episode Six*]

Wow, we really learned a lot in last night's episode, and tonight, we're going to discover more new information for you that can help you on your health journey.

We're going to explore new discoveries in the way that light affects the cells. We will also learn about a treatment that was recently used, that was selectively toxic to cancer cells, that has been shut down in a Nazi-type raid in Europe. Two experts are going to share with us the importance of water in the cancer equation, and we're also going to learn about electricity and frequencies as they relate to cancer.

But first, we're going to travel across the Atlantic ocean, all the way to London, and we're going to hook up with a doctor that was born in Lebanon that currently practices in Spain. So Dr. Raymond Hilu, I really appreciate you joining us today.

Dr. Raymond Hilu: Thank you for the invitation.

Ty: Your practice is in what areas of Spain?

Dr. Raymond Hilu: The main practice is in Marbella – that's South Spain. My second most important, or largest, practice is in Barcelona. And I have a third practice in Madrid, in the capital.

Ty: Could you talk about HRT analysis to begin with?

Dr. Raymond Hilu: Yeah, this is a higher-resolution cellular study of the blood. You just need a couple of drops from the finger. There are different ways of doing that, but the method I'm using nowadays is a special microscope built specifically for me. We magnify the sample up to 65,000 times, so I'm able to see what's happening, even inside the cells. It gives me a very good idea of imbalances, deficiencies, irregular morphologies and the contents of the blood serum. Whatever is wrong, I take note of it and try to put it right. It's as simple as that.

Ty: 65,000 times?

Dr. Raymond Hilu: Yes, that many.

Ty: Wow, just from a couple of drops of blood? That's amazing. Are you able to determine if someone has cancer from just a few drops of blood in the HRB analysis?

Dr. Raymond Hilu: Yeah, although this is not a diagnostic tool, it does help us to prevent cancer, because cancer or any other disease –call it fibromyalgia, call it chronic fatigue syndrome, call it whatever you want to call it – any disease starts off with cellular imbalances. That's the beginning of any disease. Things start to go wrong on the cellular level, and this is where the microscope becomes a very useful tool because we start seeing these irregularities before the disease appears, even cancer, years in advance. So we can prevent diseases from happening. Of course, if the patient is already suffering from cancer, we will see the imbalances that the patients are suffering and the things that are making cancer worse, and we try to correct them as well. So it's useful to treat. But mainly, I love to use this tool to *prevent* the disease from happening.

Ty: So seeing these morphologies allows you to catch it early, before it manifests.

Dr. Raymond Hilu: That's the idea. Some cancers, we can detect five years in advance, which is great.

Ty: That's awesome. Because most of what we think of as diagnostics are really not diagnostics at all. It's not early detection, I mean.

Dr. Raymond Hilu: That's too late.

Ty: Right, it's too late. So we hear about early detection is your best protection with mammograms. By the time you see it on the mammogram, it's too late typically. You want to catch it early, and that's what this allows you to do.

Dr. Raymond Hilu: We want to catch it even before it becomes a tumor. When there's a cellular imbalance that is pre-cancerous, that's when we want to catch it.

Ty: And then you got a much higher cure rate.

Dr. Raymond Hilu: Yeah. It can be even more than 95 percent, we can say.

Ty: What is the principle behind the Budwig Diet? First of all, describe it real quickly for someone that's watching that may not know what it is. And then, why does it work?

Dr. Raymond Hilu: It's very simple, in fact. Very clever and very simple. It consists of mixing cottage cheese, preferably low fat, with flaxseed oil, that's it. Banning the bad foods, the sugars, the red meat, and so on. The main ingredient is this Budwig cream mix, which is cottage cheese, flaxseed oil, two tablespoons of flaxseed oil. The amount of cottage cheese is not important, just enough to mix it well so that you can't see the oil anymore. And that's it. And you can add to the mix whatever you'd like. Use your imagination and make it—

Ty: Fruit. Add fruit.

Dr. Raymond Hilu: —nicer. You can make it go sweet and make it like a dessert or go more salty and put herbs and add it to your salad, whatever. So it's a matter of choice of whatever your flavors tell you to do. Now the scientific basis behind it, in fact, is the same scientific basis behind the work of Dr. Otto Warburg, the Nobel Prize winner, who discovered (and that's why he had this Nobel prize) that cancer cells would not normally grow in oxygen rich atmospheres. They need hypoxic to grow. In the presence of oxygen, it's difficult for them to grow. And the basics of Dr. Budwig's diet is the providing of oxygen to the tissues and the organs of the body. How is that? Well, flaxseed oil, even the industrial flaxseed oil, the one that used in paints, you use it to make quick paints, quick drying paints. So if you mix flaxseed oil with paint and you paint a facade, you paint a wall, it will dry quickly because the flaxseed attracts—

Ty: It brings the oxygen quicker.

Dr. Raymond Hilu: That's the basics. As simple as that. So she does the same thing inside the human body. She managed to do it better than others, because the difficulty with flaxseed oil, and polyunsaturated fat in general, is that it's not easily absorbed in the intestinal tract. It's difficult to absorb.

The intestinal lining has a negative charge to it, and flaxseed oil, just to put it simple, has a negative charge to it. So negative and negative, they repel each other, and it's not absorbed. Her discovery as a biochemist was that if you mix well this flaxseed oil with a positively charged protein, sulfur based in this case, like cottage cheese then it's readily absorbed. In a few minutes, it's in your bloodstream and it gets to the cells, oxygenates them, and makes life difficult for cancer cells. Easy.

Ty: While we were in London I had the privilege of interviewing Dr. Felicity Corbin-Wheeler. Now she's a pancreatic cancer survivor. One of the fascinating things about Dr. Wheeler's story is that she was diagnosed with pancreatic cancer 12 years ago. How many people can say they were diagnosed 12 years ago with pancreatic cancer and are still alive? So you really want to pay attention to her story.

Dr. Felicity Wheeler: I had been a British Red Cross nurse originally, and then I worked in the Houses of Parliament, so I have a medical, and slightly, a political background. I just realized that there were so many myths. There is so much misinformation about cancer. So I love what you were doing. I love your *Quest for the Cure* and all the work that you're doing in America.

Ty: Thank you, I appreciate it. Tell us about your—you mentioned your son and your daughter both had cancer.

Dr. Felicity Wheeler: Well, we went back to live in Jersey, which is one of the Channel Islands and we thought, an idyllic lifestyle to bring children up in. But we grow a lot of potatoes and tomatoes in Jersey. We had an old farmhouse. And the chemicals, the pesticides, and all the other chemicals that they used to grow more potatoes and more tomatoes were actually getting into our well water, and we had absolutely no idea.

Firstly, my son, he had a carcinoid tumor in his appendix at 14, and I was horrified because I had my nursing background. I'd work for one of the top London cancer surgeons called Harvey White and was absolutely shattered that my son, at 14, could produce this carcinoid tumor in the appendix. Luckily, that was encapsulated. He had a full body scan, and he was clear.

Then my daughter, six months later, was diagnosed with stage 4B Hodgkin's disease and died in two years. If my daughter had known about these cures, I'm sure that she would be here today. The oncologist who was at the Royal Marsden Hospital, when I suggested perhaps going to America and looking at DART, he said, "If you think lettuce leaves will cure your daughter, take her away and stop wasting my time." My daughter, of course, was horrified and said, "Mom, don't say things like that or he wouldn't look after me." Because she really believed that the chemo and the radiation would cure her. But sadly, it did not.

Quite unexpectedly, in 2003, I was getting a lot of indigestion, and went, and had a scan. I was by then yellow with jaundice and was told I had pancreatic cancer – a huge mass in the head of the pancreas where it's impossible to operate. So my husband, Jules, RAF, brought me to London to the military hospital here. I had a wonderful professor there who stented the common bile duct to release the toxins in the liver, which were actually killing me. I would have been dead in about six weeks. Terrible pain, I was in, and terrible nausea. Anyway, there was nothing that they could do. He just stented it and said, "Well, that will relieve the worst of it. Hospice is the thing." But, my husband took me back to church at Holy Trinity Brompton. That's my London church. And there, I mean that was the most amazing God incidence because I was prayed for by one called Emmy Wilson, who is a pastor, but also had been a gastroenterology nursing sister. And she said to me after she prayed for me, "Have you heard about B17?" And my husband, who was RAF, said, "Oh, that's a bomber." And she said, "No. Actually, it's a vitamin as well."

Ty: RAF, being of the Royal Air Force, he thought of a B-17 plane, right?

Dr. Felicity Wheeler: Absolutely.

Ty: Funny.

Dr. Felicity Wheeler: So anyway, we went back. I went and laid on the bed at the Royal Air Force Club and read my Bible, looked at Genesis 1:29-30, which tells us the right way we should eat.

Ty: What does it say in those verses?

Dr. Felicity Wheeler: It says, "Behold, I have given you every seed-bearing plant on the face of the Earth and every tree with fruit with seed in it, and this well be to you as food. And to every living thing, I give green plant." So I'm laying there in agony being sick and feeling really dreadful, thinking, "I think this is probably right. We've got to detox. I then did lots of research. I got onto the Gerson Therapy. I got B17 from Mexico from Dr. Francisco Contreras, and I got well.

Dr. Raymond Hilu: Dr. Budwig talks a lot about electricity and positive and negative charges. Part of her treatments have to do with that directly. She asks people to go barefooted and walk on grass or on sand, wet sand while sunbathing, so that electricity in the body gets corrected.

Ty: Earthing.

Dr. Raymond Hilu: Dr. Budwig treated 2,200 people only with diet, and they were cancer patients, and almost all of them were cured. Of course, I wouldn't believe that just by listening to her, so I went personally to different ones, and I interviewed them to make sure that what she was saying was true. And it was. And this was my aha moment, and I decided to use her diet to incorporate this discovery into my clinical work.

Ty: Dr. Hilu just shared with us his aha moment where he woke up. I asked him after that, what his colleagues thought about this.

Dr. Raymond Hilu: Most of them thought—and that's how they expressed their thoughts to me— that, I was nuts. Probably they were right, but I don't care. I was not very social back then, and I'm still not very social anyway. So I'm half autistic in a sense. I don't care. It doesn't bother me. Most of them did not see a good point in what I was doing. They thought that I was losing my time. I was risking my future, that I was risking the life of my patients. No matter how hard I tried to convince them, look what I'm doing has got no side effects. What you are doing, what you are prescribing on this paper, any paper that you write out to your patients, it is loaded with side effects. I never write out a prescription on anything that may have any side effects, so I don't agree.

Dr. Felicity Wheeler: That was Professor John Beard, who was an embryologist and was working at a the University of Edinburgh, and he'd also got a degree from Freiburg University in Germany, and he was promoting all this a hundred years ago, Ty, but it's all being hidden and disparaged by Big Pharma, who make all the money out of the chemo.

Ty: It's sad, isn't it?

Dr. Felicity Wheeler: It's tragic. I've lost my daughter to it. Yeah, tragic.

Ty: When you were diagnosed with pancreatic cancer, what was the prognosis from the doctor?

Dr. Felicity Wheeler: Six weeks to maybe six months.

Ty: Six weeks to six months to live?

Dr. Felicity Wheeler: But I know so many people who have had pancreatic cancer since, and no one has survived. The only people who have survived are the doctors who are cited in Phillip Day's book, *Cancer: Why We're Still Dying to Know the Truth*. There were two doctors there: one a doctor, one a dentist, in fact. And they got well with the B17, and the colonics, and the Gerson Therapy. I think, Ty, you have to put the whole thing together. You have to really detox the body. You have to restore the deficiency of living enzymes. You have to rehydrate the body with the good juices, and you have to address the stress in your life. And I'd had a lot of stress. I'm very blessed actually, because I've been elected member of The Royal Society of Medicine. I'm absolutely amazed and delighted.

Dr. Raymond Hilu: I'm not against the series of the importance of the new system. In fact, I do believe that they have a very, very important role. But over the years, I've treated many, many patients, many cancer patients, who were concentrating very hard on the immune system, taking lots of stuff to improve their immune system. Under the microscope, they had a fantastic immune system, but cancer was still growing. Because if you don't access the area that is contaminated and clean it up, even if you have the best immune system in the world, useless. Again, cancer does not depend on just *one* issue, so immune system on its own is not enough. Food on its own is not enough. Good emotions on their own are not enough. You have to do everything *simultaneously*. That's another difficulty because if you just correct the immune system and don't correct the rest, the rest will end up ruining the immune system again. If you detoxify, but you don't do the nutritional part and other things, then toxicity will accumulate again. So you will end up falling into the same mistakes again and again. That's why it's so important. That's the secret of our work in our clinics, that we do everything simultaneously.

Ty: Dr. Hilu mentioned that it's important to hit cancer simultaneously with many different types of treatments, and he does that at his two clinics in Spain with detoxification, with nutrition, with supplementation, and especially with the Budwig diet.

Another physician that we were able to interview is Dr. Leigh Erin Connealy. Now, we traveled to her clinic in Irvine, California. Let's have a listen to Dr. Connealy as she explains some of the treatment protocols that they use in her clinic in Irvine.

Dr. Leigh Erin Connealy: One of the key things in health is optimization of the immune system. I think it was 1999, a doctor or several doctors, there's actually conflicting information about who really discovered it, but that's not my deal. Anyway, there's something called Gc-MAF (macrophage activating factor). What are macrophages? Macrophages are the PacMen of your immune system. We have to have a good immune system whether you have cancer, heart disease, diabetes, dementia; we need a good immune system to take care of ourselves. When we make bad cells – cancer cells are viruses – they make an enzyme called nagalase. Nagalase poisons the macrophages, inhibiting them, attacking the bad cells.

Now, what you can actually do is you can actually measure nagalase. It's not done in the United States. It's done in a laboratory in the Netherlands, so we send our patient's' blood to the Netherlands to see what their nagalase is. Most people we know who have cancer or viruses, we know they probably have high nagalase. By the way, though, Gc-MAF has used everything from autism to Alzheimer's to heart disease to cancer to chronic viral and bug infections. We started utilizing it about two years ago.

You can actually make Gc-MAF in a probiotic, and you can actually make it in a yogurt yourself. You have to buy the starter material and make the yogurt yourself that produces Gc-MAF. You can't just buy organic yogurt on the shelves at your local store. You've got to get the starter material and you can make your own Gc-MAF in a yogurt or what we use is a probiotic suppository called Bravo Probiotic. I know it works, because every single patient that I've used it on, their nagalase levels have decreased.

Dr. Bita Badakhshan: Nagalase level tells me where your immune system is at. In a healthy patient, your nagalase level should be less than one. But if you have virus or cancer in your body, the nagalase levels tend to be higher. So I actually start on my regular, healthy patients who don't have the diagnosis of cancer, but has viruses in their body, I measure their nagalase level. If it's high or higher than one, I tell them, "Your immune system is being suppressed. Then you're going to develop cancer."

Ty: Unfortunately, as we've already seen many times in *The Global Quest*, the authorities will shut you down if you're using a treatment for cancer that works that's not approved. This recently happened with Gc-MAF, at the manufacturing facility in Europe.

Valerie Warwick, R.N.: Yeah, the Gc-MAF clinic is over in Europe, and their version of the FDA came into their lab and took all their product, all their medicine, took all their lab equipment, seized all their bank accounts, and virtually shut them down. They were helping thousands of patients reboot their immune system. They were helping kids with autism. They were an answer to cancer, and they shut them down.

Ty: So, Val, if you could talk a little bit about the details of this raid.

Valerie Warwick, R.N.: The European FDA version came into the Gc-MAF lab. Two female workers, lab technicians were in there. They came in with machine guns, bulletproof vests, and held them up at gunpoint. Took all the medicine out of the lab, seized all the bank accounts. It's really a gestapo technique to shut down any kind of alternative medicine that is not run by the Big Pharma.

Ty: Wow. It sounds like the mafia.

Valerie Warwick, R.N.: Yes. It is the mafia.

Ty: These types of raids are happening all over the United States. But, as we just heard, this is happening in Europe as well. This type of behavior is despicable no matter where it's happening because it's stopping people from getting access to treatments that could save their life. Let's go back to hear more from Dr. Connealy now.

Dr. Leigh Erin Connealy: Hyperbaric has been used over the world for many, many years. Interest in hyperbaric is growing every single day. In the United States, around the world, it's standard in the United States, and we can treat everything from cancer to wounds to diabetes to nitrogen burns, all kinds of medical problems that are approved for use for all kinds of different patients.

Autism, we have brain injuries, we have a neurosurgeon who refers those patients who have that unusual brain tumor called the glioblastoma. So, hyperbaric is a beautiful intervention for so many things.

Ty: Now what's the purpose then of the chamber, as opposed to just getting pure oxygen through a mask?

Dr. Jolly-Gabriel: It is necessary to put the patient under pressure, so that the pressure causes the gas. Any gas in that pressurized environment to dissolve into all the liquids. The prime liquid we're trying to get the oxygen to dissolve in is his blood. So we will raise the atmospheric pressure, oftentimes, up to two and a half times. This will create massive amounts of oxygen going into the blood, which creates a healing mechanism.

Ty: Dr. Jolly, what is the mechanism by which when we get oxygen into the blood with one of these hyperbaric chambers, how does that cause healing in the body? We've heard oxygen is great for the blood. We breathe oxygen. You have to have it to live. How exactly does that work to heal?

Dr. Jolly-Gabriel: Well, first of all, oxygen is the absolute essential element to sustain life. If we don't have it for a few minutes, we're gone. We can go without food for days. We can go without water for days. We cannot go without oxygen more than a few minutes. So number one, it is a sustainer of life. It is also the absolute, necessary product to begin the healing process. Without oxygen, no healing will take place. We'll develop necrosis, which is a Greek derivative for death. So cellular death can occur in a little part of the body if it's deprived of oxygen. The more oxygen you give to it, it will heal faster and you can completely heal someone who has drastic wounds from diabetes or other causes, putting them in the hyperbaric chamber 90 percent of the time when I get them at what's called a grade two, which is pretty bad, they're looking at it and saying, "Well, we may have to amputate." Ninety percent of the time, we've been able to save the limb.

Ty: Truly amazing. The hyperbaric oxygen chamber can actually save limbs. Another expert on hyperbaric oxygen chambers is Dr. David Jockers. Let's have a listen to what he has to say about these devices.

So, Dr. J, let's go a little bit further about oxygen and its role in the cancer equation.

Dr. David Jockers: Absolutely. I mean look at oxygen therapy, like for example, my clinic we use a hyperbaric oxygen chamber to help people who have chronic disease. We know with cancer that as cancer is developing, these are mutated abnormal cells. So they're no longer running off of what normal cells run off of, which is oxygen. They become hypoxic, so what happens is the core of the cancer is highly hypoxic and—

Ty: What does hypoxic mean?

Dr. Jockers: That means low oxygen environment. And that actually provides a protective mechanism against things like chemotherapy and our immune system. Because it's hypoxic in the core, that actually signals—it sends out something called VEGF, which is vascular endothelial growth factor, which then signals the body to actually start producing blood vessels, abnormal blood vessels that feed into the whole cancer tumor as it's forming. So it develops its own blood supply that's going to bring more nutrition to the core and keep it alive.

Ty: And that's what's called angiogenesis?

Dr. David Jockers: Angiogenesis is the term forming new blood vessels. That's what that means. So we pump the body with more oxygen, like oxygen therapy for example; it gets more oxygen diffusing into the plasma and into all the cells of the body. That shuts down the production of this VEGF, this vascular endothelial growth factor. Therefore, it gets the cancer. The core will have a reduced blood supply, which will weaken it and make it more exposed.

Ty: No nourishment.

Dr. David Jockers: That's right, make it more exposed to our body's own immune system, which is the greatest defense. That's the greatest military against cancer formation, and it would make it, actually, more vulnerable to chemotherapy and radiation if that person chose to go that route.

Ty: So oxygen can actually help chemotherapy and radiation work better. That's really amazing. We should be integrating this into our conventional treatments. Another vitally important subject is the issue of light.

Dr. Marcel Wolfe: We're light beings. This is actually a cross-section of the DNA. Do you know anything about sacred geometry? When I looked at that, it just made me shiver. This is actually a cross-section of the DNA. This is the DNA as we know it. It's actually the perfect antenna for picking up frequency. But this shows us here that the DNA—I call it a thing of beauty and complexity, sacred geometry – this is a cross-section of DNA revealing four billion photonic flashlights in one cross-section of DNA. What I would like to see is actually in schools and churches, let's start with children and say, "Hey look. We want you to understand that you're living in something, this human body that is miraculous. It's amazing."

Dr. Leigh Erin Connealy: Then we have a device, a new device that we've been using called the Ultraviolet Light RX.

Ty: Yeah, we saw that this morning.

Dr. Leigh Erin Connealy: Yes, and so basically in your vein is infrared light, several different wavelengths of light that are designed to kill all the bugs in your body, but it also activates your immune system, increases oxygen saturation, and it's absolutely amazing. So we've been using that for a couple of months. It's in a clinical trial, soon to be FDA approved.

Ty: So why is the ultraviolet light so important?

Dr. Suzanne Kim: The ultraviolet light has been known for a long time now to be a disinfectant, so it's able to kill viruses, bacteria, and fungus. So the ultraviolet light, in the same way, will be able to kill the viruses, bacteria, and fungus in the blood.

Ty: I see.

Dr. Suzanne Kim: And that's very important, as you can imagine, for infection. Anybody who has an infection can be treated with this treatment. But, as well for our cancer patients. We know that many cancers have their root in one of these. This is why most of our cancer patients do get this treatment. You can see, because it's light here, you can't really see the light as well, but the light is transmitting directly in.

Ty: I can kind of see.

Dr. Suzanne Kim: Can you see it?

Ty: Yeah.

Dr. Suzanne Kim: When it's darker, it's more visible.

Ty: It's a fascinating machine, the ultraviolet light machine. But what if you don't have access to that? Are there any other ways to get light into the cells?

Dr. Joseph Mercola: Vitamin D is literally nothing short of a miracle. It's a God-given miracle. It's a part of the natural plant. We were designed to be exposed to the sun. Unlike most any dermatologist you will see who will warn you and plead with you to stay out of the sun. Because of their fear of getting a skin cancer, which was a most likely—yes, people die from skin cancer, but not many. It's a small fraction, probably less than one percent of people who die from lack of sun exposure and getting other cancers, like prostate, and lung cancer, and all these other malignancies, breast cancers.

So, Vitamin D, we did not understand or appreciate its full value until this century. Last century, we didn't know. We just knew that it was available and was primarily thought to treat bone diseases, like rickets and osteomalacia. But in the late 1990s, the commercial labs became available to actually measure this. So they were able to do studies, and they found out, "Oh, my gosh. You know, 90, 95 percent of people don't have ideal levels of Vitamin D." And not only is it good for bone disease, but it's good to reduce the risk of the two biggest killers of the human race, which is heart disease and cancer. And the epidemiological studies show that you reduce all cancers by 50 percent when you have adequate vitamin D levels. I mean if that's not almost magical, I don't know what is. Now the devil is in the details, right, Ty?

So the danger that we can have is say, "Okay, let's just swallow this Vitamin D and you get our Vitamin D levels up." And that is one way that you can do it, and in many cases, it's the only way you have, the only practical option. But, that's not the ideal way. The ideal way is to follow the natural pattern, which is to go outside with very little clothing, and so I'm just going to have to be in a very moderate climate, usually subtropical or tropical, at least in the winter, and have the sunshine on your skin.

Because the sun converts a cholesterol precursor to Vitamin D, and then Vitamin D gets transferred and converted into your body to active metabolites where it does its magic. And it affects literally ten percent of our genomics. It's called an epigenetic influence, and so it optimizes ten percent of our genes.

Vitamin D is one of most profound epigenetic influences of the genetic code. There's several types of ultraviolet radiation. There's three types: UVA, B, and C. C hardly ever comes down because it's usually filtered from the atmosphere, but UVA and B. UVA is really the dangerous one, the one that causes most of the cancers. And UVB is what causes our body to make vitamin D. Well, these sunscreens, they filter UVB so your body couldn't make vitamin D. You essentially stop the vitamin D production, and they let UVA right through. So, it actually *increased* the rate of skin cancer, and that's what the studies show. You use sunscreen. You increase your risk of skin cancer.

Ty: Wow! That's worth repeating. Dr. Mercola just told us that the sunscreens increase the risk of cancer because they filter out the UVB, which our bodies convert to Vitamin D and which protects us from cancer, while they do not filter out UVA which causes cancer.

Now you may be wondering: Are there any other ways to get light into the cells? We traveled over to Amsterdam, Netherlands to have that question answered.

Dr. Henk Fransen: A healthy cell, we have equipment to measure that at the moment, is full of light. It's full of light, and it radiates a little bit of this light. This light filters through the DNA into millions of miracles of chemical processes. But a diseased cell, it contains less light. It's like it loses light. It leaks light, and a cancerous cell is almost dark. It can contain hardly any light, so the intelligence cannot filter through the DNA in the healthy processes in the cell. So I think prior to nutrition – the body, the cells, must be flooded with light. That's the first priority with cancer treatment.

Ty: Do you have a particular treatment that you use that will push light into the cells?

Dr. Henk Fransen: Right, it's exactly what you say. We teach cancer patients to flood their bodies with light. The most well-known way to do this is by taking fresh, organic foods. You could say that sunlight is accumulated in the food in greens, in fruits. When we eat this, it's like the body can open this present, take the light out of it, and then this light resonates with the light of the cell itself and makes it stronger and more vital.

Ty: We're around all this green stuff here. It's making me ready for a wheatgrass shot. Can you talk about wheatgrass?

Sayer Ji: I love wheatgrass, primarily because chlorophyll content. Chlorophyll is this amazing molecule, because it's the same as hemoglobin, the thing that makes our blood red. The difference is that it has a magnesium atom at the center of this molecule versus our blood has iron, which is what makes it attach to oxygen and turn red when it's exposed to oxygen.

Chlorophyll happens to be able to go into the mitochondria of our cells as a metabolite, and capture sunlight energy and photo-energize the Krebs Cycle, which produces ATP, which is considered the basis for the energy of our body. This new study that came out in 2014 showed that not only does it increase the efficiency and productivity of ATP to have chlorophyll in the diet, go into mitochondria, capture sunlight, but it also can keep the oxidative stress down, which then may increase the longevity of the cells as well.

Ty: So you actually can capture sunlight. It's in the plants.

Sayer Ji: We are solar hybrids. We can do that, that's what the new study shows.

Ty: Well, myself and the TTAC video team were in Atlanta filming at Better Way Health. We had a chance to go to R. Thomas restaurant, and we all got a chance to do a wheatgrass shot, and so here's Dr. David Jockers talking about that experience.

Dr. David Jockers: Bloodstream with antioxidants.

Ty: What are we eating here, Dr. Jockers?

Dr. David Jockers: We are having our winter tonic right here. We've got beets, which are one of the best methylating anti-aging foods, carrots, and celery. We've also got our wheat grass shots, which is one of the most chlorophyll-rich superfoods you can put in your body right there. So, two-ounce wheatgrass shot, a powerful blood builder.

Dr. Howard Fisher: Let's get down to chlorophyll. And the best part about chlorophyll is the magnesium is the core element – same molecules as hemoglobin. Hemoglobin has iron. Chlorophyll has magnesium, easily accepted by the body. In the reactivity series, this will start to kick out other metals. Are there toxic metals in our environment? You bet. Are they everywhere? Absolutely. They also provide nutrition, i.e. vitamins, minerals, a little glucose. All right, plant based glucose – not sugar, or GMO corn sugar, high fructose – real nutrition that goes into your body. So, love the greens. And you can live on just greens. I mean, my particular green is Moringa Oleifera. I used to love Spirulina back in the 90s, when that was the best one going that was being cultivated. And Chlorella, also very good. Mixed greens? Fabulous. I just constantly seek best. That's what I found that works best for me.

Ty: Speaking of green food, one supplement my family takes every day is called Living Fuel Supergreens. It was developed by KC Craichy for his wife Monica, and has been used by countless people to regain their health. Here's their story.

KC Craichy: You want to know a little bit about the history and how it all came to play. My beautiful bride here, Monica, she was Miss Florida and she was Miss Florida USA, and she could be the Miss America USA. You can tell she's gorgeous. This is no secret. But, I want to tell you that when we were married for three years, she came down with panic attacks, clinical depression, suicidal thoughts, and the doctors were screwing up with Xanax, and Zoloft, and psychotherapy. She was a fearless woman prior to this and this stuff made her zoned out. I think you can take it from there.

Monica Craichy: Yeah, it was pretty dark time and we were pretty desperate. I knew that the medication was kind of making even crazier. So I told KC, I said, "This is not going to be the answer." So we really dove into—he dove into the medical literature to find out what makes somebody who's perfectly healthy then fall apart like this and hit rock bottom on everything.

KC Craichy: You see it so many times. People with anxiety, and panic, and depression. It happens all the time. So, I dove in the literature and Monica was my personal clinical study of one, me being another clinical study. So I was in the literature saying, "What does the literature say about this situation?" Because, everyone is guessing. They say, "Maybe she's going to be a patient for life and maybe it'll resolve itself," but no one is ever talking about, what's the causes of these kind of things? And so we really—

Monica Craichy: And that wasn't an option for me.

Ty: It wasn't an option.

Monica Craichy: It wasn't an option, no.

KC Craichy: She flushed the Xanax and Zoloft when—I think it was in two weeks of starting it. I dove into the literature, so over a ten-year period of research and trial and error. We made great strides and fell back and strides and fell back. But the net of it is that out of that ten-year period, Monica received her healing, and we've been able to help, now, thousands of other people receive their healing. The result was this amazing Living Fuel, and my books, and the things that we teach, and so on. This Living Fuel, people look at it and say, "Well, it's a supplement and it's expensive," but the truth is it's not a supplement. It's a whole meal superfood. It's a super meal you can drink.

Monica Craichy: It's not just like having a salad or a bowl of berries. I mean it is everything from top to bottom.

Ty: Talk about the nutrient profile because there's nothing else I've seen that's comparable.

KC Craichy: Exactly. Well, you talked about it. You did a two-week fuel fast. That basically means you upgraded every one of your meals to Living Fuel for two weeks, because you knew that you were getting absolutely everything your body needs. You knew it was going to be low calorie, nutrient dense, and all those things. When you think about it, it has more protein than a half dozen egg whites and more Vitamin D than ten fillets of arctic salmon. The list is on and on and on. But the truth is, if you give your body everything it needs, but then you cut the calories – in other words, you don't have the calories required for all those foods – that you actually can bring about incredible changes in the body. People always know that all these foods – oranges do this, and omega-3 does that, and probiotics does this, but they get it from so many different sources. They really don't get it regularly on an every meal kind of basis.

Monica Craichy: it's really difficult to do that actually.

KC Craichy: If not impossible. Difficult, if not impossible. So let me feel, really, for anyone who wants to upgrade what they're doing, because any meal, you have Living Fuel. I don't care if you had a team of organic chefs putting your meal together. Any meal you did Living Fuel instead what you're going to do, is an upgrade.

Monica Craichy: And for me, obviously, I wasn't dealing with cancer. But my body was so severely depleted. His book, *The Seven Golden Keys to Lifelong Vitality*, we realized in retrospect that I was rock bottom on all seven. And usually, people are, what, depleted in maybe three or four. So I was really headed for an early grave, and it's amazing that when you give your body what it needs—I mean that's one of our taglines: "It's everything your body needs." It's amazing, the healing that can happen when we're fueling our body.

Ty: Thank you both for being on the interview.

Monica Craichy: Thank you, Ty.

Ty: I want you to know that I don't make any money from endorsing Living Fuel. I'm just telling you about it because it's good. So thank you for what you're doing.

KC Craichy: Thank you, Ty.

Ty: We appreciate it.

KC Craichy: God bless you, Ty.

Monica Craichy: God bless you. God bless you all.

Ty: As far as I'm concerned, you can't go wrong by adding Living Fuel to any nutritional protocol. Now earlier this year I was privileged to speak at the Integrative Health Conference in San Diego. And I connected with experts like Dr. Sunil Pai, Dr. Daniel Nuzum, Dr. Veronique Desaulniers, and also cancer expert Dr. Marcus Freudman. In this next clip Marcus explains why some clinics and some treatments work for some people, but not others.

Dr. Marcus Freudman: Some of them have no interest in diet. You get cheese macaroni, and whatever in their clinic to eat, and they tell you, "Don't eat sugar," but they don't care for it. In other clinics, you go in. They have no interest in hormones. Another clinic has not the slightest interest in mind of psychology or support. Others don't want to educate. Now, when you go as a patient, and you miss out on the most important area for you just because the doctor doesn't like it, you lose probably a lot of money and have no success with your treatments.

Dr. Howard Fisher: Why is it that some protocols have a lot more success than other protocols? Why is it that some protocols that are extremely successful, you've never heard of? I work with Dr. Igor Smirnov. Dr. Igor Smirnov, in 1986, when Chernobyl blew up, was one of the teams of scientists that came in to determine not why there is three million cases of cancer in this area, why these people didn't have it. And you never heard of that. Igor Smirnov went down and found there was this group of people that *didn't* have cancer. They were seeking the reason to help the others who wanted to know why these people didn't. They found it was related to the water. It gets really interesting here for everybody. The fact of the matter is the mechanism was if you can super-hydrate a cell (i.e. if you can get enough water into the cell so it functions optimally), it can basically take on almost anything.

What was happening was the structure of this water was changing by coming over the Caucasus Mountains and coming, instead of being iso-tetrahedral or pyramidal, it was coming in linear format. That in itself doesn't mean much, but it can access something called aquaporins, go into every cell, carry nutrition into every cell, bring toxins out of every cell. But still, that doesn't matter. It's allowing the cell, allowing the physiological function, to be increased. Once again, not a cure, just enabling the body to do that. No one ever heard of it. It's called Molecular Resonance Effect Technology. We didn't hear that.

Ty: And that's where you determine that the people that have lived, that have not gotten cancer. They were drinking more of this water?

Dr. Howard Fisher: They were just drinking this water. This water was allowing them to hydrate, right? And they gave a Nobel Prize to Dr. Peter Agre in 2003 for discovering aquaporins. When he found the water, he didn't know the reason. He kind of figured it out after. There are these openings that are one water molecule wide, in every cell. We knew that if you hydrated a cell properly, for example, viruses in a dehydrated cell can multiply easily. In a hydrated cell, they cannot. So, that lends itself to understanding that if you give the body what it needs to function optimally, we can defeat it with following compliant protocols. Not chemo trying to kill everything, although sometimes it works. Not radiation trying to kill everything, but of course, we know if you radiate something, doesn't it cause a tumor? Oh, I'm being silly. But the reality of that is, we know that we just have to enable the body. I think that Dr. Smirnov's technologies are something everyone should use. Is it a cure? No. Does it help your body? Absolutely!

Ty: That's really fascinating. Dr. Igor Smirnov was on a Russian team that studied why some people, after Chernobyl, didn't get cancer, and it turned out it was because of the specific kind of water that they were drinking. After the interview with Dr. Fisher, I had him call Dr. Smirnov to see if he could set up an interview with us, and he did. We traveled to California to interview him about his technological advices that he has invented and, specifically, what he calls MRET Water.

Dr. Igor Smirnov: I was involved in this in 1980s in the research related to the effect of radiation on human subjects after the 1986 Chernobyl fall out. And by chance, they found that in some areas, the group of people suffering from radiation, they were placed in different resorts. And in some areas, their rehabilitation was much better compared with the other groups. By accident, they found it was because of the spring mineral water. So we got samples. We did some studies and within a couple of years, we actually found that it's not because of the mineral content of the water, but because of the unique molecular structure of water. Then it took me probably another ten years to develop a technology how to recreate the same type of water in your kitchen.

So basically, it's a unique equipment. It actually treats the water with extremely low intensity, low frequency, electromagnetic isolation, which is kind of like resembling the earth magnetic field intensity. We did a lot of research in regards to how this water can affect human physiology, and we found it has a very profound effect. So, there was a lot of studies done in Europe, in the United States, and in Russia in regards to how this activated water, MRET activated water can affect human—

Ty: What does MRET stand for?

Dr. Igor Smirnov: It stands for Molecular Resonance Effect Technology. Two American scientists, they got a Nobel prize for discovery of so-called aquaporin channels. The main reason for proper hydration of cells is aquaporin channels. What they found is the water molecules go inside these channels one by one with the speed of several billions per second. This is how it works. So in other words, it's very important for the human body, when you drink water, to reorganize water in so-called single linear structure. In this case, it can easily go inside the cells. If the water has a different type of structure, then it requires a lot of energy for the body, for the human body, to create the proper structure, so we call it intracellular structure of the water.

After doing the research for MRET water, we found that the structure of this water quite close resembles to the structure of the intracellular water. For this reason, around so-called bio impedance testing for water, we found that the after MRET treatment, water goes inside the cells three times faster compared with regular water. So it's obviously improved hydration of the body, and we know that hydration of the body is very important. Because per ten thousand molecules of water in the human body, there is only one molecule of the protein. So the hydration of the body is the number-one mechanism, which supports the homeostasis in the body.

We conducted a lot of research in regards of how this water can affect, for example, different forms of cancer. This research was conducted at the Kyiv University, a university in Ukraine, in collaboration with Oncologist's Center. And they use mice. It was done in vivo. They used 500 mice, which means it's very good statistics. What they found was that if you just treat mice with regular, average water, their inhibition of the tumor growth is about 60 to 50 percent, compared with control groups, and the lifespan of the mice in the group which was treated with MRET water was about 70 percent higher.

Ty: 70 percent longer.

Dr. Ignor Smirnov: Longer, yeah. So, they live longer. We did a lot of so-called in vitro tests on cancer cells with this water. For example, in AltheaDx – it's a San Diego based biotech company – and they just treated the cell media with MRET equipment, because cell media is about 90 percent water. Then they placed the cancer cells, HeLa cancer cells, and regular human cells in this meteor, and obviously, there was a control cells group. What they found, number one, that on the regular cells, human cells, there is no effect of MRET water, so it's completely safe. No effect. It doesn't inhibit. It doesn't enhance growth of the cells. It's just normal. But on the HeLa cancer cells, the incubation was 52 percent.

Ty: Wow!

Dr. Igor Smirnov: 52 percent.

Ty: Not only Dr. Smirnov's special type of water, the MRET water, better hydrate the cells, it also inhibits cancer growth. And while we were there in his yard, one of the things that I noticed was these huge limes growing on a tree in his yard.

Right over there behind you is the lemon tree or lime tree actually.

Dr. Igor Smirnov: Yes, right.

Ty: I noticed over there before we started the interview that these limes are bigger than any lime I've ever seen in my life. You're telling me you're feeding the tree MRET water.

Dr. Igor Smirnov: That's right. We're doing this private experiment with my wife.

Ty: Really great information from Dr. Smirnov. Now another hydration specialist is Paul Barattiero. He's about to share with us some fascinating information about molecular hydrogen in the water.

Paul Barattiero: It's all about the molecular hydrogen, and we have over 400 studies, 40 of which are human studies. So, you've got double blind studies showing the therapeutic effects that molecular hydrogen has on 150 different human diseases and every organ in the body. So very, very, very amazing breakthrough information is coming. What we're also learning is that it has some cell signaling capabilities in the body. I was just in Japan, at the Molecular Hydrogen Symposium, the medical symposium at Nagoya University, and they were showing that 200 gene expressions can be changed. Up regulated, down regulated just for molecular hydrogen in the body.

Ty: Epigenetics?

Paul Barattiero: Yeah. One of the main things it does is—the most cytotoxic or cell-damaging free radical in the body is called a Hydroxyl radical. H2 or molecular hydrogen combines with HO to create water in the cell. So in the mitochondria, tremendous benefits in the cells of the body, where you would have that free radical, Hydroxyl radicals damaging the body. Hydrogen gets in there, combines with it, and the bi-process is water. So you're converting the most cytotoxic free radical into water molecules. Very, very powerful.

We do have studies. It's true science. It's not pseudo-science, which I think is important. It's good to be able to know what the mechanism is, and it's good for people to be drinking hydrogen-enriched water. We have a few studies on animals. A few human studies and some cell studies showing that molecular hydrogen benefits cancer.

Ty: I firmly believe in the power of molecular hydrogen. As a matter of fact, my family and I own one of Paul's echo devices in our house and that's the water that we drink every day. Earlier in the program, Dr. Hilu mentioned the fact that everything in our bodies is electric. Let's learn a little bit more about the body electric and its voltage.

Dr. Bita Badakhshan: When you have cancer or any injury in your body, that voltage of the cell goes down. It becomes like 20-30 millivoltage. Your healthy cell has 70 to 110 millivoltage. So when you do PEMF, you actually charge the body (the cell membrane) so it's always good to do pulse PEMF before any kind of treatment; IVs, any.

Ty: What is PEMF?

Dr. Marcel Wolfe: Pulsating Electromagnetic Energy Fields. Not a static magnet. Everything in life pulses. We need a pulse. On the moon, there is no PEMF, there is no pulse, and that's why nothing lives there. We have evolved and adopted, too, and now we're dependent upon energy that we weren't aware that even existed. It wasn't until we sent somebody into space in 1962, Yuri Gagarin. He was only out there for an hour and 48 minutes, but because he was beyond the reach of these frequencies in our environment, in an hour and 48 minutes, he had severe bone loss to a point of osteoporosis, decreased metabolism, loss in perception and depression, which affected him for the rest of his life. He committed suicide at the age of 37.

Now, when we expose ourselves to PEMF, you can actually flip those things, reverse them. Increase bone density. Increase perception. Increase metabolism, and increase the sense of well-being. PEMF, I'd have to say, is one of the most powerful tools that I've seen in 35 years in holistic health.

Dr. Martin Bales: The therapy is not new. It's actually first described by Tesla in the 1880s and 1890s. If you consider that malignant cells, and also damaged tissue, ride at a lot lower voltage or electrical potential, this therapy is designed to up the potential or increase the energy of the cells. So it makes the cancer unhappy. In addition, here at Center for New Medicine, when patients have IV therapies or hyperbaric oxygen, it helps drive those therapies and those nutrients to the affected area. So, we could see with Colleen here, we've placed the loop, which is one of the attachments right over her affected area. We'll run that for ten minutes, and then we'll also run the mat, which she is currently lying on the mat here for ten minutes to help the electrical potential of all of the cells in her body.

Ty: So this is actually pulsing good electricity or good frequencies. Is that what it is—through the body?

Dr. Martin Bales: It is. It is. We hear a lot about EMF and we know the dangers of the very high frequency EMF. The very low frequency is actually beneficial. It's similar to the earth's magnetic pulse, which actually, we're losing the effect of.

Laura Bond: In 2011, the FDA approved a machine using electrical fields for brain cancer. The way that they describe the way that works is by interrupting cancer cell division, so it's kind of interesting. I think this area of electrical nutrition – I know that's what Keith Scott-Mumby calls it – is really exciting. These machines are becoming more and more affordable, which is great news.

Ty: How many doctors know that there's actually an FDA-approved electronic device for treating brain cancer? I wonder. Now Dr. Bales has mentioned dirty electricity. When we think of dirty electricity we think of EMF, electromagnetic frequencies, cell phone towers, radiation, and that's what we think of when we hear the term "dirty electricity."

Every time we step outside we're exposed to a toxic slew of dirty electricity, especially in the United States today, where cell phone towers being everywhere. You may be wondering, is there any way to mitigate the radiation from cell phones? I've seen many different chips, and gadgets, and little things that you stick on your cell phone, things that were supposedly holograms, and just all kinds of weird stuff that supposedly stops any danger from occurring from cell phones. Now, I had one on my cell phone. I don't usually carry it in my pocket here, but this is just for you to see. It's a little device here, and it's called the MRET device. It's developed by Dr. Smirnov. Now, we're going to listen to him describe how he developed this technology, but first, we're going to hear a brief clip from Dr. Leigh Erin Connealy.

Dr. Leigh Erin Connealy: If you walk outside, you're exposed to lots of different challenges, and we don't know. We talk about electro smog. We don't know everybody—there's lots of stuff written on it, but we don't know exactly what our cell phones, and EMF, and cell towers and all of this electricity, what that is doing to our body. Some people think it's the single biggest threat we have to mankind. Because people think that we're just this physical person that we're seeing, but no, you have this bio-energetic electrical field that is probably more influential than what's just the 3D morphology that you see right now.

Ty: As you can see here on my phone, I've got a little device here and this is called an MRET device.

Dr. Igor Smirnov: It's MRET nylon device, yeah.

Ty: What does this do? I've got it on my phone because we know about the dangers of cell phone radiation. I've had this on my phone ever since I learned about this technology over a year ago. What is this and how does it work?

Dr. Igor Smirnov: It basically works the same way like MRET water machine because it's based on this so-called generation of the low frequency, low intensity, so-called noise field, magnetic field, which might close resemble natural geomagnetic field. Probably within the last 150 years, there's a lot of distortion of this electromagnetic field because we developed a lot of manmade electromagnetic pollution around. So in order to protect human body, we have to recreate the same noise field, natural noise field to protect the human cells.

When manmade electromagnetic field affect the cells, they shut down their membrane, so-called hardening of the cell's membrane mechanism. It's a natural mechanism, the same way cells behave when—kind of like a chemical poison can be introduced to the cells. The only difference is that you can easily remove, because of the flash and human body activity. The chemicals can be easily removed out of the body. But when you are exposed to the electromagnetic—you cannot remove it. You cannot stop it. You continuously exposed to this pollution, especially after interaction of Wi-Fi.

Ty: And the cell phone towers.

Dr. Igor Smirnov: Right, towers, yeah.

Ty: This recreates the noise field that we're used to for our bodies.

Dr. Igor Smirnov: Exactly. That's right.

Ty: So how does it protect us?

Dr. Igor Smirnov: When it generates this noise field, extremely low intensity noise field, the noise field can be superimposed on the microwave signals, manmade electricity. It's kind of like it's a piggyback. It's carry this noise field frequency. The microwave signal carry this noise field frequency. In other words, when it hit the cells, the noise field kind of like masks the microwave signal, so cells cannot recognize microwave signals, and they don't shut down their membrane. It's a polymer material. And when you expose this polymer material to electromagnetic microwave radiation, it's kind of like creating excitation in the molecular structure in the polymer.

Ty: And then it—

Dr. Igor Smirnov: This is how the polymer generates low frequency.

Ty: Wow. Do I believe in this technology? Let's just say that I have one of these little MRET devices on every mobile device, every handheld device that my family owns. There's been a direct correlation shown in the research between cell phone radiation and brain cancer. While we were in London, we interviewed a man, Rob Olifent that lost his father to a brain tumor. His wife, Sue, is a cancer conqueror, and we're about to hear their story.

So your story begins back in 2008, Robert, with your parents being diagnosed with cancer? Can you tell the viewers about that story.

Rob Olifent: Both of them, they got cancer at the same time and they died within three weeks of each other, which was quite a horrendous time.

Ty: What kind of cancer did your parents have, Robert?

Rob Olifent: My father had a brain tumor. My mother had it everywhere, pretty much everywhere. I witnessed quite a few things that I was really uncomfortable with in the medical paradigm, and it just got me asking questions. I went into researching quite a lot. Sue wasn't on board at all, but I researched for two-and-a-half years.

Sue Olifent: I thought he was crazy [chuckles]. Video after video, after DVD after all—

Rob Olifent: And reading stuff all—

Sue Olifent: Yeah, just constantly researching. I didn't see him at all really. He was always upstairs. Weren't you?

Rob Olifent: I didn't think I was that bad, but then maybe I was [chuckles].

Ty: Robert, what did you find in your research on cancer?

Rob Olifent: I wondered why like one in two people are going to get cancer in their lifetime, and yet the media was saying, "Well, we're winning the war on cancer. Just give us more money." I wondered why they had chocolate bar dispensers on every oncology ward. I wondered why they had coke machines, fizzy drink machines containing sugar on all these wards, and why they gave my dad and mom, and uncle, who later died of cancer, apple pie and ice cream. It just didn't make sense. So I did all this research.

But then two and a half years down the line, Sue got very poorly, and she lost a stone and a half in weight [*approx 20 lbs*]. And every time she ate, she had tremendous stabbing pains in the stomach, and she couldn't eat particularly acidic foods. She had a scan, and they found a two and a half inch tumor in the liver where the tubes are coming out, and it was strangulating the tubes. That's the position that we're in. She also got three smaller growths on the pancreas. We basically had to throw everything in because the doctors said, "I'm so very sorry. I've never seen a cancer this type, in a woman of your age." We were left in a position where he said, "There is nothing we can do. We can't do anything. It's such a sensitive area." She went out and bought 25 pounds worth of goodbye cards. It was quite a horrendous time.

Ty: What was the year, Sue, that you were diagnosed?

Sue Olifent: 2011.

Ty: 2011?

Sue Olifent: Mm-hmm.

Ty: Okay, so four years ago?

Sue Olifent: Yeah. I was on my own when I was diagnosed, but I didn't want to—the time Robert himself was quite so—after losing his parents, he was struggling. He had to be off work, so I didn't want to put any pressure on him. He really wasn't well at that time, so I decided to go—I had a feeling that it was going to be bad news when I went because of the way the receptionist spoke to me on the phone the night before when I'd rung up. When I did go in, it was just like normal. It was like it was a haze, like it wasn't happening, and I just kept thinking, "I can't tell Rob. It will make him ill." I didn't know what to do. I just got on a bus and went into town in this daze, and then found myself in the card shop. But, then I realized I had to tell him in the end because when he walked in the door, I was shaking from head to toe. I thought I'd hold it together, but I couldn't stop crying. The thought of telling my 16-year-old son, my head was all over the place. It was really hard.

Rob Olifent: But, we had an advantage because I'd done quite a lot of research involving this and because we had nowhere else to go, basically. They said there was no hope by medical standards. We threw everything into what we'd learned, what I'd learned. We started instigating an anti-cancer protocol, and were quite strict. We started having lemons first thing in the morning, juicing with green, leafy vegetables. Maybe include an apple in there to sweeten it up a little bit. A little bit of ginger, celery, cucumber, things to liven up the taste of it. Because sometimes when you have green juices on their own, they leave a little bit to be desired on the taste factor, so we included other things in them. Apples are great because they're low sugar, low glycemic, and they just lift the flavor of that a little bit.

So we got organic veggie box delivered every week. So we made sure that what was coming inside us was pure. That it didn't have toxicity or these things that are going into mass farm production today, which are pesticides, larvicides, fungicides, and the rest of it. So, these are part of the protocols. We took out milk and dairy products. We still did have bread, but we didn't have white bread. We've since learned—because it's a progression of learning, and there's better things like the ancient grained bread, which is far better for you.

I think there was a time, which I remember in the kitchen, and it was a really positive time where we were discussing all what we're doing, and we decided to go on the apricot kernels when we were discussing those, and I got my arms around Sue, and I said, "We're going really to do this. We're going to—this is going to be okay." I felt really positive at that time, and I think that was a change around for Sue as well. I think you saw the apricot kernels. I mean there's no silver bullet, as such, because cancer is a holistic thing, and you have to deal with everything: emotional, and psychological, and nutritional, hydration, detoxification. But that was a moment which was a step forward.

Sue Olifent: I think to me, each time I put them in my mouth, I was feeling they were the medicine. They were what we're going to break this cancer down.

Rob Olifent: It's crazy that cancer organizations actually state that if you have these products, these apricot kernels, that you'll have a long list of things that happen to you. You'll get nauseous. You'll vomit all over the place. You'll get hives. You'll get headaches. You'll get migraines and then ending in death. I've read the Cancer Research UK website, and this is what it says. Well, it's not my experience, and I've heard thousands of them. It's not Sue's experience. She's still alive, without cancer. I know various other people that are taking these things, and they're still alive, without cancer.

We shout this from the rooftops, all about the information that we have gained, and we put on meetings. We set up a little support group – it's just me and Sue – and we put on meetings every month, and I explain to people the principles of what we chose to do. But we're seeing people that don't have cancer anymore through this. Some people that have been written off by the cancer industry, societies, that truly they don't have their cancer anymore.

Sue Olifent: We've been watching them every month getting better and better and better.

Ty: Very encouraging story from Rob and Sue. They radically changed their diet. They stopped eating the things that were making them sick, specifically Sue, and she healed.

Ard Pisa: Look at this world. We can get on every corner, also in Amsterdam here, unhealthy food. If you want healthy food, you have to search for it. You have to search for it. That's just not only nutrition. We have to feed our system, not only with nutrition, but also with emotional well-being. There is a lot of stress. Look at Amsterdam. What is speed in Amsterdam?

Ty: Fast-paced.

Ard Pisa: Fast. 24/7. So much stress, and look at the people. You see the mouth?

Ty: Frowning.

Ard Pisa: Frowning. Not happy. They are surviving instead of living. We have to live.

Dr. Francisco Contreras: There's a study, very interesting study that shows that for every minute of anger, you will depress significantly and measurably, of course, the quality and quantity of your immune system. One minute of anger, six hours of depression. One minute of laughter will boost, significantly, your immune system for 24 hours.

Dr. Patrick Quillin: I found a textbook from the New York Academy of Sciences called *The Biological Foundations of Music*, and this is a hundred dollar textbook from all these academically affiliated MDs and PhDs. What they found is, they showed when you play music, and actually, you can show things when you sing too. Music in general is therapeutic. Singing and playing is even more therapeutic. Just listening to music that relaxes you is good for you, and it can have extraordinary healing capacities.

The studies are beyond argument now that the music that you are listening to, making, singing, or playing, actually changes the way the brain works. Hans Selye and his incredible work. Dr. Selye was the grandfather of stress. And there's many others in the field who have clearly proven that stress is a killer, and music is a healer.

Ty: Stress is definitely a killer. And when you're sick with cancer, the last thing that you need is more challenges to your immune system, because it's your immune system that actually heals you. Unfortunately, many of the traditional treatments, specifically the chemotherapy, is devastating to the immune system. Here's a few poignant quotes on that topic.

Dr. Matthias Rath: In this case, the unfortunate decision was taken to apply it for the alleged treatment of cancer. In fact, as Dr. [?] pointed out, it is a business model, it's not a treatment. The intention is to give the impression that something goes away, and it may go away for a few months. But the real mass megadeath in the field of cancer patients is happening after six months or nine months, when this initial effect of doing away with the tumor breaks down, and the cancer comes back massively. Even more than before because now the immune system is dead. And no one talks about that.

Dr. Russell Blaylock: I always tell cancer patients, when you go talk to your oncologist, number one, when they start talking about how, "Oh, we are getting really good response in this drug," ask them the most important question. "What are the chances this will cure me?" Not make me feel better, not make the tumor shrink for a little while. What are the chances they will cure me? Because then he will say, this blank look come over the oncologist's face, and he will say, "Well, most people will die of this cancer anyway." This might make you feel better or live a month or two longer or six months longer. So it's deceptive. It's not being truthful when they talk to these cancer patients. So I tell them always to ask that question.

Ty: Any other questions that cancer patients should ask the oncologist?

Dr. Russell Blaylock: Well, you want to know, what are the complications of this? What is the known death rate from using this chemotherapy? A lot of patient's don't understand that a significant number of cancer patients are dying from the treatment itself, and not the cancer. It can vary between one or two percent to as much as 10 percent to 15 percent that are dying from the treatment. A lot of patients have to stop their treatment because their treatment makes them so sick, they die if they keep doing it, and they found if you have to interrupt the treatment, the cancer grows a lot faster, and they're less likely to live.

All of these things, patients need to ask their doctor, and the doctor is not going to volunteer it, because he's trying to sell the protocol. He's trying to sell you to take his $500,000 treatment. And if he says, "Well, there's a 15 percent chance you could die. It's probably not going to cure you. You'll only get a few months. It's really going to make you sick. It's going to destroy your immune system, and these are known to cause heart failure, that it's incurable. And this will destroy your lungs," and these are all things known with chemotherapy. Well, not many people would do it. Most people will say, "I don't think I want to do that if it's going to destroy my lungs, if it's going to destroy my heart. I'll go into progressive heart failure. I don't think I want to do that."

Dr. Roby Mitchell: The overwhelming majority of physicians who treat cancer with those therapies depend solely on the radiation or the chemo. And the consequences of that is a weakened immune system. So the very system that you're depending on to cure cancer, we kill that off. And that's why so many people with cancer, they die of the treatment, rather than the cancer.

Dr. Matthias Rath: Once you define a business as an investment business, you have to define the return on investment. In the pharmaceutical industry, these are patent fees, royalties. Then the next step is, "How do you get a patent?" You only get a patent if you do something new, and most of the patents in the pharmaceutical industry, therefore relate to synthetically defined new drugs – artificially created. In other words, the body doesn't know them, these molecules, and treats them as toxins. And in many cases, our organs are not able to detoxify them, and there you have it. As a result of this business model, of being an investment industry, you have this avalanche of side effects factored into this business model.

Dr. Sunil Pai: The reason why I'm angry is because I feel that at least it's negligence, that's what's happening in the conventional medical care – particularly with oncological patients and cancer treatments. If you go further, it almost could be thought of as criminal because we're letting people die unnecessarily. We're giving people lower -quality lives and lower outcomes, but we're pushing profits every day.

With our Hippocratic Oath, which most physicians have never read, the first thing says, "First, do no harm." We always have to go back and saying, "Well, are we doing harm," number one. Number two, is it also says, just further down in the Hippocratic Oath, is, "I will not give a poison, a deadly poison." Most of the drugs that we give, particularly in oncological care, has a black-box warning, which means that more people often end up in the black box.

Dr. David Brownstein: When we graduate from medical school, we take the Hippocratic Oath, which says, in part, "Above all, do no harm." I can tell you, a lot of conventional therapies are harmful and toxic to the body.

Dr. Darrell Wolfe: *"Whenever a doctor cannot do good, he must be kept from doing harm."* What happened to the Hippocratic Oath? I think the only thing that's left is called the hypocrite.

Pam Pinney: In 2007, my husband and I, Harry, we did a 40-day fast, and I lost 25 pounds. So, I was laying in bed one day, and I laid my hand on my chest, and I noticed this pea-like thing in my chest. I was like, "Huh, that's interesting." I went in. They did testing. Biopsy said it's stage I invasive ductal carcinoma. So, I had surgery. There was this urgency - have surgery, have chemo, have radiation. I quickly did the surgery out of fear and—

Ty: And you removed the little pea-sized—?

Pam Pinney:: Removed the lump, had a lumpectomy. They said, "You need to have chemo and radiation." Actually, there was mixed—some days they said, "We don't know what to do with you." Other days, "You're going to die if you don't have it." So, I prayed about what to do, and I felt the Lord said, "Every good and perfect gift comes from above." He said, "Chemo causes cancer. Why would you do that?" And so, I thought, "Well, I'm just not going to do it."

Announcing that to the family, it didn't go well. Everybody –it's not just you and your fear – the whole family gets in fear. So I didn't do chemo or radiation. We began making lifestyle changes because I didn't want my parents to see me pass before them. They're 82 and 84. And I thought, "They've lived a long time. No way do I want them to bury me." I'm going to fight—

Charles Daniel: Same here.

Pam Pinney: —and go to their funerals, even though I'm not looking forward to that. But that's the way—yeah.

Charles Daniel: The same.

Ty: What's the most important question you can ask if you're recently diagnosed?

Sissy: I know what my most important question was. I started having a lot of reactions to the chemo that I hadn't had before. I just sat across from my oncologist and looked at her, and I said, "Cancer is not going to kill me, is it? Chemo is going to kill me." And she went, "Mm-hmm." And I walked out and never went back.

James O'Neill: When I was first diagnosed, the doctors I was dealing with were so sterile, emotionally. There was such a disconnect, and I guess as a patient at the time, I felt like, "Well, they must have to do that, to deal with so many patients and tragic situations that that's part of it." But I felt lost. Like lost at sea without a compass. And I was not being offered anything except for one very narrow path, that my heart was just saying, "You cannot go down that path. It is not going to go well."

Mary Lou: I know one question that I don't think that they should ever tell you, and that is—or you should ask is, how long do I have? I think when they tell you that, that can really set the mind in a tizzy. You really have to try to overcome that, and I don't think any oncologist marking the bottom of my foot, "You're going to expire on such and such date. I think they're playing God sometimes. Only God knows when he wants you. He's going to come and get you.

Dr. Veronique Desaulniers: I'm living proof, and thousands of women around the globe and hundreds of thousands of people who've healed cancer in general. We know there is a cure. The cure lies in our food, in detoxifying our body properly, balancing our energy, in dealing with our stress and our emotional wounds, making sure we don't have dental toxicities, using food and plants to repair our bodies, and then staying on top of everything, making sure that you can prevent cancer in the future. Because traditional medicine will use certain markers, but they're very, very gross and very ineffective markers. There are markers like the PHI enzyme, or the cancer profile, or the Oncoblot test that can determine cancer when it's only a few million cells in the body, instead of a tumor, because it take five to eight years for a tumor to develop. Thermography is also a great tool to be able to access the physiological changes that's going on in the body. So yes, there is a cure, and yes, you can prevent it.

Ty: I'm so thankful that during this episode you've been given the understanding of how you can heal cancer with clean electricity. It's an area of cancer prevention and treatment that's ignored by many professionals. Today you've seen the science and even the conventional medical community's approval of this technology and related devices, due to the remarkable success in treating cancer, even the most challenging forms including brain cancer.

You've also seen the information we've covered concerning unique water that contains vital keys to protecting the body from cancer, and even healing a body that already has cancer. I hope it's a good incentive for you to make sure that you're consistently hydrated with clean water.

You've seen how the sun and its ultraviolet light, which we have been misled to believe is always bad for us, and that this mixes with the cholesterol in our skin to form Vitamin D. Now Vitamin D is essential each day for your health and happiness, and it's even been shown in multiple studies to drastically reduce the incidence of cancer.

And again you've witnessed the incredible power of combining superfoods and that these rich nutrient supplies are glad to replenish your body every day, fueling you with nutrients that bring your body energy, aid in detoxification, strengthen the immune system, and equip the body to fight and fend off disease, including the vanquished foe – cancer.

In the next episode, we're going to be traveling to the Netherlands. We're going to stay here in the United States, and we're going to go to Mexico as we interview three renowned medical doctors that are treating and beating cancer with innovative, scientifically proven approaches. It's an episode you do not want to miss. In the meantime, have yourself a great rest of your day. Get some rest and we'll see you tomorrow. God bless all of you.

[*credits roll*]

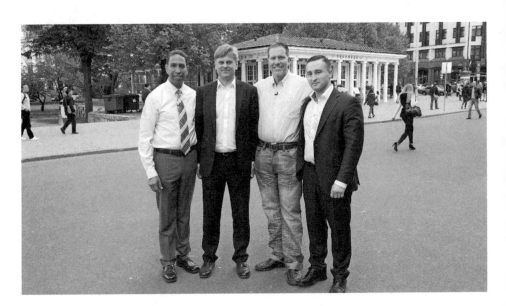

With Dr. Antonio Jimenez, Dr. Kaspars Losans, and Andreji Repisevski in Riga, Latvia

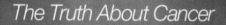

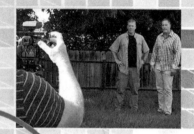

The Truth About Cancer
A GLOBAL QUEST
Episode 8

Cannabis, Nature's Epigenetic Switches, Peptides & Healing with Micronutrient Therapy

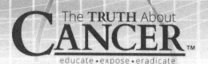

Ty: Welcome back to *The Truth About Cancer: A Global Quest*. I am so glad that you joined us for this episode, but just in case you missed any of the last episode here is a brief recap for you.

[*video plays: Summary of Episode Seven*]

Ty: In this episode, we're going to travel to Mexico, just south of Tijuana to learn about the Gerson Therapy. We're going to take a trip to Houston, Texas, to the Burzynski Clinic and learn a little bit more from Dr. Burzynski about the Antineoplaston treatment that he has been so heavily persecuted for. We're going to talk a little bit about hemp as a treatment for cancer. But this episode begins with a trip across the Atlantic Ocean to Heerlen, Netherlands, for an interview that we did with Dr. Matthias Rath and Aleksandra Niedzwiecki to discuss their protocol which focuses on micronutrients to treat and beat cancer.

Dr. Aleksandra Niedzwiecki: Our study shows that the underlying cause of majority of chronic diseases – diseases that develop over years or even decades – is the long-term deficiency of micronutrients. Vitamins, trace elements, some amino acids, or other active components which cause cellular dysfunction that, with time, turns into disease, organ disease.

Dr. Matthias Rath: Generally micronutrients comprise vitamins, minerals, trace elements, certain amino acids, phytochemicals or phytobiologicals as we call them, extracts from plants – small molecules that have a distinct metabolic role in the cells of the body. We are not looking at individual types of cancer, but we are looking at the key mechanism that unites them all. Cells, many cells migrate within our body at any time. White blood cells, the police cells, they need to leave the bloodstream and enter, for example, the lung to fight pneumonia or any other organ. We have the egg cell in the monthly cycle of the woman that leaves the ovary and migrates into the Fallopian tube.

All these processes are extremely tightly controlled because they involve destruction of connective tissue. Meaning destructing of tissue that surrounds the cell at that moment – mostly collagen or elastin. And this destruction happens with the help of an enzyme or a group of enzymes which, for simplicity, we can call collagenases, collagen-digesting enzymes.

Under normal circumstances, this mechanism is tightly controlled. Cancer cells use exactly that mechanism, exactly the same group of enzymes to make their way through the body, to migrate through the body. First in their environment – we call this invasion. So the tumor grows and spreads, let's say, within the organ of the liver and then ultimately to migrate into other organs and we call that step metastasis. In each case, it's the same type of enzyme that paves the way of the cancer cell or cancer cells to migrate.

It's probably like an expeditionary corp in the jungle with a machete. They pave their way through the jungle.

And what we found out is that we can block these collagen-digesting enzymes, and we understand today the key micronutrients that are able to do that. Not chemotherapy – natural substances that are able to block cancer cells from doing harm to the body. Therefore, the approach that we are going to talk about a little more, is not related to an individual type of cancer like breast cancer or prostate cancer. It is a common mechanism that we understand today quite well, and that we have developed and tested a composition of micronutrients for in over 50 human cell lines. In other words any commercial human cancer cell line that is available currently we tested those micronutrients and they are effective in each and every case.

Dr. Aleksandra Niedzwiecki: Our studies have shown that this composition of micronutrients is effective in inhibiting key mechanisms that cancer uses in our body. So these micronutrients can inhibit proliferation or growth of cancer cells; inhibit formation of tumors. They can also inhibit the invasion of cancer cells in the tissue. They are effective in inhibiting metastasis. We tested in several cases that metastasis can be inhibited by 70, up to 80 percent. And also they are effective in inhibiting formation of new blood vessels that feed the tumor.

Interestingly, this mixture of natural compounds is also able to work at the genetic level in cancer cells and convert them from cells which are immortal into cells that start dying. And so these micronutrients can induce natural death of cancer cells called apoptosis, and we also published a lot of studies supporting this type of finding. So if we can—what is the beauty of using nutrient synergy is that several mechanisms that are involved in certain pathologies can be affected at once, making in case of cancer more difficult for cancer cells to escape this control.

Ty: What are these nutrients that have the—

Dr. Aleksandra Niedzwiecki: Components?

Ty: Synergistic effect like the orchestra? What are the components of this—?

Dr. Aleksandra Niedzwiecki: Yeah. This is vitamin C, you know, for simple reasons since we are targeting the stability and integrity of connective tissue. Without vitamin C, connective tissue cannot be produced. The other compounds of this synergy, a very powerful component, is amino acid lysine. Lysine is inhibitor of those collagen- digestive enzymes, but also lysine is a component of collagen. One third of amino acids in collagen are lysine and proline so it is important that they are included. And lysine, similarly to vitamin C, is not produced in our body. It only comes from the diet.

We are also having other components like n-acetylcysteine, we are having trace elements including copper, selenium. And we are having the active component from green tea called epigallocatechin gallate or EGCG for short, and quercetin.

So this is the mixture of several components. You can find the information on our website. This is what we tested them. We tested individual compounds and also we combined them in the synergy. So there are components acting on different mechanisms in our body, including what we see they also have anti-inflammatory effect. And what we know from one site, inflammation is associated with cancer and also long-lasting inflammation is the triggering factor for developing cancer. And these micronutrients are also effective in addressing this important aspect. So this is this pleiotropic effect of micronutrient synergy that we are working with.

Ty: I love the way that Dr. Niedzwiecki puts that – the micronutrient synergy. But this isn't just theory. Drs. Rath and Niedzwiecki have literally thousands of patients across Europe that are treating and beating cancer with their micronutrient protocol.

Dr. Matthias Rath: We have, mostly here in Europe, more than 10,000 patients who are using the synergy program, and some of them have survived the predicted death now for 15 years. We have x-ray documentation of many of them, etcetera. And we've summarized this fantastic work that Dr. Niedzwiecki and her team were leading in a book called *Victory Over Cancer*. So anyone who wants to get more details we were just explaining that it is available for free online. Everyone can read it anywhere in the world.

There are, to our knowledge, to our understanding, there is no more precise mechanism that has been identified as being critical for the control of cancer than the one we just described.

There's no program that we are aware of in the field of natural health that is more effective in controlling cancer in vivo in humans. We're not giving a guarantee obviously. That would be not what we ethically should do. But we know that there are no science-based programs in natural health that are more effective as we speak. Micronutrients give – in layman's terms now – give the cancer cell two options. Either you think about how you operate properly and become a healthy cell again or you die, you commit suicide. And this is this process that Dr. Niedzwiecki said – apoptosis.

That happens at a genetic level, and we understand quite a bit about the regulation, how micronutrients go directly to the core of a cancer cell, to the DNA, and challenges the very inner sanctum of this cell into this process.

Of course it is not an intellectual deliberation, it is a forced biological interception. Either you function properly or you commit suicide. And that's really powerful. That is something that no chemotherapy drug or no synthetic drug can do. And, of course, that again is a sign for the real power of natural health. These regulatory processes, they didn't appear in a reagent glass or a petri dish in a laboratory of the pharmaceutical industry 20 years ago or five years ago. These are processes that nature developed over millennia, and this is why they function so distinctly.

One of our first patients – that is now almost 20 years ago – who went on the program here in Europe, he had lung cancer and he was given half a year to live and put his affairs in order. And he decided to go on this program, and I think six, seven months later he came back and x-ray was taken and there was no more tumor.

So the doctor apologized. He said, "You know, sorry, you have to come back a week later. We need to repair our machine. It is apparently kaput, as they say in German." So the gentleman said, "Sure, I understand. I come back in a week." And they redid the x-ray and it was the same picture. And then the doctor started to try to find other excuses because, this was a female doctor, she had not seen anything like that. But our patient, he said, "Well, I don't think I need to come back. I know what I've been doing."

I'm not telling that to add an episode to this conversation. I'm telling it to underline the transformational time that it is inconceivable for health professionals, for doctors, educated people, that cancer can disappear in a natural way. Just go away.

Ty: I agree with Dr. Rath. This is inconceivable for most doctors because they've been miseducated about natural cancer treatments. Back in episode one, we had a little history lesson about why doctors don't know and why they don't believe in natural treatments.

Dr. Matthias Rath: Ty, "If we are not learning from history," and I'm quoting a philosopher, "we are sentenced to relive it again." And I wasn't born as a historian. I was a scientist, a doctor, and after publishing these initial new concepts on cancer and heart disease with Linus Pauling, I felt the world will embrace us. They will say, "This is great." The fact is we were being fought for every single advance in natural health. There are more than 100 lawsuits that the status quo, the pharmaceutical lobby, has been bringing against myself, Dr. Niedzwiecki, our research over the past 15 years.

More than 100 times we were dragged into the courtrooms for one goal: these interests did not want us to talk today or, for that matter, to inform you what we have found out about the most common diseases can be greatly reduced, maybe eventually largely eliminated, with the knowledge we have today. The fact that we are doing this interview now shows they didn't succeed, and the main reason why we succeeded, actually summarizing it in one word was: science.

Ty: These interests did not want us to have this conversation, but we did. And, yes, Dr. Rath's protocol has mountains of scientific evidence to support it, but these same interests that have persecuted Dr. Rath and Dr. Niedzwiecki are attempting to stifle science-based innovative cancer treatments across the globe.

Another scientist that has been persecuted by these same interests for using outside-the-box type treatments is Dr. Stanislaw Burzynski out of Houston, Texas. He uses a treatment that's called antineoplastons. Now antineoplastons are basically like a missing link between proteins and amino acids. And he realized that cancer patients are typically deficient in these certain types of antineoplastons.

While we were in Seattle, I was able to sit down with Dr. Gaston Cornu Labat, who learned about the antineoplaston treatment from Dr. Burzynski. And he shares some of the behind-the-scenes happenings of the persecution of Dr. Burzynski and his treatment.

Dr. Gaston Cornu-Labat: It's very unclear exactly what's going on between the FDA and Burzynski except that every step he tries to take with the antineoplaston therapy, there's some kind of roadblock. So at that time the roadblock, in my understanding, was that the FDA was looking into—the Burzynski Clinic started clinical trials. However, any patient outside of the conditions of the clinical trial that needed treatment, it could not be done in the Clinic. So they needed somebody outside of the Clinic to run antineoplaston therapy. And I said, "Okay. I'll do it."

So I went to Houston, I spent a couple of days there, I started getting acquainted with the therapy. And from then on, started developing all the necessary knowledge to be able to start implementing the therapy in our clinic. Now, each patient that was referred to me for antineoplaston therapy needed to go through a process of approval of Investigational New Drug application Expanded Access. So that's an IND application. The second patient was a 4-year-old kid from Florida.

Ty: Four?

Dr. Gaston Cornu-Labat: Four years old.

Ty: Okay.

Dr. Gaston Cornu-Labat: With what's known as DIPG, which is sort of a kind of an advanced brain stem tumor.

Ty: Diffused intrinsic—

Dr. Gaston Cornu-Labat: Pontine glioma. Yes. And DIPG is well-established, it doesn't respond to anything. So these kids—it's common in children and these kids die from it. Burzynski has documented cases. Not every tumor responds, that's for sure, but he has documented cases of significant response, of significant prolongation of life, and documented cases of cures—of complete response. Complete remission of the tumor.

Ty: With DIPG specifically?

Dr. Gaston Cornu-Labat: With DIPG, yes, which is the only therapy right now that can claim some percentage of total response. There's no other therapy that can claim that. Period. Nothing in the literature that says, you know, we have cured one patient or two patients.

Nothing. Actually Burzynski is the only one that can claim that. There's patients 20 years ago that's still running around.

Ty: I've seen the pictures on his walls.

Dr. Gaston Cornu-Labat: Right.

Ty: Okay, so just to recap to this point. There are children with brain tumors that are untreatable by any conventional methods. Dr. Burzynski's antineoplaston treatment has proven to cure these types of tumors that are untreatable, but because of the onerous FDA regulations he is not able to treat them. So Dr. Cornu-Labat has learned from Dr. Burzynski how to do this antineoplaston treatment. He completed an IND, which is an Innovative New Drug application, and then that's where our story picks up.

Dr. Gaston Cornu-Labat: When I moved ahead with the application for the second case, they spent about four weeks back and forward picking on little—"Oh, this word here doesn't fit. This word here doesn't fit. What are these charges? What?" So it was picking on nuisance, if the expression is correct, for about a month and a half. This kid was a very advanced case, deteriorating on a daily basis almost. And then after about a month and a half, they said, "Okay. The request is on hold, on clinical hold." Which means it's in limbo.

Ty: In limbo?

Dr. Gaston Cornu-Labat: Because we're not denying it.

Ty: But you can't do it.

Dr. Gaston Cornu-Labat: But you can't do it because it's on hold. And, okay,   "Why?" "Well? Because we think that the risks outweigh the benefits." The kid's going to die.

Ty: This is with a terminal brain cancer patient that has no options?

Dr. Gaston Cornu-Labat: Well, the kid's going to die.

Ty: Other than this?

Dr. Gaston Cornu-Labat: Right. "Well, we really can't disclose the information we have to complete this."

Ty: So the risks are greater than the risk of death? I mean, how can you have something that's more risky than death?

Dr. Gaston Cornu-Labat: I have no explanation whatsoever. We could not make sense. The family was totally devastated. My participation in this was, you know, tell them I think it's absurd. I think you are responsible if this kid dies, you are responsible for this kid's death. Not because he was going to be saved for sure with antineoplastons, but because he had the possibility. And the best evidence that we have, and Burzynski has collected a lot of scientific—he's very—he's by no means esoteric, natural, voodoo, nothing.

Ty: He's a scientist.

Dr. Gaston Cornu-Labat: Tremendously scientific. And all stats collected pointed out to the fact that antineoplastons is the only therapy available today that could give a possibility to this child of having an improvement or even a small chance, but chance nonetheless, of a cure. Now the FDA considered, in writing, that the risks of doing this therapy outweighed the benefits. Of what? I don't know. I can't wrap my head around it.

Ty: That's insane.

Dr. Gaston Cornu-Labat: It is very, very profoundly absurd. Now, after that—that was kind of a disheartening experience. There had been a lot of work. I'm not the significant one in this. This kid ended up dying. The family totally devastated. I don't think the family ever initiated any kind of legal actions or anything on this. They were running, getting into debt with everything they could on trying to collect money to treat this little kid that was dying. And they were so broken down afterwards that it just hushed, and it went to oblivion.

Ty: That's just...

Dr. Gaston Cornu-Labat: It gets forgotten. How do you sleep at night after condemning a 4-year-old to die?

Ty: This is criminal, folks. Children are being condemned to death because they don't have access to these innovative treatments that could save their life. How do these bureaucrats sleep at night? And the doctors are handcuffed because they can't use the treatments.

Dr. Stanislaw Burzynski: It's not easy to treat these advanced patients because you are continuously being harassed for doing this, okay. It is incredible! We should be awarded! We should be set as the example! We are saving the lives of people who have sentence to die. No, we are mercilessly harassed by lawyers, by people who know nothing about treatment, who are stupid puppets of the guys behind who know very well what we can offer but are directing these guys like in Nazi Germany. They are simply obeying orders because they are programmed this way. Okay? I think maybe a time when they used some type of Nuremberg trials where all of this white collar, nicely dressed lawyers and clerks who are chewing the money of taxpayers they be held accountable for what they do, because many people died because of their actions.

Ty: Now one such child that died because of these despicable actions is Thomas Navarro. I had the privilege to interview his mother and father, Jim and Donna. And Thomas was diagnosed with a terminal type of brain cancer. They wanted to take Thomas to Dr. Burzynski's clinic and this was about 20 years ago, but because of these onerous regulations at the FDA and the fact that they require the children to go through chemotherapy and radiation first *before* they can use Dr. Burzynski's treatment, they forced Thomas to do this. And in 18 months, Thomas was dead before he could get to the antineoplaston treatment. And on his death certificate, one of the reasons for death was toxicity due to chemotherapy. The treatment actually killed him.

Dr. Stanislaw Burzynski: Recently randomized, controlled clinical trials have been completed by my Japanese colleagues on antineoplastons in colon cancer which spread to the liver. They proved that they can increase the survival, median survival, by about three years. Median survival is about five years, by about three years. Three years versus three weeks or versus three months. Because the usual standard for FDA approval for the new drug is to extend median survival from three weeks to three months. Here we got about three years, okay.

Ty: And they're still having issues?

Dr. Stanislaw Burzynski: No. No. Now they're saying, "The risks does not justify the benefits." Okay?

Ty: Well, my question is this: If you look at risk versus reward—

Dr. Stanislaw Burzynski: Oh, the risk is death, okay, because—

Ty: The risk is death.

Dr. Stanislaw Burzynski: Obviously, liver cancer—well, colon cancer with liver spread practically everybody dies for it, okay?

Ty: Dr. Burzynski just shared with us about controlled clinical trials on colon cancer and they are having great success with his treatment. Case in point, here's one of Dr. Burzynski's patients that was diagnosed with colon cancer eight years ago. He went to Hermann Memorial in Houston and also MD Anderson in Houston and both of those hospitals and all the physicians there told him that his only option was surgery. But then he learned about the Burzynski Clinic.

Arize Chris Onuekwusi: I have relatives here in Houston, and everybody was saying, "What are you waiting for? Go for surgery. Go, get your surgery and then you can talk about the Burzynski Clinic later on, but you need to do the surgery. That's what the doctor says." My older brother is a doctor. His friends are doctors, and just the pressure was too much. But you know what, I was a little bit stubborn. I said, "You know what? I'm going with him. If that's where it's going to end, then that's where it's going to end. But I'm not going to the surgery. I'm not going to do radiation and all that stuff."

So I called him up. So I came on down here and they said, "Okay." And they took me through what they going to do, their treatment protocol. And they laid it out for me, and said they'll have to do blood work and map my genes and then see what kind of treatment would be best for me. And I really liked that, you know.

Ty: Individualized treatment.

Arize Chris Onuekwusi: Individualized. That's really one other thing that made me say, "Hmm, this guy is different." So after three months, I went for a checkup – another PET scan and check-up. That was on a Friday. The result came back, and the tumor was gone. Can you believe it?

Ty: The tumor was gone?

Arize Chris Onuekwusi: The tumor was gone! The tumor was gone. If I had gone for surgery, because my tumor was right at the junction of the small and large intestine, and there's a valve there they call the secum valve that regulates the flow of nutrients from your small intestine to your large intestine, and that could have been taken out during surgery. And so I would have been a candidate for a colostomy bag. So I would have been carrying a colostomy bag, and I wouldn't have met you because I'd be dead by now, you know?

Ty: So this treatment saved your life?

Arize Chris Onuekwusi: It did. I feel great.

Ty: Yeah? You look great.

Arize Chris Onuekwusi: I feel great!

Ty: That's awesome to hear Chris' testimonial, and it's so good that Dr. Burzynski is having success with his treatment but that doesn't mean that it's any easier for him to prescribe it for his patients. And one of the main reasons is that the decisions on which treatments are available for use are not being made by medical doctors. They're being made by attorneys and by bureaucrats.

Dr. Stanislaw Burzynski: How the doctor can select the best treatment for his patient if the only treatment he can give is up to the lawyers, up to the nurses who never treated such things. Okay? They don't have any idea how to treat advanced cancer. And this is the system which is punishing the doctors to be inventors, to be discoverers. And the name of the game is the big money because if you have many doctors who are inventors, it's no good for the large institutions. The inventors should be awarded, not punished. I am being punished now by Texas Medical Board for saving lives of the worst cancers you can get—pancreatic cancer.

We have a patient who survived over six years with pancreatic cancer which spread to the liver, okay? I am now investigated. I have to go to court. I may lose my license because the Texas Board is harassing me, because I used my invention to save the life of this patient, okay? This patient obviously was sentenced to die. Everybody dies from pancreatic cancer. It's one out of a million cases which lives a little longer, okay? Usually people who have pancreatic cancer spread to the liver, they are dead within a few months. I have a number of patients with very long-term survivors like over 20 years, approaching 20 years. And within the last year or two, we have a number of weddings to which we are invited and these are the weddings of the patients who we started as little children and now they grew up, didn't have cancer. They live normal life, and they live highly productive life. They don't have long-term adverse reactions. They tolerated treatment well. They live normal life.

Arize Chris Onuekwusi: What I liked about the clinic was when I came here it had a full-time dietitian that I had to see that guided me as to what to eat to help me with my treatment. And I came to realize later that nutrition is a key component of your treatment. You get the food that Mother Nature gave you and your body can take care of itself. I believe that 100 percent.

Ty: I do, too.

Arize Chris Onuekwusi: I don't care what it is. You got to eat, baby, you got to eat.

Ty: Eat clean foods, right?

Arize Chris Onuekwusi: You have to eat real food, and you will be okay.

Ty: The first doctor that you visited, Chris, did he have any kind of a nutritional plan over at MD Anderson?

Arize Chris Onuekwusi: No.

Ty: No?

Arize Chris Onuekwusi: No, no, no, no. They never talked about nutrition. The first doctor that I went for a colonoscopy, right?

Ty: Yeah.

Arize Chris Onuekwusi: And then at first he said it was surgery. So he didn't say anything about nutrition or anything else. And said it didn't matter what opinion I got, it was going to be surgery anyway so I went to MD Anderson and they tell me—as a matter of fact they scheduled surgery about three days after I met them.

Ty: Really? They were in a rush—

Arize Chris Onuekwusi: And I hadn't even told me family, you know, that I had cancer and now here you are scheduling me for surgery? I've got to go home and tell my family first. So there was nothing about nutrition whatsoever. If anybody has cancer, if you have the money – unfortunately it's expensive and there are some companies that will not pick up the tab – but if you have the money, come on here. And that's all I'm saying. Come on here.

Ty: Thank you, brother.

Arize Chris Onuekwusi: You're welcome.

Ty: Awesome. It's great to hear the rest of Chris' testimonial and I have to agree with him— nutrition is the key. As a matter of fact, food can be epigenetic. Let's listen to some more of our experts discuss that topic.

Joel Salatin: Trust me. If you're sick, it's not because you're pharmaceutically disadvantaged. It's probably because there's some underlying thing. Now it might not be food. It might be stress, it might be something else. And certainly there are genetic propensities. But what we've now learned already through epigenetics is that we can actually move our diet to a profoundly elevated nutritional plane enough to actually override our genetic propensity. Through epigenetics realign in a healthy fashion those genetic propensities and start over. Now, whether you say you can start over completely we can argue, but at least you can give yourself a new shot at it. You're not just inevitably programmed for whatever grandma, or mom had or whatever. We can absolutely change that epigenetic code through care and attention to our body's fuel.

Dr. Nalini Chilkov: I always tell my patients to eat the rainbow, because every pigment in fruits and vegetables actually enters the nucleus of the cell and interacts with your genes, which is why it matters what you eat, right? So if you just eat the rainbow, and half your plate is colorful fruits and vegetables – blueberries, spinach, kale, carrots, tomatoes, persimmons, pomegranates. If you eat color you are going to also get these phytochemicals. Also you have a medicine chest in your spice rack in your kitchen: oregano, thyme, ginger, turmeric – all of the culinary spices not only aid your digestion, but they also have these powerful chemicals. Carnisol is found in rosemary for example – a very powerful anti-cancer chemical.

So we can easily make our diets talk to our genes really easily. Anybody can do it. It's actually more powerful to turn on what we call the apoptotic switch which is a signal, an intelligence, wisdom in cells that tells them they're not healthy cells, they should die and recycle themselves. That is lost in tumor cells so not only are they growing but they're failing to die. And so a better solution is over here, and there are so many botanicals and phytochemicals that turn that apoptotic switch back on. So that's really powerful. Resveratrol, curcumin, ECGC in green tea – those are examples of common phytochemicals used in cancer that do that.

Dr. Jonathan Wright: It's nature's medicine, and has been that way ever since there's been people. The wise grannies, and some of the wise grandpas learned that this herb or that thing helped with this problem and they passed it down and passed it down and passed it down. But it's medicine that's derived from our planet. Now the reason why that's so important it's derived from our planet is that our bodies are made up of the substance and energy of planet. Unless you're space aliens and that's a different story.

Ty: Maybe the FDA is space aliens.

Dr. Jonathan Wright: I don't know. One wonders sometimes. If we are regular people, substance and energy of planet Earth. And the molecules are all from planet Earth and the energies are all from planet Earth. So what's going to work best in your Chevy if it's broken? Chevy parts! If the body is broken, do we put in original body parts which are original molecules and original energies? No! We take them and we twist them a little bit so we can patent them, and of course they don't fit quite right any more if it's a molecule. Or we use an energy that isn't natural to the body, and we expect the body to heal with that?! The best it can do is cover up symptoms. So you get to buy it for the next 40 years while you're covering up your symptoms.

Chris Wark: You cannot cut a tumor off or shrink a tumor or poison a tumor and expect to stay well and stay healthy, because you're not addressing the real problem, you are only addressing the symptom.

Dr. Rashid Buttar: If you took your car to a mechanic and there was a flashing check engine light on your car, and the mechanic says, "Yeah I can fix that," and takes the fuse out, okay, and says, "Okay. Now your problem's solved." Or, "I've got a knocking in my engine." "Okay, well here, turn up the radio. Do you hear it now?" "Well I can kind of still hear it." "Here, put some earmuffs on." "Yeah, no, now I don't hear it." "Okay, perfect." You haven't done anything to the engine.

Ty: I would fire the mechanic.

Dr. Rashid Buttar: Exactly. And that's the question that when you ask a person, their logical answer is, "Yeah, fire the mechanic." But then why aren't they firing the doctors because that's exactly what the doctors are doing.

Ty: Don't smash your body's check engine light. The tumor is a symptom. Unfortunately, most modern oncologists don't look for the *cause* of the cancer. We're only treating symptoms. But what if you're already on chemo? The good news is that many of these spices and herbs in nature's medicine chest can have a positive effect and actually help chemo be more targeted.

Dr. Sunil Pai: We are able to now with conventional therapies, with natural therapies like I mentioned at the conference here – the Bosmeric-SR, the curcumin, the Boswellin, the ginger, the black pepper, there's a lot of data that will show with the top 15 chemotherapy agents we can help sensitize a tumor. Meaning it takes a toxic agent and makes it more targeted and it also has a protective effect of say oral mucosa damage, heart damage, kidney damage, lung damage, so we are protecting the healthy tissues. So sometimes most people, like we talked about yesterday, most people are going to be getting conventional care. Most people are already in the treatment right now. What can we do to help improve their outcome?

And now the data will show that if you had a physician who actually did some studies, or if you told your oncologist to go on PubMed and look up curcumin or these other chemotherapy agents, you will see now the data will support that using it in conjunction will have a better outcome than just using chemotherapy alone. The fear of chemotherapy is the side effects, right. So people lose weight, they have cachexia, diarrhea, hair loss, you know all these other—the fear of chemo.

Ty: The direct effects of chemo.

Dr. Sunil Pai: The direct effects of chemo, right? And the common effects of chemo. And so everybody is uniquely different when they get chemo. Some people can get chemo and not have much problems, and some people they don't survive even the treatment. And so we want to improve everybody's outcome. And so what the studies will show again—but when we take things like Bosmeric, right, which has a curcumin C3 complex. It has Boswellin-PS, ginger, and black pepper in a special delivery form. During the treatment, in fact, people will do better.

And in fact with our patients we always improve outcomes. A lot of people will call us and say, "I'm already in my sixth round and they are expecting to do another six more. What can I do?" So we're looking at giving natural anti-inflammatories, but these all work on the same pathways, but they also work on preventative and protective pathways. Some of these ingredients like curcumin will increase genetic expression of what we want to turn cancer cells off. So we are not just talking about suppression of cancer growth, we are looking at turning on your own immune system – the inherent ability for the body to heal itself, which is there.

Ty: So is that also considered part of the epigenetics in turning on as well as turning off the expression?

Dr. Sunil Pai: Yeah. Western medicine we have only just to turn off. And that's why when we give some of these agents, they're very good at doing what they're doing. They're turning off certain cells, like cancer cells, but the side effects is they also turn off a lot of normal cells, right? And through that process there is also damage that some of those cells can then become more resistant to chemotherapy over time and they can also genetically change where they start creating more cancer, or secondary cancers, or other chronic conditions down the line.

Ty: Now one treatment protocol that focuses heavily on the diet is the Gerson Therapy, often times called the Gerson Diet. We had the privilege of traveling to Mexico to the Gerson Clinic of Northern Baja, and we interviewed Dr. Patrick Vickers. Now, Dr. Max Gerson was called the greatest genius in medical history by Nobel Peace Prize winner Albert Schweitzer. And the Gerson Therapy relies heavily on the production of energy at the cellular level. Let's have a listen to Dr. Patrick Vickers explain how juicing, which is a staple of the Gerson treatment, fires up the immune system and produces cellular energy.

Dr. Patrick Vickers: When you eat raw fruit, raw vegetables, you're drinking raw juices. Do you know if you tested those juices with litmus paper before they went into your body, they test acidic? They test acidic with litmus paper, but when you drink it that gets broken down into an alkaline ash called potassium hydroxide. The hydroxyl molecule literally goes into your body. Now chemically written a hydroxyl molecule is OH- (oxygen, hydrogen, negative charge). What's hydrogen? The acidic nature of hydrogen is a positively charged hydrogen ion (H+). Imagine what happens when that juice gets broken down into hydroxyl ions (OH-) and reacts with the positively charged hydrogen ion. What reaction do you think takes place? You have an OH- and an H+: two Hs and an O. That reaction forms water. Water is neutral. You neutralize that acidity.

You've now changed the charge at the level of the cell membrane, and you've now just allowed your body to properly oxygenate tissues making the sugars in these fruits and vegetable juices and the natural fruits and vegetables they get at our clinic – they can now be easily converted to massive amounts of energy. And that is what ultimately fires up the immune system and that's why we have the storied history of reversing these advanced diseases.

One of the biggest portions of the therapy is the detoxification procedures of the Gerson Therapy. And the Gerson Therapy has made these famous, and that's the coffee enema. Now, we're talking about the juicing and how the juicing neutralizes that acidity and forms water. Well, if you're forming massive amounts of water in the body like that, what do you think is happening on the cellular level? The toxins are getting flushed out of the cells into the bloodstream. And those toxins, they have to get released.

The coffee enema. Now, people say, "Come on. Now I've heard everything. The coffee enema? I prefer to take mine in the morning first thing when I wake up."

Ty: With cream and sugar?

Dr. Patrick Vickers: With cream and sugar. [laughter] But it's ingenious. Let me explain why. There's a lot of reasons why, but the main reason is this: your liver produces an enzyme. It's called glutathione transferase. Glutathione transferase is the most potent detoxifying enzyme in the human body. The liver produces it. What the liver uses is palmitic acid as the chemical base to produce glutathione transferase. Properly roasted organic coffee – it's lightly, lightly roasted. It's not a drinking coffee. It's a particular bean that's not a drinking bean, and it's also roasted so lightly that you don't denaturize it like you would a drinking coffee. But properly roasted coffee is loaded with palmitic acid.

Studies on coffee enemas have proven that when you do one coffee enema, the production of glutathione transferase by the body goes up 600-700 percent greater than normal. And our patients, they're getting five a day.

In 1959, Gerson wrote a book right before he died. And he theorized the direction he wanted to take his therapy in. He mentioned the word *Coleys*. He mentioned William B. Coley. William B. Coley was a Harvard oncologist. Back in the late 1800s, actually, he discovered that when his patients came down with staph or strep infections their cancers got better, reduced, or went away completely. But once the infection was gone, they started to come back. So what he did was he began to culture the toxins that staph and strep bacteria make, and he began injecting them into the connective tissue of his patients. And he got the same fever response. The patients would break out in fevers and their tumors would reduce.

Laetrile is one of the darling therapies that people come to Mexico for, and they have been coming for years. Laetrile is vitamin B17. It comes from apricot kernel, right? Apricot kernel pits, and its active agent is cyanide, ultimately. And it causes immediate cell death of cancer cells, but it really has to be done in conjunction with hyperthermia. Hyperthermia is—it's been shown that when you do Laetrile with hyperthermia, its effects go up nearly seven to ten fold.

When Thomas Edison said, "The doctor of the future will give no medicine, but will interest his patients in nutrition and caring for the human spine," he was talking about a chiropractor and a Gerson therapist.

Ty: He was a pretty smart fella.

Dr. Patrick Vickers: He was.

Ty: The Gerson Therapy revolves around detoxification, optimizing the immune system, and massive amounts of nutrition. It reminds me of one of my favorite quotes from Chris Wark, who, when he was diagnosed with supposedly terminal colon cancer over a decade ago, he decided that rather than poison his body with chemo, he would "overdose on nutrition." Let's listen to what Chris has to say about nutrition and the immune system.

Chris Wark: The only permanent cure to cancer is your immune system, and nutrition gives your immune system the firepower it needs to keep you well. So without nutrition, you're fighting with no weapons. Without your immune system, you're fighting with no army.

Dr. Jonathan Wright: I picked up that book and went to the University of Washington library. That book had a lot of nice footnotes to the medical studies. And I started, "Oh my gosh. Look at all this stuff about vitamins and minerals and herbs that I never learned in medical school, and it's right there in the medical journal! How come I never learned it in medical school?"

Ty: Dr. Wright never learned this because medical schools do not teach nutrition. But perhaps there are certain things that are self-evident. Perhaps if we really opened our minds we would realize that almost everything in nature is medicine.

Mike Adams: You can't even walk through nature without encountering medicine everywhere. There's an ancient fable in traditional Chinese medicine where a Chinese teacher challenges his students to go out into nature, walk into the forest, and try to find anything that *isn't* medicine. And the students point to the rocks and they say, "Well those rocks – those aren't medicine." And the teacher says, "But of course they are. They're made of minerals. The right minerals with the right treatment can be very medicinal, can be very healing. So, yeah, those can be medicine, too."

And the students point to, "Well the tree bark. That's not medicine." Well of course tree bark is medicine. Where does cinnamon come from? Cinnamon helps regulate blood sugar. It's part of traditional Chinese medicine. Many of the medicinal substances come from bark. Even aspirin is derived from white willow bark that was originally used by the American Indians. So, yeah, of course the tree bark is medicine.

Well the students point to the dirt, "Well, the dirt can't be medicine." "Ah, but the dirt is full of probiotics, living organisms. The right organisms can actually, if you ingest them, enhance your health and protect your health. So those can be medicine, too. Everything around you – what about the sunlight? That's a medicine. What about the tree leaves – that's medicine. What about the air that you're breathing?" Well you can breathe therapeutically. You can reduce stress. You can change your physiology by breathing in the right manner. The water in the stream, not just the water in the stream but the sound of the water in the stream is medicinal.

Ty: Isn't it insane that people sometimes have to risk going to jail to treat their cancer the way that they see fit? Now one substance that people do risk going to jail if they are caught in the possession of the substance is hemp, or cannabis. Sometimes referred to by the slang term marijuana. It's not commonly known that the hemp plant is not only medicine, but it's a super food. And as we are about to hear from Dr. Patrick Quillin who is the former Vice President of Nutrition for the Cancer Treatment Centers of America, he calls it the most useful plant on Earth.

Talk really quickly if you will about the medicinal effects of the hemp plant, or cannabis?

Dr. Patrick Quillin: Hemp cannabis is arguably the most useful plant on Earth. If you do a history of it, you look at canvas which is what our ancestors used for the conestoga wagons and for their clothing—canvas comes from the word cannabis because cannabis was the material that they used to make all of their clothing and canvas. It lasts longer than cotton or polyester. If you go back and look at your history, it was around 1937 when DuPont got its patent for polyester and that was the beginning of the witch hunt to get rid of cannabis because it was competition.

You can use it for paper pulp, for clothing, you can eat it. The food, the seeds are high in omega-3 fats, high in protein. The oils from hemp oil is delicious, nutty-tasting, and high in omega-3s. And then there's the medicinal parts: the cannabinoids. There are many studies that have been done. One of them for instance, the DEA – the Drug Enforcement Agency – decided they wanted to prove how unhealthy marijuana was. And so they went to a major researcher at UCLA, University of California at Los Angeles, and said, "We want you to prove that smoking marijuana causes lung cancer." He said, "Shouldn't be a problem." They did a huge study, a prospective randomized trial. And he said, "Not only it doesn't cause it, it actually helps to prevent it." THC has an anti-cancer property.

I'm not telling people "You should smoke marijuana." I'm telling you that we need to have a rational discussion on marijuana, hemp, cannabis because there's an abundance of data now that says that it's nontoxic and has therapeutic benefits. The CBD – the cannabinoids – apparently there are cannabinoid receptors in the human body. And it's almost as if nature designed—here's lock and key and this fits in and it improves—it's a adaptagen not unlike ginseng or garlic or substances that just make everything work a little bit better.

Dr. Robert Scott Bell: We're learning what's known as, what we all have, an endocannabinoid system or endocannabinoid receptors or cannabinoid receptors within the body. There are certain foods that contain these cannabinoids. There are certain abilities to produce some from within as well. But these receptors are present almost everywhere in the body, particularly heavily entrenched in the gastrointestinal system, the liver, the brain, the nervous system, interestingly enough. And what we're finding, the impact of the two key cannabinoids that are not the only ones: the cannabidiol which is CBD, the non-psychoactive component it's considered and the THC, the tetrahydrocannabinol which you say all so well. And those two aspects, which the THC is considered the psychoactive component and alters the state of the mind, and that's been argued as the dangerous addictive drug. Which now doctors like Sanjay Gupta and others say, "Well, maybe it's not really that addictive at all and in fact it might have benefit."

And we're finding out in relation to certain cancers, not just one or two, but many cancers a tremendous benefit. Some to stimulate the apoptosis, right? The cellular death. Others to address protection of cells, neurological cells, brain and nervous system cells from cancer. A lot of epithelial integrity relying upon the impact of these cannabinoids. We talk about gastrointestinal recovery. Seizure disorders in children and adults – a lot of it is actually sourced right there in that second brain, in the gut. And in these cases we're seeing the use of CBD, sometimes THC, or both together are reversing these cancers and reversing even seizure activity, seizure disorders.

Ty: So are there studies that have shown there's effectiveness of this CBD and THC against cancer?

Dr. Robert Scott Bell: Oh, yes, an incredible amount. It's almost too much to go through if we talk about the references that we have here for breast cancer, colorectal cancer, prostate cancer, stomach cancer, skin cancer, leukemia, lymphoma, lung cancer, uterine cancer, thyroid cancer, pancreatic cancer, cervical cancer, mouth cancer, glioma, brain cancer, and biliary tract cancer.

So we've got a tremendous amount of scientific research. A 2007 Harvard Medical School study published in *Science Daily* showed that hemp's THC decreases lung cancer tumors by 50 percent and it significantly reduces the ability of the cancer to metastasize. I mean, this is huge. Again, this is just one of many things.

Ah, here it is: Cannabinoids – this is directly from a United States patent. This is the shocker. Cannabinoids including THC and cannabidiol promote the re-emergence of apoptosis so that tumors will stop dividing and die. This is a profound—now I'm not one that says there's one panacea that does everything for everyone, but if there was a plant to look at, you know. One plant that does so many extraordinary things, this cannabis plant which is sometimes wrongly referred to marijuana is the slang, or hemp as well, in many forms has so much from a nutritional value but now we learn more and more about its specific value in reversing cancers that are active, much less in their prevention.

Dr. Patrick Quillin: It's not a gateway to more drugs, it's a gateway to health. And, you know, I'm not smoking it, I'm not using it. I think it should be legalized and available and taxed and regulated so that we have standardized concentrations of it. If you compare it to the $280 billion a year drug industry and, according to an article in the *Journal of the American Medical Association*, at least 100,000 Americans die each year from the on-label use of prescription drugs, find me the deaths from cannabis.

Ty: They're not there.

Dr. Patrick Quillin: They aren't there.

Ty: While we were in London, we also had the privilege of interviewing a gentleman named David Hibbitt. Now in July of 2012, he was diagnosed with stage 3 aggressive bowel cancer. He did a couple of rounds of chemo, and he was told twice that he was cancer-free, and that is where our story picks up. The first time that you were told that you were okay, you probably believed it. The second time, were you a little bit more skeptical in light of the fact that it had already returned once?

David Hibbitt: Yeah, well obviously I had that in the back of me mind, but I wanted to believe that I would be okay so I suppose at the time I tried to not think about it too much. And especially just coming out of the chemotherapy as well, and how bad it made me feel I just wanted it to get better. You know, and Christmas was coming up as well, so—

Ty: Right. And you're a young man, so this—How old were you when you were diagnosed?

David Hibbitt: Thirty. I'm thirty-three now. And what happened was it was soon after Christmas when it came back again for the third time, again in the lymph nodes. This time, though, this is when they told me that I was terminal and there was very little they could do.

Ty: What kind of an emotional blow was that, to hear that after the first two—you know, you go through the two rounds of treatments and you were told you were cancer-free twice, and now they say, "Well, actually, it's terminal"?

David Hibbitt: "Can't listen to this." Devastated, completely devastated. I mean I got a little boy who was three or four at the time, and it was just—I couldn't accept it from them. I couldn't believe it, but I struggled to see how I was going to get through it after them telling me, though. And obviously me family, you know, me mum especially—it was devastating for everyone, it really was.

Ty: Where did you go from there?

David Hibbitt: Well, I was actually—I went with the treatment that they offered me. I went on with the chemotherapy. I did that for three months.

Ty: Even though they said it was terminal?

David Hibbitt: Yeah, yeah. Because they told me that this could possibly extend my life. If I didn't start the treatment, he was saying that I had about six months to live and with the treatments, depending on its success, I could have 18 months. And so to me at the time, I thought an extra 12 months with me little boy, "I'll do it." And three months into the chemo, I had another scan and it had been reasonably successful. The tumors had shrunk a bit, but he was still giving me the same prognosis. And it was then, because I started to get a lot more sick three months into it, it was then I was thinking, "You know, I'm not going to last 18 months anyway. My body is telling me, You can't go on no more."

And I'd been told about certain alternative treatments by people leading up to this point, but to be honest with you I didn't actually believe them back then. But it had just come to a point where I knew I had to try something whether I believed it or not. And I looked on the internet, and there was one particular thing that kept coming up more than anything, and seeing a tremendous, insane amount of research done maybe not on humans as such but in a lot of laboratories, so I went ahead with this treatment. Well, it's done really well for me, it really has.

Ty: What did you decide to do?

David Hibbitt: It's cannabis oil. It's extracted from a cannabis plant, and so it has high THC content. It's something that I take orally. I just put a little bit in my mouth and let it absorb. I took this alongside chemotherapy initially for a couple of months, and it made me feel a hell of a lot better just on the chemotherapy. And my hair stopped falling out. The pins and needles that I got from the last chemotherapy, which I was told I'd have that for the rest of my life, actually have disappeared. It started to disappear when I started taking this oil. And I actually started missing chemotherapy sessions then. I only went once a month for the next couple of months, and then eventually stopped at the beginning of August.

I then went on to have favorable scans and the fear of it growing or spreading that the doctors thought was going to happen never happened. They've gone on to remove me lymph nodes. Now the measurement when they took the lymph node out was actually a little bit smaller than what it was after I stopped the chemo. And after the operation, I just changed my diet. I was very healthy. They couldn't give me radiotherapy because I had had the legal amounts already. I didn't want more chemotherapy, so I just carried on with oil and a good diet. This time, the three-month scan was clear. That's the first time this happened for me.

Ty: Now, here in the UK, how do you get hemp oil? Do you have go to the doctor to get it prescribed or?

David Hibbitt: It's actually illegal in the UK.

Ty: Is it? Okay.

David Hibbitt: Yeah, it's illegal medically. It's illegal recreationally. It's not seen as having any medical use in the UK at the moment.

Ty: It's illegal in many states in the United States, too.

David Hibbitt: Yes, yes, I believe it is.

Ty: It depends on the state, but many states it's illegal as well.

David Hibbitt: Yes. A lot of other countries it's still illegal, as well. So I had to—I made some myself by purchasing the cannabis illegally, and I also purchased some oil from what I suppose you would call a local drug dealer.

Ty: Isn't it absurd, David, that you have to go to an underground drug dealer to buy a plant that can heal your cancer?

David Hibbitt: It's crazy. Absolutely crazy. I just don't understand this. I really don't. Now I've gone back to the doctors, who have looked at me records. They are actually telling me to continue doing what I'm doing.

Ty: They're telling you to continue? That's great.

David Hibbitt: Yeah. I've not got it in writing, unfortunately, but if the doctors are willing to say that to me then I can't understand why it's classed as an illegal drug, if you know it's being used for medicinal usage. It just does not make sense. If you looked at me, you know, three months before taking cannabis oil and then looked at me now, the difference, I look ten years younger. I mean, it's truly amazing. My family have commented on it a lot. I personally didn't realize, and then I looked back at photographs and I saw for myself. You know, I was shocked. I really was. It was crazy, but I looked like an old man.

Ty: So after you go through your first scan that is completely clear, and you go home and see your boy. I mean, emotionally, contrast that with how you felt before when you had the diagnosis.

David Hibbitt: Oh, man, I don't know.

Ty: You can't even describe it?

David Hibbitt: It's—it makes me emotional now thinking about it. Honestly, after being told that and then in such a short time as well to get told pretty much the exact opposite it's unreal. And, you know, the journey I've gone through as well in taking the oil. You know, my friends and family didn't want me to do the oil and stop the chemotherapy. Nobody wanted me to because even if you thought it might work and we all hoped it might work, nobody knew. So it's been an emotional roller-coaster and, you know, to get that news! Oh, it's just…

Ty: I bet it was fantastic!

David Hibbitt: Amazing, yeah, surreal. It's…

Ty: And now? Your friends and family now?

David Hibbitt: Oh yeah, yeah, yeah.

Ty: How are they now?

David Hibbitt: Yeah, they're all for it now. And they're backing me to try and get this available to cancer patients should have in this country, I've started off with me own little petition. Because the fact that it's illegal for a cancer patient is just absolutely crazy. And if you want to try it, you should be allowed to. I've even spoken to the police. I won't say the police person's name, but they've told me that if it's for medicinal reasons they don't want to arrest anyone for it. Why would they? The high is a side effect so, you know, if you're not taking it to get high but you're taking it to make you feel a little bit better, I could say, "How could you arrest someone for that?"

I was told I was terminal, and now I'm told I'm not so there is hope there. There's just not me as well, there's plenty of other people that've gone through it. If I can, well they can, too.

Ty: Wow! These stories really give you hope, don't they? One of the things—well actually a couple of things that David was not able to share with us because they hadn't happened yet was number one: he recently had another scan and he was told that he was cancer-free. So that's two scans that he's gotten and he's completely cancer-free. And then, probably even more exciting to David at this point, is just a couple months ago in August of 2015, he got married. Think about how ironic this is. Hemp is natural and it heals cancer. Chemotherapy is synthetic and artificial and often times it kills the cancer patient. It reminds me of a quote from Sir Albert Howard.

Joel Salatin: Sir Albert Howard said, and he is of course the godfather of modern scientific aerobic composting and in his iconic book *An Agricultural Testament* in 1943, he said, "When we feed the soil with artificials" – that's what he called chemical fertilizer, artificials – he said, "when we feed the soil with artificials it creates artificial plants which make artificial animals which make artificial people who can only be kept alive with artificials." If you eat things you can pronounce and you eat things, plants and animals from sources that honor the distinctives, the glory of those beings, the chances are it will honor your place and your glory, as well.

Dr. Darrell Wolfe: If you walk into a grocery store, 90 percent of the groceries in the grocery store are toxic and they'll cause cancer – 90 percent. You know what, if it's not from a farmer it's not worth eating.

Ty: Well, what's your take on the ketogenic diet and cancer?

Dr. Joseph Mercola: Well, I believe it has great value, and in my view should seriously be considered as an adjunctive therapy in the treatment of most malignancies. And you might say, "Why?" Because of the basic understanding that we have of the physiology of cancer cells. And Otto Warburg was awarded a Nobel Prize, I believe in the 30s, for the understanding that the primary fuel for cancer cells is glucose, or sugar. And our non-cancer cells have the ability to use glucose or fat – those are the two primary fuels. And cancer cells seem to have lost this ability, so when you—the unfortunate challenge in contemporary Western countries is that most of us are not very well-adapted to burning fat effectively. And this is an artifact of the way we eat, and the timing of the food that we eat. Primarily it is both. Many people don't understand the timing. We'll talk about the timing in a moment.

So the problem is is that we eat regularly, pretty much three meals a day and then snacks in between, and about the only time when we aren't eating is when we're sleeping. So our body can store sugar as glycogen in our muscles and in our liver, and we have about a 12-hour supply. Some people less and some a little bit more, but in that range. Not a very long supply, where our fat stores can last us for months. So if we're given sugar all the time and we have that fuel available, then there's really limited reason for a body to have the ability to burn fat so it suppresses those abilities of those enzymes and we just eventually forget how to burn fat efficiently or effectively.

So when we shift our diet throughout—primarily through restricting processed foods and especially processed sugars, and change the timing of the food so we have these regular periods when we're not eating for a while – something called intermittent fasting – then we up-regulate those enzymes that burn fat and we can really shift away from having high levels of sugar in our blood which also has the additional benefit of improving insulin resistance. And insulin resistance may be, many experts believe, may be at the core of many of these degenerative diseases and many malignancies. So it's really a challenge to treat a cancer if you have high insulin resistance, so how do you know if you have insulin resistance? Well typically clinically if you are overweight, if you have high blood pressure, diabetes, or if you are taking a statin drug that's a good suggestion, or high blood pressure.

Ty: And how many people? That's like 70 percent of people.

Dr. Joseph Mercola: Well, it's about 70-80 percent and the other way to know for sure objectively is to draw fasting blood insulin – not blood sugar but blood insulin level – and if that's below three then you're fine and if it's above four or five then you probably have it and the higher it is the worse it is. So a simple test to do, very inexpensive, available at any commercial lab across the world, and to me it should be the standard of care in the treatment of anyone with a malignancy to understand what your fasting insulin level is and to control that. Because if your fasting insulin level is low, then that's going to be highly correlated with your body's ability to effectively metabolize fat as a primary fuel. And that's what you want to be able to have that metabolic flexibility, to be able to burn fat or sugar, not just be able to rely on sugar. Because that's going to potentially, and more than likely, feed into the growth and the acceleration of the malignant cells.

There are a number of good studies that show that it's quite effective in treating certain types of malignancies, specifically brain cancers. But they're probably generally used for most malignancies, but the typical strategy one would do is to really focus on the quality of the food and the timing of the food. I like to call it the 3A3, so that is basically don't eat for at least, *at least* three hours before you go to bed. Sleep for eight hours, because sleep is another crucial component for healing and if you're only sleeping four or five hours a night, your body's immune system is not going to be optimized to fight these malignancies.

When you produce energy in your body. It doesn't occur there magically. There's this process that occurs, and you take these substrates – the fuels that are broken down to either the carbohydrate or the fats – and it combines it with the oxygen. There's usually some—like when you're burning any fuel for energy there's by products, right? There's waste products. When you are converting hydrogen to fuel, that's a pretty innocuous by-product, but in our own mitochondria they produce—you have the potential to produce excessive electrons and when you do that your body has to compensate for that with antioxidants.

If you're using the energy, then it's no problem because you generate it, you use it and it flows and there's very little excess waste products. But when you don't use the energy, if you're not being able to burn fat and you have just a lot of sugar that you're building up, then you have this excess energy. And then these electrons build up. It causes massive amounts of free radicals, which can damage your tissues, your cell membranes, your DNA. It can actually prematurely kill your mitochondria, and certainly prematurely age you.

There are many experts who believe in the whole mitochondrial theory of aging, so we want to preserve the function and health of our mitochondria and one of the best ways you can do this is by simple strategies like delaying the time—or not eating before you go to bed. Simple concept, right? But we didn't know that if you eat right before you go to bed, it's one of the worst things you can do because you have all this excess energy that is generating. You don't need energy when you're sleeping, that's when you recover and repair. Your body is more than enough fuelly-compensated for that. When you have extra and surplus energy going around, you actually cause free radical damage.

Ty: Dr. Mercola explained the value of the ketogenic diet coupled with intermittent fasting. Now again, the ketogenic diet is very high in fats, moderate in protein, and very few carbs. But not all fats are created equal. You must have high quality fats. But what exactly are high quality fats?

Dr. Joseph Mercola: High quality fats. An example would be avocados, coconut oil, grass-fed pastured organic butter, ideally raw, olives, nuts would be another good source. And you want to be careful to have relatively low-protein nuts so macadamia and pecans would be the two best because they're high in the fat and very low in the protein. Olive oil would work, too. You want to be careful of avoiding other oils – the omega-6 oils, the processed oils, the industrialized oils.

Ty: All the vegetable oils that people think are healthy because it says "vegetable."

Dr. Joseph Mercola: Oh yeah. That is absolutely the worst because the other factor that is a variable that is really important in the treatment of cancer is something called the omega-6 to the omega-3 ratio, omega-3 being the good fats, of course, like fish oil and ALA from flaxseed and chia seeds. These are beneficial ones, and normally that ratio should be anywhere from 1-to-1 to 5-to-1. The problem is when you have a processed food diet, which is loaded with these Omega-6 industrialized oil, that ratio can go to 20-to-1 to 50-to-1, literally 75 to 100 times what it was last century, around 1900, all because of this industrialization process that allowed us the opportunity to have access to this food. You could not create that food prior to that time. This is really an artifact of modern industry.

Dr. Russell Blaylock: Eliminate things like omega-6 fats, which are cancer fuels: corn oil, safflower oil, sunflower oil, peanut oil, canola oil. They all oxidize. They're all powerful inflammatories, and they promote cancer growth. And that's been proven. It's all through the literature. They make cancer grow faster.

Ty: So omega-6 oils actually make cancer grow faster. Please think twice before you buy another gallon of vegetable oil. Dr. Mercola shared the value of intermittent fasting, but what about fasting in general? Here's Dr. Boris Grinblat from Russia.
So, Boris, talk about the importance of fasting – that fasting might play in overcoming cancer. Because it's very popular in the United States and I know in Russia you mentioned that fasting is done as well.

Dr. Boris Grinblat: Yes, in Russia, it doesn't take much money. Well, cancer cells they differ from regular cells. And we can play on those differences. And one of the differences, they don't take as well heat as normal cells and they cannot survive without food for them, which is usually mostly glucose. So in fasting they suffer more than normal cells. Even for normal cells, it isn't good. They kind of detoxify themselves so nothing bad happening to them, but cancer cells they die. So this is reason why it's good. So it's a plus for normal cells, and it's a minus for cancer cells.

Ty: So the fasting eliminates the food for those cancer cells, but you also mentioned that they don't respond well to heat, so hyperthermia.

Dr. Boris Grinblat: Absolutely. In Russia what they do—it's a famous Russian banya or sauna—so in the clinics it's hyperthermia. So you can do it a double-whammy. You can do fast, and then you can do this hyperthermia in Russian banya. So you can use this normal physiological difference of cancer cells and kill them with heat and with fasting.

Ty: Speaking of fasting, someone recently told me that the only way they could afford to be healthy was too fast. They couldn't afford to buy organic food. That seems extreme. Is it true?

One of the things that I hear a lot is, "You know, I can't afford to eat organic food. I know I should, but I can't afford it." So what's your response to someone that says that?

Joel Salatin: Sure. Well, there are several answers. One is that if you buy in volume, you can save a lot of money. So get a freezer, alright—I mean, you know, we're in the animal business so I'm thinking frozen beef and chicken or whatever. But you can get a huge price break if you buy in volume. Number two, look in the mirror and ask yourself, "Is there anything that I'm buying that I don't need?" And whenever anybody says that, I want to grab them and say, "Okay, take me to your house and here's what we're not going to find, I'm sure, at your house. We're not going to find soda. We're not going to find lottery tickets. We're not going to find $100 designer jeans with holes already in the knees, coffee, alcohol, Hot Pockets, frozen, microwaveable dinners, french fries. I mean you can go down the list, okay?" And the truth is there aren't very many households that don't have those things in them, and none of that is actual nutrition. None of it.

I went to New York City's Union Square Green Market, arguably the most expensive farmer's market in the world, and I asked my hostess, I said, "Could you take me to the most expensive potato in the New York City Union Square Green Market?" She said, "Yes, I know just the guy." So she elbows her way through, and we go up and we get to this potato guy. And he's got, you know, about 30 potatoes out there. There's red ones and white ones and blue ones and green ones and orange ones and fat ones and long ones and skinny ones and all this stuff. So I looked through all the little boxes there and I find the most expensive one. It's an heirloom Peruvian blue fingerling potato. And it's $1.99 a pound. But that whole market is surrounded by supermarkets with 100 feet of fluorescent-lighted, handicapped-accessed retail floor space selling french fries and potato chips for $3.00 a pound.

Sayer Ji: In some cases, organically produced produce will have 100 times higher polyphenols, so when you look at the ultimate price you're paying, you know, maybe it's 50 percent more for organic but you're getting 100 times more value as an anti-cancer nutrient. It's clearly a better value, especially since when you price cancer you're talking about $1 million and financial bankruptcy, not to mention all of the suffering that it causes.

Ty: And Sayer is right, folks. These conventional treatments, they do create a lot of suffering. And nobody wants to see a cancer patient suffer. I can't imagine what it would be like to witness the suffering day in and day out, but many of the practitioners that we interviewed that's exactly what they do. They've dedicated their lives to helping to alleviate the suffering. And we got insight into one of those doctors when we were in Mexico, Dr. Patrick Vickers. And in this next clip he shares with us some heartfelt emotions about the suffering and helping cancer patients.

Dr. Patrick Vickers: Well people come into our clinic for three weeks, and they live with us, and we bond with them and they bond with us. And then they go home, and they continue their therapy at home. And so, you know, when you're dealing with that kind of, I don't know what you would call it, you would call it gravity. That kind of gravity, you know, the perspective on life as you and I know it, it changes. And we live our lives a lot of the time to satisfy ourselves and be entertained, but when this is happening in front of you, things tend to take on a more serious nature. And I think that's how it's changed me the most is

I don't really live anymore to please myself. I live to save these people's lives, and my staff live to save these people's lives.

It's an incredible responsibility, first of all. Like I said, they're coming to us as a last resort, as a last resort of hope to save their lives and so when I hear the children—really, what really touches us the most is when we have these young couples come in and they have children. And they'll have two, four, six-year-old children. The ones you saw were 13, 15, 17, and 18. But Katrina who was also there with us, she has a two-year-old, a four-year-old, I think an eight-year-old. I mean, when you consider the fact and the gravity of what happens if they don't make it and who are they going to leave behind, it just makes our job that much more important and that much more vital to their story.

It's a deep burden for us. We don't take these things lightly. We know what's going on behind the scenes in their life. We know what they're fighting for and what they're living for and it just takes on that added burden to what we're doing. And, quite frankly, you do feel a heavy weight on your shoulders. Not to feel like a martyr or anything, that's not what we do. That's not how we feel, but it's a sincere burden that we feel and we know, especially when there's children involved like you experienced because, like I said, those children they know what's going on and they don't want to lose their parents.

Every day. Every day. Every day I feel that burden, but you can't walk away because nobody in the world knows what we know. And to walk away from that would be walking away from your creator, which is what you were intended to do.

Karen Berrios: My family and I went to Peru last summer on a family trip. I'm originally from Peru, and so is my husband. And it was the first time that we were taking the kids. And the first place that we stopped was up north, north Peru, to visit my dad. He insisted that I would go and see a doctor because I usually have this tendency to break out, and he said, "Let's go and see a dermatologist up there." And so I did, and so she recommended for me to see an endocrinologist. And so the doctor there checked me completely, and she said, "I feel a lump on your neck." And she sent me for an ultrasound, and it was really funny that the radiologist is the one that did the ultrasound. It's not a technician like in the US. So when he was doing the test, the scan, he was really freaked out. He was afraid. And I knew something was wrong then.

I walked away from the office and I decided to put it on hold, since we were there for three weeks. I came back to the US, and I had a biopsy, and it turned out to be thyroid cancer. The word cancer is usually tied into death, you know, pain, brokenness, oppression. I knew right away that was not me. That's not where God wanted me. And that's why he led me to find it, and from then on I don't even know how to call this – intuition. I knew I did not want to do anything conventional. Although I didn't know that this whole new world of holistic existed, you know. I didn't know you could cure cancer with nontoxic treatments. But it was the beginning of this new journey of discovery, and that's how it all started.

I was told that I needed surgery right away, radiation, and I said no. And it's not that I was afraid. I just knew that it wasn't for me, that's not the path for me to heal. As you see, the ocean right here. If we allowed our emotions to lead us in our healing path, we are going to be going back like the waves, back and forth. Right? I don't want to be like the waves back and forth. I want to be still and continue taking one step at a time into my healing, towards my healing journey which is my ultimate goal.

So when I was first diagnosed, the doctor couldn't tell me whether or not after surgery the cancer could come back. So I chose to follow this nontoxic treatment approach. And it was pretty scary, because again you're going against the flow. Everyone around you tells you you're crazy. But that was what I decided to do, and I've never done anything like this. I didn't know what to expect. But even the doctors don't know what to expect. They don't know, they can't tell you. There are no guarantees. But I chose this path for me, and it has worked. It's working. It's working. So my—the tumor. The tumor has shrunk dramatically and my lab work shows, reflects that the tumor markers have decreased approximately 65 percent in the past five months, which is amazing. And it will continue, it will continue to decrease until it's gone.

Ty: Wow! What an episode we had for you today. Now this was a bit of a roller coaster, I know. But I also know that you gained a lot of insights through the topics covered and through the incredible experiences of our experts. How amazing it is that the small things in life really mean the most. Perhaps many people are unsuccessful in treating their cancer because they are looking in the wrong places.

For instance, nutrients are perceived as small things, when in reality they are of paramount importance. And speaking of small, micronutrients are some of the smallest things, but it's these micronutrients that are some of the biggest allies in winning the battle against cancer. You've seen that micronutrients actually aid the body in stopping tumor formation (angiogenesis, which is the formation of new blood supply), metastasis (proliferation of cancer), and they even induce apoptosis, which is programmed cell death. You've learned that rather than perceiving cannabis as the "devil's weed," maybe we should think of it as "heavenly hemp" due to its plethora of medicinal uses and that it's best understood as a friend, rather than a foe when it comes to cancer treatment.

You've again seen the devastating reality of the brave heroes that have undergone heartache and loss, sacrificing their own personal assets and security, for the sake of their patients' lives.

Missing peptides like antineoplastons have successfully been used to heal a multitude of so-called terminal cancer patients. And finally, you've seen that no matter what your background or family lineage, you are not destined to end up with the same disease as your parents. You've seen that the science of epigenetics proves you have the ability to choose your own path and cultivate your own health and healing, irrespective of your genetic predisposition.

We have good news for you in this moment. You *are* free. And the prison of death and disease is behind you. You and your loved ones are free to step outside the cancer box, which is full of lies and confusion, into a beautiful world which beckons you with all the things you desire and deserve.

We covered a lot of ground in this episode, but we know from experience in our last documentary, the next episode the final episode, is going to be the most inspiring and it's going to give you hope. Why? Because the next episode is totally dedicated to sharing cancer conqueror stories and that's what you're going to get. So thanks for joining us, and I know we are going to see you again tomorrow. Have a great evening, and God bless all of you!

[*credits roll*]

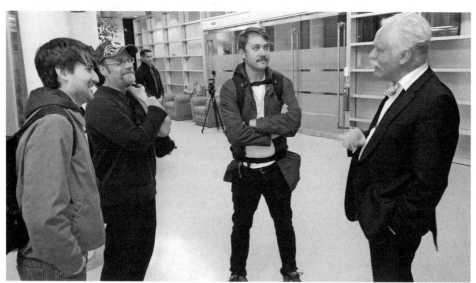

Zach, Alan, and Travis with Dr. Gorter at his clinic in Cologne, Germany

The Truth About Cancer

A

GLOBAL
QUEST
Episode 9

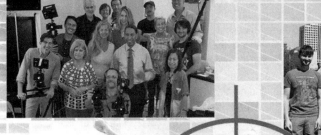
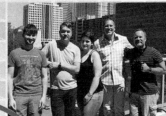

Cancer Conquerors & Their
Powerful Stories of Victory

The **TRUTH** About
CANCER ™
educate • expose • eradicate

Ty: This episode is going to inspire you and it's going to give you hope. Oftentimes, when a person is diagnosed with cancer they're afraid, but it doesn't have to be that way. These stories are going to show you that there is life after a cancer diagnosis. These cancer conquerors are actually healthier and happier after they've made it through cancer. This episode will inspire you. It will give you hope. This is our gift to you. So, sit back and enjoy the episode.

Michael Stephenson: I don't think I have the ability to put it into words. It is so amazing, so humble, so awesome to go. I have been blessed, I have been given a second chance. I took the road less traveled, and that has made all the difference.

Dr. Antonio Jimenez: And he really took it. He walked the walk, walked the talk and made the changes, changed his lifestyle and he went for it 110 percent.

Michael Stephenson: I can tell you this, he may have been two-years-old, but if you say Dr. Tony, he knows exactly who we're talking about. Because Dr. Tony is a hero, and revered in our home. That's pretty amazing, huh? You know, a two-year old. You know you have arrived when a two-year old remembers you and goes, "Dr. Tony. Oh, yeah. Dr. Tony in Mexico." He does know when you were there getting treated because you were sick. He doesn't know the cancer, he doesn't know the gravity of it, but he knows that you were really sick. His grandfather passed away and had cancer, and it was horrible, but he got to go the way he wanted to go, and he didn't get treatment. It was a sad situation. But, what we tell Dylan, because this is what he can't understand, when his granddad passed away, he flew away with the birds and one day we'll fly away with the birds and see him, and that he can understand. So, it is putting it into words. It's so heartfelt, it's so emotional for me to go. When I walked in here today, I walked around and went outside. That's how it felt, and then we just thank you. Thank you.

Jared Bucey: I didn't really know too much about cancer or chemo, and I didn't think that there is much of a cure for cancer. I thought cancer pretty much is my death right on the spot. I did one round, one full cycle of chemo and then all the side effects were just so severe. I had really bad mouth sores throughout my whole GI system. I had really bad bone pain. I couldn't stand, I couldn't walk. My parents had to help me walk to the bathroom and back. I could barely use my phone or the TV remote because my hands were cramping from the bone pain.

Eventually, I just felt, in my heart and soul that I was going to die in the next round because all those side effects were killing me. We went in to get the pick line taken out and then I said that I was done and I didn't want to do chemo anymore. They explained to me how it would be like to die if I didn't do chemo. They said that it would feel like I was drowning underwater. So, they asked if I ever – I felt like I was holding my breath under water, and they said that it would be like that except I won't come out for air.

Ty: It sounds like they trying to scare you—

Jared Bucey: Trying to bully me.

Ty: —and to bully you into doing chemo after you told them you don't want to. Telling you if you don't, you're going to eventually suffocate like you're drowning, if you don't do chemo. So, you decide against chemo, and that's you know now as Jared the kid against chemo. That's how we first learned about you, was on Facebook, kid against chemo. So, you decided not to do any more chemo, and what did you do at the point you said, "I am not going to do chemo, but I am going to do this"? What did you said to do for your cancer at that point?

Jared Bucey: I just do all alternative methods from vitamins, supplements, infrared sauna, all organic juice, and all raw vegetables.

Ty: Sounds kind of like Chris Wark.

Jared Bucey: Yeah, exactly.

Ty: That's what Chris did.

Jared Bucey: Exactly.

Ty: But, you're out now, how are you feeling?

Jared Bucey: I feel great. The last blood test we took, all my cancer markers were normal. All my blood tests were normal, and everything was just normal and great.

Jordan S. Rubin: I started in my journey in a natural health from day one. I was born at a naturopathic university. My father was a naturopathic student at the National College of Naturopathic Medicine outside of Portland, Oregon. I like to say I was born with a silver sprout in my mouth. So, in the 70s, eating healthy, cleansing, detoxification, chiropractic was not common place. However, my parents were non-conformists, I guess you could call them hippie health nuts in the 70s. They started in Kansas and then moved to Oregon to follow the school, and my dad was all about natural health. I think for fun, they would all take activated charcoal and measure each other's transit times. You know what I'm talking about.

This was way before anything was accepted. It was definitely outside of the norm, so to speak. I was born in a naturopathic university, wasn't vaccinated, was really ushered into the natural health movement. But as a child, I only thought about what I couldn't do, what my restrictions were. The health foods, back in the day, were very limited. I think we had seaweed, there was wheat germ, brewer's yeast, and all manner of soy products, nothing like today. No big health food stores, everything was small and niche.

However, growing up having a healthy constitution was part of my life. When I was 15 years of age, I was threatened by my school that if I was not vaccinated for measles, mumps, and rubella, I would be suspended. My father said, "Take the suspension, it's not worth it." One little needle and a second time may have contributed to my diagnosis of Crohn's Colitis three years later. It was in the midst of a very fun and successful college career that I was blindsided by these digestive and immune system issues. I went from 185 pounds at nearly 6'1" – college athlete, just on fire for God, on fire for life to being bedridden, suffering for two years with now 18 medical conditions. I had diabetes, I had symptoms of rheumatoid arthritis, parasites, fungal infection, bacteria, a lot of what is now implicated in the disease that we collectively call "cancer."

Nearly a year later, I met a man who taught me how to eat and live like the Bible says. It's really the Bible meets history, meets modern science. Out of that experience of 40 days, just living and eating the way my ancestors did, I overcame my diseases in just 40 days, of what I later called *The Maker's Diet: The 40-Day Health Experience*. I not only got well, but I had a new mission in life. I went from having a certain path, to knowing that my life was going to be about helping others either overcome disease, or better yet, avoid it.

Out of that, I started a company called Garden of Life, where we manufacture whole food nutritional supplements. Later, I would write 25 books on health and wellness. Recently, I became an organic farmer, and now I'm really on a similar quest as you. I would love to see this disease – this group of challenges and attacks on our body – that we call cancer, be ameliorated. I believe we can, but nothing prepared me for the shock in 2008 that I received. Now, I had written books, not only *The Maker's Diet*, but an entire series on specific health issues and diseases including *The Great Physician's Prescription for Cancer*. I helped my own grandmother have a great result with cancer. I've coached thousands of people over the years. But in 2008, due to a surgery that I should have had at birth, at least my parents should have considered it, I was led into something in 2008 that, once again, changed my life forever, and it was a cancer diagnosis.

Ty, I was really at a crossroads because here I was helping, in my mind, be part of the solution and all of a sudden I was not only dealt the blow of a cancer diagnosis, but I had to deal with, like so many others, the waiting game of, "Have we gotten it all? Has it spread?" I had what they call an exploratory surgical procedure in my pelvic cavity, thinking it was a hernia, and it ultimately was an advanced form of embryonal testicular cancer. Now, the reason being for me is I had an undescended testicle that was never operated on that lodged in my pelvis, not knowing there was a thousand-fold increase in cancer risk. Here I am, thinking it was a surgical procedure for an inguinal hernia or what they call a sports hernia, and instead I was given a cancer diagnosis.

The doctor walked back in. My wife and I were sitting there and he said, "You have a fast growing form of cancer." He said, "There are treatments now that can help you. Years ago, this cancer killed *everyone* who was diagnosed with this progressive state." I said,

"Doc, God is going to heal me and I need time. I need time to attack this." He said, "I was afraid you would say that. I looked you up online. I know who you are." He said something I won't say on camera, but he said, "Don't [blank] around with this. If you wait for conventional treatment, you will be dead within three months. 100 percent chance."

Jill Schneider: I just looked at the doctor and I said, "I think this is something that I need to do some research on and begin a program of nutrition." He looked at me as though I was completely off the wall and he slammed the door in my face. I just walked out of the doctor's office, and I knew I never wanted to see that person again. That evening, I had to perform – I'm a singer/songwriter/guitarist – on a radio station. From the time I had the appointment, I found out that I had malignant cervical cancer, until I sang that night because I knew I couldn't sing if I had fear, I gave it up, gave up all the fear. What point would it have in my life at that moment?

Shortly after that, I quit a job that was very stressful. I knew I had to leave the country just to have the time to take care of myself. So, a month later – after a month of acupuncture and herbs – I had another test, it had already gone to a number three. I said, "I'm clear. This is a piece of cake. I'm off to South America. I'm going to hang out in the jungle for a while and then go down to Peru and do some hiking, Machu Picchu, 1975."

Ty: So, you already saw progress within a month, and then you left.

Jill Schneider: Yeah. Then I left to go and really have a real health vacation. I went to hot springs, I hiked in the mountains, I ate their food, I lived. Immediately, as soon as I got home, I was responsible. I went to the doctor, and it went from a five to a one in five months, and two and a half years later, I had a child, and now I'm a grandmother of two little girls.

Ty: Wow. Congratulations!

Enoch DeBus: 2009, I came down with basal cancer. It was on my—

Ty: You had basal cell carcinoma?

Enoch DeBus: Yes, I did. On my cheek, between my eyes, and on my arm, they did a biopsy and came back positive. When I went to the dermatologist—I knew I had it in 2009. I didn't go until 2010. The one in between my eyes wouldn't stop bleeding, so I went to my chiropractor friend, Linda Force – fantastic woman, I've known her for many years, precious woman of God, and she's one of the best chiropractors I've ever been to. She's got a big practice in Canton, and her name is Linda Force, and she's got the force, I tell you. To work with people in chiropractic, and she loves the Lord. She says, it's where the force comes from, and I agree with her. I'm sure you do, too. But she says, "Enoch, you need to get that checked out." She said, "I think you have cancer." I said, "Yeah, I know it is. I can't imagine me getting cancer," but I said, "You know, I've had so many poisons all throughout my life, all these toxins, so it's probably hit me."

Because I was going through a stressful time, 2008 the bottom dropped out. I had been audited with the IRS. They did some things to me that we won't repeat. I went to the dermatologists that Linda recommended – was a friend of hers – and she looked at me, she had me take my shirt off, she checked my body over. She says, "Normally, I have my clients come in once every quarter," she says, "You're going to be coming in every three weeks." I said, "I'm that bad?" She said, "You're that bad," I said, "Wow, you got me by surprise." She said, "Let's send these out, see what it is." So, I went back, the test was positive, and I said, "What can I do to help?" She said, "Not a thing," she said, "Basically, this is from all the sun you've got over the years."

Ty: So, she said nothing you could do?

Enoch DeBus: She said, "There's nothing I can do." She said, "The damage is done." I asked, "What happens if I don't get the surgery?" She looked at me very seriously. She was a young gal, a little-bitty thing, and she had a nurse in there, she says, "If you don't get this done in six months, you'll be totally blind, and 12 months from that you'll be a dead man." I said, "For sure?" She says, "Yeah," and I said, "Thank you," and she set up an appointment for the surgeon, I said I would go see him. I walked out of there and I shook my head, I said, "I'm not buying it."

I went home and I got on my knees. I said, "Father, you know the results of the test and everything," I said "You're in charge of everything, you created me." I said, "I am not going to have them cut up my face," I said, "I'm ready if you're ready. If it's my time," I say, "I've been ready for a long time." I said, "I enjoy living, and I enjoy sharing the good news, and I enjoy—I love people, you know that," I said, "But I'm not going to be cut up." I said, "So, either please give me the wisdom, what I can do on my part so you can do your part."

Right after prayer, all of a sudden I had ginger came to my mind. Ginger and hot peppers and all that, and nobody's ever told me about this. I went and I got a bunch of organic ginger, I got habaneros, jalapenos, and there's other a couple of other hot peppers at the time, tabasco pepper, and another one. I took them, cleaned them, chopped up the ginger. I had no directions, no recipe, and I put that in as soon as it hit a boil, I turned it down to brew, just simmer. After 30 minutes, I found myself putting these peppers in there, and I cleaned them and I chopped them up, seeds and all for about 10 minutes and then I stopped it, let it cool off. I put it in a blender and I ground them all up, and I took off the lid and it about blew me back. I mean it did really took my breath away. It was powerful.

So, I put that in a jug, and I had about a half a gallon of it. I filled it up with filtered water and I tried it, about burned my tongue off. I cut it and I added some other stuff to it. I put cilantro in it, but I put it in as I drank it. I had that as a stock and I'd take it and cut it each day when I use it. Basically, I would take it for my workout – I go to the gym – and I noticed that it gave me a kick.

Ty: Kick 'em juice.

Enoch DeBus: I named it right then and there. I said, "Man, this is kick 'em juice."

Ty: So, this kick 'em juice, is this what you attribute to curing your cancer?

Enoch DeBus: So, this kick 'em juice is what I thought the Holy Spirit inspired me to make, and the bleeding stopped within days. It healed and filled up completely. I had just started taking it, within two days. I went to the surgeon because I was scheduled to go there, and he was a tall – about 6'8" – young Jewish man. I really respected him. He was very respectful. When he came and he said, "I'll be right back." The nurse came and I said, "What a doctor, he's really fantastic." She said, "His wife's just like him when she comes here – precious people."

So, he came back in, he measured me, and he tried to prepare me in a gentle way. He said, "We'll do this at first and maybe we won't have to do radiation, or chemo, or that, you know." I said, "How long do I have that I can wait before we start to do this?" He said, "Well, I wouldn't go more than a month." I said, "Okay, I'm going to take that month," I said, "I'm trying something new." He said, "Okay, you'll survive for a month," and he said, "We'll contact you in about a month." So, sure enough, they contact me a little after a month and I said, "I won't be coming in, I don't think I'll need it." I said, "It's all calmed down, I don't have any problems, you know." I said, "I think the good Lord touched me and healed me."

Pamela Bost: When the doctor came in and said, "Jonathan, we're going to go and we're going to put a port within you, you've got cancer and you need to be hospitalized for the next few weeks." He confidently walked over to me and said, "Mama, don't let them do this to me. Mama, don't let them take me away." I don't know if you have children, but I know that any mama or papa that is listening to my words now, I know they can identify with that feeling of helplessness. Imagine looking at your son, he just got the notice that he had cancer just moments before, and there's nothing I can do. There's nothing I can say that will change the outcome whatsoever.

We had a choice at that point, but I can't emphasize to you enough how very much it felt like we were just cattle being processed through the system. I live seven miles from the Mexican border. Every day, I wondered if I cross over, could I change and have a positive influence in the outcome of the situation that my son at five years old is facing? I have seven other children besides Jonathan, and I'm afraid it's the greater of the whole, if you will, at this point than it was for the one individual. And, at some point, I always felt like there was a hope. Quite honestly, I didn't believe that the doors were closed as shut so tightly as they were.

I truly thought that I would have a voice. I knew about integrative medicine. I knew there were herbal remedies and options. I did not know that pediatric cancer was so different. It is completely a different animal. It is a nightmare. You have no voice. You have no say. Every day, when I go in and I hand my child his chemo, I have to remember that it's me that signed on that dotted line, that form that they make you sign, and it's me that's handing it to my child every single day. I know the end result is that my child will come out. Our hope is that our child will come out a healthy individual.

Is there a way that we could accomplish this without violating everybody involved? I understand that they are experts in the field that they are experts in. I understand that they speak a language that is different than me. But should it be that I don't have a voice, that we don't consider other options that we don't listen to other people? That we listen to Jonathan? It's a horrifying, helpless experience that I wish on no one.

Dr. Morten Hekneby: I got very high inflammation and CRP.

Ty: C - reactive protein, sure.

Dr. Morten Hekneby: It was really high and my blood pressure went down, and I was resuscitated one time in the hospital. Just one week after, they let me go from the hospital.

Ty: So, they thought you were gone a few times. Did you ever get the family together and say, "Hey, Dad's not gonna make it?"

Jacqueline Hekneby: We were not aware. We never thought about death. I don't know why, but in six months, with him being 55 and never been ill before, we actually didn't think about him dying. It wasn't until two days before Christmas, they called wanting him for a meeting when they said that this could be literally only three months to live. So, it complicated his body for many years, because it really came up on the PET scan all over the body. They literally said, "Well, we'll call you in a week's time and see the result, tell you the results of the PET scan." They called 8 AM the next morning to get to the doctor before 9.

Dr. Morten Hekneby: And it was lightening up all over my body, except the brain. So, they thought I had metastasis all over, in the bone marrow, lymph system, lungs, all over. It was very serious.

Ty: How is it that you're standing here with us in Amsterdam today? Why are you alive? What happened?

Dr. Morten Hekneby: [chuckles] You can tell that story because you are the reason for it, and you are actually a reason for it [indicating Ty] too. You're the main reason actually.

Jacqueline Hekneby It's quite crazy really, because the doctors basically gave up. Morten was just getting worse and worse over that period when he was in their care. After last visit to the hospital with a biopsy, it's just was really bad. You weren't producing enough white blood cells, you didn't produce any hormones, your heart was beating irregularly.

Dr. Morten Hekneby: I got chronic obstructive lung disorder. I have that now. I got jumping heart, atrial fibrillation, and a lot of diagnosis.

Jacqueline Hekneby: He had no energy at all, absolutely no energy. He couldn't take a single conversation, couldn't walk down the stairs, nothing. He said walking down the stairs on Christmas Day was like running several kilometers. That's when it hit us that Morten was dying. It hit so hard. I had no idea. I wasn't prepared, so the first day I just screamed like a pig that had been stuck with a dagger, and the kids were just clinging to me. The second day, I went out in the garden, and I just prayed because I've done it before when I had a crisis with you before. I said, "Lord, I just need you. You're just going to have to guide me." I felt the Lord say, "Put Morten in a chair and get the family to pray." So, I gathered the family, and we're quite a big family. Everyone laid hands on Morten and we prayed, and we all felt peace, which was very strange in that situation. When you have peace, you're able to think straight.

Then, I remembered your book, and I hadn't thought about that for the whole six months when Morten was ill because the doctors were taking care of him. When they were out of the picture, I picked up the book and—you tell me if I'm wrong, but I picked it up and I opened it up and I read, "If you've been given a diagnosis to terminal cancer, you've still got a 90 percent chance of survival." I've never found that again since. But when I read that to you, it's like the blood came back into your veins, it gave hope. I just started by saying to Morten, "Okay, I want to give it a go, give it a shot. We'll start with no sugar today, and no alcohol, and keep off the white flour."

That was two days after Christmas and then the shops are opened. I literally took everything out of the cupboards - all the food, all the skin products, hair products – and I put them on the front door and I put on Facebook that if anybody wants them, they can come get them. I went down to the health shop and I re-stocked with everything organic. Our second daughter, Ann, she just dropped everything to be my right hand, and I admit that it took two people full time job to do this. People need to know that it's a lot of work. Then I remembered what you had to do with the food. So, I made a list for my daughter of the food that was supposed to be cancer-fighting, like garlic and ginger. Ann made a plate of lovely food. We started with a Budwig diet in the morning. Then this plate of raw food that you had to chew. She made it look beautiful, but it was pretty awful, some of it. Then in the evening, she made an Indian curry out of all these ingredients that were cancer-fighting. So, I started to talk to this Dr. Mike Farley. I don't know if he likes his name mentioned or not.

Ty: That's okay.

Jacqueline Hekneby: I learned a lot from him. He just gave everything to help me with Morten. He made a herbal mixture.

Ty: Yeah, Dr. Farley developed LifeOne.

Jacqueline Hekneby: Yeah, LifeOne was—well, it had cured over 3,000 terminal cancer and AIDS patients in eight years with that, and he thought he was going to get a medical prize for it, but he wasn't very popular when he made it. It took about a month to get it into Norway because the toll system. It's really, really strict in Norway.

Dr. Morten Hekneby: But it worked.

Ty: It worked, didn't it?

Dr. Morten Hekneby: And he was a fantastic support,

Jacqueline Hekneby: It was amazing.

Dr. Morten Hekneby: We were talking sometimes, and he was—

Jacqueline Hekneby He was amazing.

Dr. Morten Hekneby: He was an amazing person.

Jacqueline Hekneby: We're still in contact with him. But basically, really honestly, four days after I changed the products out, you started to feel stronger, less pain, breathing easier.

Ty: Really? Four days is all it took to see a difference?

Jacqueline Hekneby: Yeah.

Dr. Morten Hekneby: More color, strength, yes.

Jacqueline Hekneby: We all saw it, and you felt it, but your eyes were still really yellow. At the time, Morten said, "Are my eyes yellow," and I said "no," because I knew that if he knew his eyes was yellow he would understand the seriousness of his situation. So, I didn't tell him, but I didn't know if I had the time. I could see it was working, but I really didn't know if I had the time. So, every night when we went to bed, I wasn't sure Morten would be awake in the morning. It was that bad. We didn't get in LifeOne for a month, but basically this process, Morten went back to work in two months.

Dr. Morten Hekneby: The core in it was the information from your book, and that strengthened you up. You strengthened me up, and we changed the diet totally.

Jacqueline Hekneby: Totally, 100 percent straight.

Dr. Morten Hekneby: That made me get—go from 3 or 4 percent energy to 20 percent, but that was huge difference in four days and I knew I would live.

Jacqueline Hekneby: By two months, you were about 60 percent, I think, if I remember correctly.

Ty: And within two months, he was back to work?

Jacqueline Hekneby: Yeah, he wasn't 100 percent at all, but he was probably up to about 60 percent. I was thinking, "There must be more to this. We can do more than this." That's when you called me in May 2013 and told me about the Moringa product. It takes time to understand that product, even if you know a lot.

Ty: It's a product that has just amazing amounts of nutrition.

Jacqueline Hekneby: That's right, and the body can take it up 99 percent. I got in the country and I saw the difference it made in Dr. Morten Hekneby, and I started taking it myself, and it completely changed my life as well. Morten has never had any medication since I took over. It's now going how long, two and a half years?

Dr. Morten Hekneby: I was thinking if I had taken chemotherapy or cortisone, I think I wouldn't live today.

Chris Pederson: March 2009, my husband brought home a book that I read cover to cover and it was Verne Verona's *Nature's Cancer Fighting Foods*, and I embraced everything in that book. The next day, after I had my cry-pity-party, "I can't do this," I changed my diet the next day. I'm very disciplined, I got that from my dad. I'm very disciplined, so I stuck with it, just all kinds of vegetables. I'd cut up vegetables and I'd make my own dressing. I didn't even have lettuce in it either. I would just cut up a variety of vegetables and eat those and that was my main meal, my main thing. Then I would juice and blend those, and do all different things.

Ty: You were getting serious nutrition.

Chris Pederson: I was getting serious nutrition. I also added some, very few, but a few supplements and an herbal combination. B17 I took that. So, I took these things and then went through those, still removing the polyps. About a year onto my whole diet, big regimen change, I had zero polyps.

Ty: Wow. That's amazing. How did that make you feel?

Chris Pederson: That made me feel great. It was really a blessing.

Ty: The fruits of your one year labor of being so disciplined and strict eating paid off quickly.

Chris Pederson: Very much. I was ready to shout it from the mountain tops because I had beat genetic cancer. To be honest, when I started out, I wasn't sure, but I had been doing tons of research on my gene to figure out what it was and what it was all about. It had only been discovered in 2002. I wasn't really sure what the effect would be, but I started looking into this new science called Epigenetics. Epigenetics simply said it's being affected by your environment to change your genes. Well, the first thing that you can control about your environment is what you put in your body, and so I was doing that. I started feeling like, "Okay, this can probably work." When it did work, I was just thrilled.

Now, the interesting thing is the doctor who did that colonoscopy, I thought he would be, "What did you do? Tell me all about it," because I told them that I was doing a diet. I was really making big changes there. He walked in, handed my husband the pictures of my colon, he just said, "You're clear," and walked out the room. That's the only words he said, and I was still reeling from the anesthesia, but I wanted to scream at him, "Don't you want to know about what I do so you can share that with your other patients?"

Ty: What's your message to cancer patients that may have been told they have some kind of a genetic cancer? What is your message that you want them to take away from this interview?

Chris Pederson: Well, I tell friends of mine who complain about, "Well, you know, the genes in my family," and I just shake them off and say, "Look at me. Look what I did and you can do it, too. You just have to make some changes in your life."

Jordan S. Rubin: I immediately began a program that involved spiritual, mental, and physical health. I want to be very clear, spiritual is first. I did end up really attacking my diet. For the first few weeks, I was on an all raw diet. I postponed the Boston trip – I did go. I wanted to be responsible. So, 40 days, I went to my team at Garden of Life and I told them what had happened to me. They we're freaked out. I said, "Listen, God has already paid the price for me. I am healed, you're going to see it, but I need to step away from work. Six weeks, you won't hear from me, no emails, no texts." For me, Ty, that's a miracle if I can go 30 minutes without that, much less six weeks.

I did the opposite of what most cancer patients do. You see, cancer patients go and basically submit themselves to the convention, and it's easy, "Well, what do you mean, it's easy? You have side effects and hair loss." No, it's easy because you let someone else tell you what to do. You let somebody else tell you how your side effects are going to go, what's going to happen, what your outcome is going to be, what your prognosis is. They can do radiation, chemotherapy and surgery, but they're doing it. You don't have to think for yourself. There is no individuality, you're just a number. But I said, "You know what, I'm doing this, I'm going to go after it in every way."

Twelve to 14 hours a day Ty, spiritual, emotional, healing, nutrition, and detoxification. I started with spiritual. I had written a prayer that really was a combination of scripture and some great teachers, and I quoted it three times a day out loud, and I honestly felt like the demons in hell were holding their ears like a dog whistle to a dog. I mean, I was storming the gates of hell to get well here. Some people will say, "But Jordan, I don't share the same faith as you." All I can tell you is if you're desperate enough, you will find God, on your knees, because I believe in essence, cancer is a spiritual disease. Cancer attacks the spirit like nothing else.

I'll give you an example. You go in for a physical, and you're told you have terminal cancer. You walk out of there different. I mean you literally—it's like your body and your spirit have been hijacked. When you have a headache after a cancer diagnosis, it's not a headache, it's spread to the brain. If your elbow hurts, you don't have a bruise or a broken bone, it's cancer, it's spreading. You wake up every morning like you're looking behind your back, over your shoulder, "When is this disease going to kill me?" I believe, Ty, that people who are diagnosed with cancer, they either make up their mind immediately that they're going to conquer, or they begin to die that minute.

I didn't say the word cancer very much during those 40 days. I didn't call myself a "cancer victim." People go around and say, "My son's autistic," "I'm diabetic." If you're going to have a title or a label, don't make it that. It's as if you're saying and believing and receiving that. I didn't receive it. I spent 40 days working my rear end off. I literally was in a sauna, an infrared sauna, two hours a day. I was doing amazing raw food cocktails, phytotherapy or herbalism, consuming an all raw omnivorous diet. I went after it, but you know what I didn't do? I didn't suffer in misery. I had more joy and more peace during my 40 days of healing than most people have with all the money and all the stuff in the world. I was facing a death sentence, 100 percent chance, and I decided to live.

I chose it from the beginning. I walked it out. I prayed those three times a day. I went back over every memory that I had in my life – this is work – starting from two years old and anytime anyone hurt me or I had hurt them, I wrote the experience down and I prayed until I felt peace. Ty, I'm talking about when I was ten years old and my baseball coach told me if you strike out again, I am going to do something terrible to you. We actually store cellular memories, emotions, and failures or unforgiveness that turn to bitterness, and we store it – in my mind – like our body grows cancer cells. I felt like if we fear a malignancy, we should fear unforgiveness and bitterness much more. I dealt with issues, it took me days, and I dealt with everyone. I'm talking about thousands of memories, and people say, "Well, Jordan, what does it have to do with my health that someone turned me down for the prom when I was 16?"
Well, what did it make you feel like? Did you say, "You're worthless"? Did you decide weren't good enough? There are people out there, Ty, that have had marriages with infidelity. They've had their spouse divorce them. They've had their parents tell them they don't love them. These are serious, and we store them in our body like a virus on a hard drive computer. If we don't take care of it, they'll eat us away.

Todd Jones: It's something where you just—everything just blurs. Your energy just leaves your body. You're in shock. It's traumatic, and you look at each other and you don't know what to say. It happens to so many parents now, it's horrible. I guess it's one of the fastest growing segments in the hospital, child oncology is. It's growing and out of control. So, you're speechless, and I called my boss. I was supposed to be at a trade show and I was bawling. I said, "Man, we just got some bad news." One of the first things we grabbed on to was the LifeOne product for enhanced immune system support because that has such an amazing track record. I think it was Dr. Michael—

Ty: Farley.

Todd Jones: Yeah, Farley, and his oncology surgeon partner from Florida.

Ty: Dr. LaRochelle.

Todd Jones: Yeah, LaRochelle. Those guys put it together I think, right?
They just had ten years of use and just amazing results. So that, with LivingFuel together, we said, "Okay, we're going to help little Janae's immune system right away." Because what happened was we were told she had to get into treatment, but we knew she had to get something done. We also had no track record or experience like any parent. Nobody knows. So, we said, "Okay, let's get her on the treatment," and the treatment is an intensified treatment for 30 days where they use vincristine chemotherapy and steroids, and that little child just got loaded up with that stuff daily.

Ty: You have mentioned earlier about the difference between Janae when she was going through treatment and then the other kids in the ward.

Todd Jones: Right. For us, it was a tell-all right there. We were watching the other children and we could see what was going on in the hospital. For example, the food. Right away, if you're a parent, you need to pay attention to this because most hospitals just have hospital food, and that stuff is french fries and hamburgers. It's corn dogs and chips and chicken strips and canned green beans and homogenized pasteurized milk.

Ty: With ice cream for dessert.

Todd Jones: With ice cream for dessert, or jell-o or canned fruit chunks with corn syrup and GMO; everything. You really want to pay attention to just not letting the children who are being treated just have that stuff. As you know, we talked about the steroids that create a desire for salty food. So, parents are just wanting to keep the child happy or satisfied during this horrible treatment period, and so they get that salty stuff and all that denatured junk food.

Even the hospital staff, doctors, the hematologist, "Oh, they need that because they need something. They're going through all that, just let them have it." I'm like, "This is not the kind of advice I really feel good about." That's why we got these big syringes, and we fill them with LivingFuel. We put stevia in it to sweeten it up. I mean we stayed clean.

Ty: So, you were putting LivingFuel in syringes and giving it to Janae orally?

Todd Jones: Yeah. She was just sucking it up, and she loved it. We prayed about it, too, by the way. When you're in a situation like that, there's so many moments where you don't know what to do. If you know the power of prayer, you have to use it in these times. You have to just say, "Lord, we need your help, guide us on this," because this is how you help other people, when your conviction in your faith is involved. We were blessed because, in this very challenging moment, we were demonstrating that we could make a difference, too.

Ty: You said you were using LivingFuel and syringes, did you use LifeOne as well?

Todd Jones: Same deal, you bet. We kept that going on, alternatingly and—

Ty: During her treatment, during her chemo?

Todd Jones: Absolutely, during the chemo. I have to recall here, she did get it during her chemo for sure. She got it throughout the whole three-year treatment. But after the first month, and I shared this with you, too, we made a decision that we wanted to—since the cancer was so far down, in remission as they say, and they told us themselves, that we were just like, "Okay, you know what? Thank you for your business, we're good now. We're going to go ahead and build her up naturally. Now that the cancer and half of her system has been "chemoed," chemically cleansed, we're going to go in and put in the natural good stuff now, and see how we can get her to respond there." Well, the hospital didn't like that.

When that happened, it wasn't three days later, and there was that very, very, very loud, aggressive knock at our door. I'm thinking, "Hmm, that doesn't sound like anybody I know. Nobody knocks like that. It almost sounded like a boot." I went to the door and it was the Office of Child Services. They came, and they said, "Look, the hospital called. You have taken your child out of treatment and you need to bring your child right back to treatment." I'm like, "Well, we're finished with that treatment. We're just going to continue on with another treatment, all right? I'm the parent." I even looked up the Alaska statutes. Parents have a legal right to decide how their children get treated.

What I didn't know is, it doesn't matter what the statutes say. The administrative truth about that is that the child is a ward of the state, and so you don't have that decision to make. It got kind of dicey at that point as well, because I certainly wasn't into causing more stress than my wife and I had already had. We're really still in trauma with our little one here, but we were very hopeful because the cancer was down and we were getting things going in the right direction, as far as we were certainly concerned and convicted about. But the officer at child services told us right up-front, "We will take both your children and they will both go into foster care, if you do not get that child right back into the hospital."

Ty: Take both of your children?

Todd Jones: Both of them. So, I'm thinking, wow, these guys are making the statement pretty hard, right up my face, right up front. I remember calling you that night saying, "Dude, this is what's happening, you know," and I remember you weren't impressed either. I made a decision there to not rock the boat and cause more dismay. I could never imagine my two young girls in the care of other people. I went to two lawyers and got very well-informed about this. They said, "Yeah, we can get your daughters back. Eight hundred grand and two years later is pretty much what you can count on, because of all the BS that—"

Ty: And who has that kind of money?

Todd Jones: That's right. I mean, it's already bad enough when you're stuck in this treatment program for three years. So, we got her back into treatment, and we continued with the regimen. We continued to replace a lot of hospital food with stuff that we would bring from home.

Ty: So, you continued on chemo?

Todd Jones: Yeah. We're continuing on, because it's a three-year regimen. Well, actually two and a half, and then it kind of sort of fades into three. It seems like forever. So, we would observe the children and we could see that our daughter was very resilient, because there were episodes where she would get heavy dosages and then the steroids on top. You could see how it really wipes out the whole—the natural state of the child was very low energy and just depleted, but she would bounce back quick.

As this evolved in the treatment time, we noticed that the other children weren't eating at all anymore. They had to get feeding tubes. You could just count them. It was like all of a sudden in that month, there are three or four more kids who are getting feeding tubes. Well, guess who didn't have to get the feeding tube? Because she was still doing it and she didn't need it. She was doing LifeOne and LivingFuel and whatever else we could get in there. The pharmacist though came up and said, "What are you guys giving her?" I'm like, let me think, how much am I going to say today. But we were pretty cool, we shared and it was because it's all natural and it's all food, they can't really say much. We weren't doing isolated, synthetic vitamins and minerals, and stuff like that. That's junk anyway. We were doing the full-fledged flavonoid, fennel spectrum, if you will.

So, she stayed on that, and did great. Praise God, our kid made it and we saw a couple that didn't, and that just makes your heart break. That's why I was happy when you shared with me that you were doing another docu-series, and I was more than happy to show up and say, "Hey, Ty, man, this is what we did. And hopefully we can help some other parents keep the faith, and you keep doing the right things, and you take care of your child as much as you can."

Ty: Well, you're, what, four years later now?

Todd Jones: Four years, yeah.

Ty: She's six now?

Todd Jones: She'll be six this September. We're a whole year since treatment. Last spring was the last part of the treatment. So, we're a whole year now and a couple months out of treatment. She's playing tee-ball, and she jumps on the trampoline with her big sister, and she runs all over the place, and she's at school. She's doing great, yeah.

Ty: That's awesome. Well, so glad she's doing well. I want a picture.

Todd Jones: Yeah, you're going to get a picture. I'll give you one of her sport pictures with an autograph.

Ty: I want her to sign it for me [laughter].

Todd Jones: That's right.

Ty: Tell her to autograph it.

Todd Jones: She'll know someday that you were part of that support network, and that'll be a beautiful thing.

Ann Fonfa: I was diagnosed with breast cancer when I was 44 years from my left arm without my express or informed consent, I just felt really uncomfortable with the way they were doing it. They had told me on a Thursday that they had an opening for surgery on Monday, which I understood to mean, "Uh-oh, you have the worst cancer in the universe." I didn't know that that's what they did with old women or men with breast cancer, rush us into treatment.

So, I saw an oncologist, and the oncologist said to me as I walked in, "Oh, we'll start you on chemo next week," and I said, "You know, doc, I have a problem." He said immediately, "Oh, it doesn't matter," and I said, "No, I just have to tell you what it is. I'm chemically sensitive. I respond badly to every kind of cleaning product, anything people are wearing on their neck or their hair, their laundry detergent, everything bothers me. Wet paint will cause me to fall to the ground," and he said, "Oh, it doesn't matter." I was like, "Oh, goodbye, doc, you know—

Ty: You're still going to do it?

Ann Fonfa: —I have to go." It was great. I walked out and I decided that's not for me, and I started to explore what else I can do. I was astonished—

Ty: You fired the doctor about that?

Ann Fonfa: Exactly. He probably would have fired me, but he was an idiot. I mean, it doesn't matter? Well, it's my life, it matters to me. When I met a Chinese herbalist at the San Antonio Breast Cancer Symposium in 1998 of December, and he said, "I think I can help you." So, by April of the next year, I said that I need help, and I went to see him. In the first prescription that he gave me, I made a tea. When I drank that tea, my entire body turned into a hive, a giant hive, every inch. So, of course that was scary, but three days later, I realized my chemical sensitivity symptoms had completely changed, and the intensity had reduced by about 65 percent.

So now, I have a normal life. I can function like everyone else. I'm not going to pass out if you were wearing fragrance 40-feet away from me, which was what my life was like. In addition to that, over time, I never got any more tumors. I've had an MRI when I started the herbs because I wanted to prove something. At the end of the time, I had another MRI, and by then I was completely proven cancer-free. That was September 2001. Ironically, I got that diagnosis September 12, 2001 in New York City. No traffic, no cars, no buses, no taxis. I walked to the hospital, and my doctor came from New Jersey, and she said to me, "We can't find anything of cancer, we're going to call you 'No discernible disease.'" They didn't give me NDD, which is the usual diagnosis, because I didn't do chemo, I didn't do radiations. We don't know how you're really doing. I knew how I was doing. I was going to live.

Carol Smith: Travis is an engineer and he said to the doctor—

Trevor Smith: Well, I said to him, "There has to be a different way, another way to do things," and he said, "No, this is the way." So, it's like, I'm going to get my way, and that was the driver. But everybody believes somebody in a white coat has the answer and it's not necessarily so.

Carol Smith: So, we asked how long if we didn't do the operation, and we were told 18 months to two years, at the most.

Trevor Smith: No, it was 18 months. It was like less than that.

Ty: 18 months or you better act now?

Carol Smith: Yeah.

Ty: So, they instill the sense of urgency to undergo their protocol.

Trevor Smith: But one thing about it, we had somewhere to go instead of staying in England.

Carol Smith: Well, all of the family were pushing us to go for chemo, get the blood out, especially Travis' family, "No, he needs to have chemo. He needs to do what the doctor is saying."

Trevor Smith: So, taking a step back, we were able to go back home and take some time away from everybody.

Ty: Back to Dubai?

Carol Smith: Yes. Yeah. I made some decisions even there, with the doctors there.

Carol Smith: But first, we spoke to our sons, and we told them our decision to take the 18 months. We started giving away money to our sons and—

Ty: Did you?

Carol Smith: Yeah, we were going to live our lives. I was going to go with him. I was going to take some time—

Ty: Tell me that story.

Trevor Smith: What I said was that I'll take the 18 months and celebrate, live life to the full, do things that we always said we wanted to do. For me, I was going to walk straight into the desert, if it got to the point where it was painful or something I couldn't do. I was going to walk straight into the desert and not bother anybody, and that's the way I was going to do it. But my wife decided, "No, I'm coming with you, not mainly straight into the desert, but I don't want to be left around without you."

Carol Smith: I just got to work and then I started meeting people that have cured their own cancer online. My computer saved his life. It wasn't me. It was the computer. It was the Internet. It was the Facebook pages. So, I kept the journal basically for emails for my family, and then when I realized what was happening to him, he lost 19 kilograms in weight. He never was sick for one day and he got better and better and he got fitter and fitter. He was playing eleven-a-side football.

Ty: What were you—what did you decide to do?

Carol Smith: We changed his diet, first off, completely cut out all processed foods. He only ate organic chicken, fish, vegetables, salads, fruits. We juiced every day. He drank smoothies, nuts, dried fruits.

Trevor Smith: Basically, what I wasn't eating, I changed my whole diet, greens—

Carol Smith: We got a naturopathic doctor on board and she did the tests, and found out it was completely—

Trevor Smith: That was a big turning point.

Carol Smith: Yeah, it was completely depleted—

Trevor Smith: We went through a point where—there's all blood tests of everything. They covered all different spectrum and they found out what was depleted. So, the high doses came into vitamin C or—

Carol Smith: We didn't know what we were doing. We're just taking it off the Internet. If I've had your input, I would have known exactly what to do, but I found other sources. Ten months afterwards, I came across cannabis oil.

Ty: Cannabis oil?

Carol Smith: Cannabis oil.

Trevor Smith: But you know what, that's not quite true because we were way past it when we came across it—

Carol Smith: After six months, we came across it and I was trying to figure out how could I get it, and I sourced somebody in Spain. Then I was trying to figure out how could I get it. I wasn't going to take it to Dubai, how I could I get it to the UK. So, I was going to break the law and fetch the cannabis oil myself. But then he was getting better, so we didn't need to do it then.

Trevor Smith: But there was that one thing that was said to you, if—

Carol Smith: Yes, one guy said to me, "I can bring it to you but if I'm not prepared to risk imprisonment for—if you're not prepared to risk imprisonment for somebody you love, why should I?" That made me realize, I need to risk it. But I knew if I went to prison in England, I'd get out. I'd have a slap on the wrist and I'd get out. But I knew if I tried to do it to Dubai, there's no chance. I wouldn't get out of prison there.

Ty: Did you make it yourself?

Carol Smith: No. It was made by a legal cannabis oil maker, and she also wrote the foreword—because eventually, I publish my journal that I was keeping for emails for my family. I self-published it because I knew that we were onto something, and people needed to know what we'd done and how we'd done it, when the doctor said there was no other way.

Ty: So, what is the name of the book that you've published?

Carol Smith: The book's called *Taking Control* by Alicia Sade. Alicia and Sade are my two beautiful granddaughters.

Ty: Did you take apricot pits or apple seeds?

Trevor Smith: No, B17 capsules.

Ty: Oh, the capsule, B17, okay.

Carol Smith: And high doses of Vitamin C, 20,000 milligrams of vitamin D—

Ty: We just had our vitamin D here at breakfast [laughter].
We're taking it everywhere we go. Yeah, we do. So, the combination of the changing the diet, the vitamin C, vitamin D, the hemp oil, the vitamin B17, all of that in combination and keeping a positive mental attitude—

Carol Smith: And having lots of love and support.

Ty: Oh, I can see that. It's evident.

Trevor Smith: Support is big. It's key, yeah.

Carol Smith: And he's well. He's two years now cancer-free.

Ty: Yeah. You look really healthy.

Carol Smith: He does.

Trevor Smith: My weight, initially, I think was just under 100 kilograms.

Carol Smith: He started looking younger and younger, and I started looking older with the stress [chuckles].

Trevor Smith: Not at all [laughter].

Dr. Robert Gorter: Well, I'm originally from Holland, Amsterdam, where I did my medical training. Then I did extra training in oncology in an anthroposophical hospital in Basel, in Switzerland then I started my own clinic. But, almost on day number one, I was diagnosed myself with a very far advanced called germ cell carcinoma. They usually start in women from an ovary or men from a testicle, and they grow very, very fast. When I was diagnosed, they said, "Well, three months with some luck, maximum of six months. We'll do a chemo, we'll do this, we'll do that." I said, "No, no, no, no, no," because I knew, as a doctor, what I would go through, and I thought, "Well, even if it's true that I'll live six weeks longer, but on the blood of others—I'm not afraid of death and I'd rather die than statistically, a few weeks earlier."

They all decided I was crazy. But, then I said, "No, there are other options." I also had this idea that the root of cancer is an immune suppression, so I should improve immune function. So, I did. I treated myself with mistletoe injection. I got hyperthermia, so I went in a hot water bath. My temperature was up to 40 degrees, and I did those few things. Remarkably, I got better and better. Probably about a year and a half later, I was free of cancer because I didn't check every day, because if I have to die, I'll die so I won't change anything. But it wasn't clear that after about a year and a half, when I really checked myself, nothing could be found. I was perfectly back in order.

Ty:　　How many years ago was this? What year was that?

Dr. Robert Gorter: 43 years ago.

Ty:　　Did you ever go back to see the doctors that told you that you were crazy?

Dr. Robert Gorter: No, because they all had died by now. They were nothing and just started as a doctor. These were big professionals who were all in their 50s and 60s, and when I said I didn't want chemo, they're like—though I was like how stupid I was. But probably, I was right and they were stupid. But anyway, who knows? I don't feel I should show any revenge or any—that I did better. I went my way, and it worked.

Lourdes Colon:　　I loved sugar.

Ty:　　Who doesn't love sugar?

Lourdes Colon:　　Oh, my gosh, mine was extreme. I would eat—95 percent of my intake was of sugar. It was like if I had breakfast, I would have 12 sandwich ice creams for breakfast because I felt I'm skinny, I don't gain weight, I'm good, and not realizing the destruction I was doing to my body. Then we go out for dinner and he would have a meal—and as my husband had his meal, I would have my brownie with ice cream on it, and that's what I would have for dinner. That was like day in and day out, and then it really took a toll.

Ty:　　When you were diagnosed did your oncologist suggest that one thing you might do is to give up this sugar?

Lourdes Colon:　　My advice when I was diagnosed with cancer – because I was really really skinny and, again, I didn't know that I was losing so much weight because of the cancer – was, looking really skinny, go out, eat as much ice cream as you can, enjoy yourself, put on the weight. When she told me that, it was interesting because I thought, "Well, no, sugar feeds cancer, so I'm not going to do that." I didn't tell her that, but I was like, "Wow."

Ty: That doesn't make sense.

Lourdes Colon: No. Here, they're not telling me, "Get out there, start eating healthy," they were like, "Eat the sugar, put on the weight." I pursued completely non-toxic treatments. Anything that is said to shrinks tumors, fight cancer, I took. It had to make sense. If it was something you had to achieve, I wouldn't do it. But, if it was all about detoxing, cleansing up the cells, getting the body back to normal. When it started making sense to me – like this makes sense, this is what I'm going to do because—it's interesting because everything I searched out, every last one of them was all about detox, vamping your body, getting the stuff that's in there that's been there forever out. I read this book called *Killing Cancer – Not People*. I had so many books I read—

Ty: Is that Bob Wright?

Lourdes Colon: I think so.

Ty: I think Bob Wright wrote that.

Lourdes Colon: Yeah. I have so many books at home, and I did so much reading, like that's all I did on a daily basis. There was one that talked about doing a colonic on a daily basis. So, I went and got the colema board, and I started doing the colonics every day. I noticed the moment that I did that, I did start feeling a difference. Because before that, they did PET-CT scan and it was still—even though, they say it's out of your body after 45 minutes or whatever, so not true. I continue feeling the process of the growth in the cancer. I finally got the colema board and started doing it daily. It started flushing things out and I didn't feel the pain, I didn't feel the swelling, I didn't feel the agony. I felt that it's shrinking. I learned about wheatgrass.

Ty: Wheatgrass?

Lourdes Colon: Yeah. Wheatgrass was a really big part of the things that I did in fighting cancer.

Ty: When you were diagnosed with cancer and you were a sugar addict before, and now you've changed the way you're eating, give me a kind of typical day in the diet of Lourdes Colon.

Jordon S. Rubin: I was doing essential oil therapy. I was on infrared heating mats. I was trying to exercise the best I could on a mini trampoline, 20 to 30 minutes a day. Everything you can think of, everything that I knew, I put together in that program. You know what else I did? I found a doctor, Dr. Emil Schandl in Fort Lauderdale, Florida. He would give me not only one blood test, but tested three ways, every two weeks, and then there was the 40 day CT scan with contrast. So, I could do it exactly the same way, same radiologist, although he didn't realize I wasn't under an oncologist's supervision at the time. So, the first two weeks, program hardcore. I go get my blood drawn. I'm praying the whole time.

Now, remember my number was about 278, so to speak – my HCG – which is typically the pregnancy hormone, but in testicular cancer, oftentimes it is elevated. So, I took the blood test three days later, which was the two- week mark, I was going to get my results.

I see my phone ring, Dr. Schandl's name comes up and I begin to shake. Now, I had a lot of peace and a lot of faith, but man, when you're going to hear those results, "Look at what was riding on this." So, I answer and he says, "Jordan," and I said, "Yes." He says, "I got your results. I tested three ways, but you said you were in the 260s, 270. I'm getting 32, 20, 26." And I said, "Praise God," and then I told my parents, I told my wife. Then I said, "But wait a minute, what if he tested in a different way? What if it's not comparable with the methodology?" Doubt began to creep in. But, no time for that. Two more weeks of hard core spiritual, emotional, mental and physical nutrition, detoxification, healing. I go get my blood drawn again, praying, praying, praying, wanting this to be a positive result. I got a call. It was on a Friday afternoon. See Dr. Schandl's name on my caller ID. I answer. He says, "Jordan," and I said, "Yes?" He said, "I have your results." He said, "I'm getting zero, zero, zero." It was time for celebration.

A couple days later, I had my CT scan. I went in, and I don't know about you, but if you've ever had an enclosed CT scan or MRI—I guess I'm more claustrophobic than I thought. That was awful. But, I prayed the whole time. I don't believe in getting radiation or contrast fluid, or drinking barium, or any of that nonsense, but I needed to show the world what God was going to do in my life. Three days later, I was going to get the results, and I look, and I see normal, normal, normal, normal. I dropped the packet. I started to weep. I hugged my wife, and I couldn't believe it, but yet I believed it. It's like nothing I could ever explain. I was free. This disease that I never claimed was a part of my life, was now officially gone.

I called 20 or 30 people that I shared this with, and they were the best phone calls I've ever had. I mean, to be able to tell them what a miracle had happened in my life. Some of them admitted to me that they were really concerned. Some of them were overjoyed and said that they knew all along, but it was an awesome day for me. My son, Joshua, who was four or five years old at the time, I said to my wife, "Hey, can we pick up Joshua from school and take him to Toys R Us and buy him anything in the store" and she said, "Why?" I said, "I can't explain to him what miracle I've just experienced other than telling him, 'You can get any toy you want.'" Of course, he was excited and he asked me why, and I said, "Dad's experienced a great gift – myself. God gave me a great gift today."

As I stand here today, Ty, I am convinced that what you eat, the supplements you take, IV therapies, hydrotherapy, certainly far infrared saunas, various exercises, and various machines can make a difference in your health, can help you build your immune system. I'm convinced that emotional health is critical, but I can tell you something that probably no one else in this series will. Cancer starts with a spiritual disease, and if I were to be with somebody for 20 minutes after their diagnosis, I bet I could predict if they're going to live and thrive, or suffer and die. Don't own the disease. Cancer is not who you are, and I think you've realized after all these interviews, cancer isn't one disease. How could it affect somebody's blood, another person's bone marrow, someone's colon? How could it be a solid tumor in one person and not in another and be the same disease? The name "cancer" is evil, but it's evil for different ways than we think. You decide if you win or lose, and I think you're going to find the common denominator in people who are survivors or conquerors, as I like better, are those that decide to go after it and win. Don't sit back and let somebody tell you what to do. Make the most important decisions of your life.

You know what's crazy, Ty? If you try natural health with cancer and you die, they killed you. If you go conventional and you die, we did the best that we could do. How is that possible? We lost loved ones. You've lost loved ones. You know what? I'm writing a book. I'm writing a book soon. I think the most appropriate title is, *To Hell With Cancer*. That's where it came from, in my opinion, and I want to help send it back. I do believe that if somebody, if anybody wants to overcome this dreaded disease, you start by making the decision that cancer will not win. Cancer will not own you. You are not a cancer patient. You are more than a conqueror. Frankly, next time I hear somebody get diagnosed with cancer, my first encouragements is going to be: you say it, "To hell with cancer."

Henry McElligott: I was told that I had base of tongue cancer tumors that had spread to my lymph nodes on my neck, and they were worried that it had already spread to the rest of my body and my organs. So, they put me in a room with about 34 oncologists that is major hospital, and put a camera down through my nose to have a look at the tumors that were at the base of my tongue. A copy of the tumors all appeared up in the screen behind my head and my wife saw them, and she said, "They look scary." The head oncologist came to us, and he said, "You need to start radiation and chemo immediately," because they're worried that it's spreading", or else I would not survive.

We were in total shock at that time. We lost words, and we just looked at each other. A few days later, I went to see another group of 11 oncologists at another hospital near my home, and they said the same thing. They said, "Immediate radiation and chemo or you will not survive very long, because this is a very dangerous type of cancer. It's already spread to your lymph nodes. We don't know where it is at this stage without the PET scans, MRIs, things like that." So, I went home with Joy({wife), and just in total confusion, hopelessness, despair, sat in for a few days, we didn't know what to do. I decided to start looking on the Internet. What are the side effects of radiation and chemo and what exactly is chemo and radiation?

I discovered on the Internet Ty Bollinger's *Quest for Cancer Cures*, and I listened to all his interviews with various cancer specialists all over America, and I was especially intrigued by some of them. I learned so much. For treatment with chemo and radiation, for the type of tumor I had, I would need a tube to breath and a tube—they wanted to insert the tube in my stomach for food. So, I rang the hospital and sent them an email, both hospitals, and I said, "I refuse the chemo treatment and the radiation. I'm going to do some research myself and seek a natural alternative to the chemo and the radiation." That was it for the couple of days, and then they started ringing me and creating fear over the phone, saying things, "You won't live very long."

I went on total vegetarian food. I had a lot of fruits and nuts to eat. I went on a three-week fast, just water and taking these vitamins. After the three-week fast, I had lost about ten or 15 kilos. However, I was feeling good. What I noticed after taking these products for about six weeks, the swelling at the left side of my neck began to decrease in size and the swelling on my right decreased, and I was able to swallow much more easily. My tongue was not swollen so much, so I got really encouraged by this because I had no doctors care whatsoever. I continued this treatment until March. At that point, I decided are these tumors decreasing or has the cancer spread already? That was major concern. My blood test went to Germany at the end of April, and I got a call from the doctor's secretary on the 8th of May. She said, "Your results are here from Germany, would you like to come in and see them?" I said, "Of course, I do." I got really excited.

When I got there, I had to wait in the room for about 20 minutes for the doctor to see me. It felt like the longest 20 minutes in my life. I just kept wiggling my thumbs. So, eventually, he called me upstairs to his office and he opened this envelope, and he looked at me stunned. I said, "Doctor, what's the result, I'm sweating, what is the result?" He said, "Henry, this is a miracle." He said, "I've been a doctor since 1979. You are the first person that has come to this clinic that hasn't been messing around with chemotherapy radiation or surgery as a cancer cure." I said, "Am I?" He said, "These are marvelous results," and he said, "This report is a miracle." He said, "It says, 'Numerous fragmented, dead cancer tumors floating all over the blood.'" Then he said, "It is the same result as if you've been having chemo and radiation treatment for the last six months." I was in total shock. I just relaxed in the chair, and I said, "What does that mean, Doctor?" He says, "Your cancer marker is barely registering on the scale – on the radar scale." He said, "I'm very shocked," and I said, "Well, what will I do now, Doctor?" He said, "Whatever you're doing, just keep doing it for the rest of your life, and you'll live another hundred years."

Alan Ray: When we went to San Diego this past spring, we had people coming up to us, to Ty, because they recognize him. These are people who had had cancer, who had gone to the oncologist, chemotherapy, and been told, "There's nothing more we can do for you. Get your affairs in order." Then they say, "But we saw *The Quest for the Cures*, and we found out about a treatment or a doctor, and I'm alive today because of what you did in your series" and, man, it brought it home in a way that nothing else could.

Tara Mann: It's validation. Going through what I went through and being so unsure and jumping off the cliff, going from making over $100,000 to making nothing, and putting myself out there. But to have someone like Ty and Charlene and Cancer Truth say, "We approve. You're doing a good job and we want you to continue," it means so much. Charlene sent me a message and said, "Oh, we're going to donate to Cancer Crackdown." I didn't even know, and it was $10,000. What's so amazing about *The Quest For The Cures* is that you have all these real doctors that everybody trusts, and that will go to and let them take over their life and their health, that are telling you that it doesn't have to be that way, and

I know, I'm a doctor. I know because I was trained as a doctor, but I also have learned these other things, and that is so valuable to people. It's doctor after doctor after doctor telling you what you need to know to empower yourself and to take control of your own health. The value in this series is invaluable.

Dr. Gaston Cornu-Labat: Eventually, medicine will come to terms. Humanity will come to terms with the fact that healing comes from within. That us, the doctors, the clinics, and the medications are the ones that facilitate that process of healing, so it doesn't belong to us. It belongs to you as a patient. My true role as a practitioner is to empower and facilitate that healing within.

Dr. Nalini Chilkov: The Big C word is *never* a death sentence. There's always a path, there's always a path. Some people are living with cancer as a chronic illness, right? So, that's fine. It's the same as living with diabetes or high blood pressure or high cholesterol. If we can manage it and keep it at a microscopic level, you carry on with your life. It is not a death sentence.

Ty: Wow. Isn't it incredible to have heard these cancer conqueror stories to have experienced it with them and to be uplifted and filled with hope? That's our message. Cancer does not have to be a death sentence. There's always hope. I want to thank you from the bottom of my heart for joining us these last nine days to watch *The Truth About Cancer: A Global Quest*. This is the culmination of a lot of blood, sweat, and tears. This is our gift to you. We hope that you've enjoyed it. Thanks for joining us. God bless all of you. [credits roll]

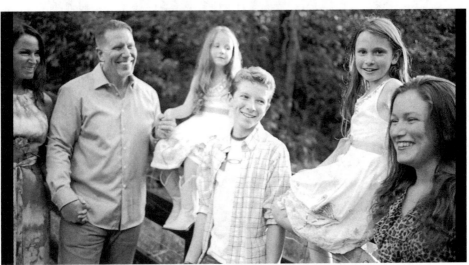

The Bollinger Family – (from left to right)
Charlene, Ty, Charity, Bryce, Tabitha, Brianna

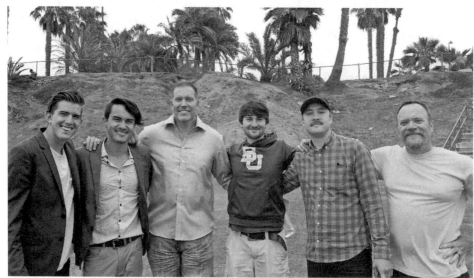

The TTAC Audio Visual Team – (from left to right)
Eithel Krauss, Jonathan Otto, Ty Bollinger, Zachry Karisch, Travis Jones, Alan Ray

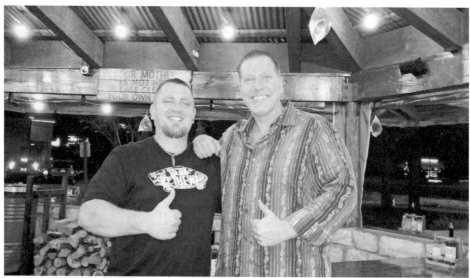

TTAC Founders – Jonathan Hunsaker & Ty Bollinger

THE EXPERTS

Dr. Matthias Rath, M.D.
Founder of Dr. Rath Research
Institute (Netherlands)

**Dr. Josh Axe, D.N.M.,
D.C., C.N.S.**
Nutrition Expert, Author &
Founder of DrAxe.com

Dr. Russell Blaylock, M.D.
Neurosurgeon, Scientist & Editor
of the Blaylock Wellness Report

Dr. Joseph Mercola, D.O.
Founder of Mercola.com,
New York Times Best-selling
Author

Sayer Ji
Author, Lecturer, National Health
Federation Advisory Board

**Dr. Jonathan V. Wright,
M.D.**
Medical Director and Founder -
Tahoma Clinic (Washington, USA)

**Dr. Véronique Desaulniers,
D.C.**
Breast Cancer Conqueror,
Author, Physician & Lecturer

Ocean Robbins
CEO of Food Revolution
Network, Author, Speaker
& Facilitator

Mike Adams
aka "The Health Ranger" - Food
Scientist, Author, and Lecturer

**Dr. Stanislaw Burzynski,
M.D., Ph.D**
Scientist and Biochemist, Founder
- Burzynski Clinic (Texas, USA)

**Dr. Leigh Erin Connealy,
M.D.**
Medical Director - Center for
New Medicine (California, USA)

**Dr. Patrick Quillin, Ph.D,
R.D., C.N.S.**
Author, Lecturer & Former VP
of Nutrition - Cancer Treatment
Centers of America

G. Edward Griffin
Author, Lecturer, and Filmmaker

Dr. Roby Mitchell, M.D.
aka "Dr. Fitt" - Orthomolecular
Medicine Physician

**Dr. Francisco Contreras,
M.D.**
Oncologist and Surgeon

Jeffrey M. Smith
GMO Expert, Filmmaker,
Researcher & Lecturer

Dr. Sherri Tenpenny, D.O.
Author, Lecturer, Consultant
& Vaccine Expert

**Dr. Edward F. Group III,
D.C., N.D.**
CEO - Global Healing Center,
Speaker, Author & Educator

**Dr. Tullio Simoncini,
M.D., Ph.D**
Oncologist, Pioneer in Sodium
Bicarbonate Therapy

**Dr. Ben Johnson, M.D.,
N.M.D., D.O.**
Author, Lecturer, and Researcher

**Dr. Joel Wallach,
D.V.M., N.D.**
Founder of Youngevity,
Biomedical Researcher,
Best-selling Author

Desiree Rover
Medical Research Journalist,
Author & Radio Host

Dr. Bita Badakhshan, M.D.
Integrative Medicine
Physician - Center for New
Medicine (California, USA)

Dr. Boris Grinblat, M.D.
Naturopath & Medical
Researcher

Dr. Elias Gutierrez, M.D.
Medical Director -
Biomedical Center (Tijuana)

Suzanne Somers
Cancer Survivor, Author,
and Actress

Jonathan Emord
Constitutional Attorney
"The FDA Dragonslayer"

Dr. Sunil Pai, M.D.
Integrative Medicine Physician,
Lecturer and Researcher

Dr. James Forsythe, M.D.
Oncologist and Homeopath

Dr. Robert Scott Bell
Author, Lecturer, and Syndicated
Host of the "Robert Scott
Bell Show"

THE EXPERTS

 Dr. David Jockers Author and Lecturer Exodus Health Center

 Burton Goldberg aka "The Voice of Alternative Medicine" Author and Lecturer

 Dr. Nicholas Gonzalez, M.D. Lecturer and Author

 AJ Lanigan Author, Lecturer, and Immunologist

 Dr. Rashid Buttar Best-selling Author

 Chris Wark Cancer Survivor, Author, and Lecturer

 Bill Henderson Cancer Coach, Lecturer, and Author

 KC Craichy Author and Nutritional Expert

 Dr. Linda Isaacs, M.D Lecturer and Author

 R. Webster Kehr aka "The Cancer Tutor"

 Dr. Keith Scott Mumby, M.D., PhD Author and Lecturer

 Dr. Darrell Wolfe, Ac. PhD Author and Lecturer

 Jason Vale Cancer Survivor

 Charlene Bollinger Researcher & Health Freedom Advocate, Co-Founder of www.CancerTruth.net

 Dr. Daniel Nuzum, D.O., N.M.D. Toxicologist, Professor, Scientist and Researcher

 Dr. Murray "Buzz" Susser, M.D. Integrative Physician and Lecturer

 Dr. Tony Jimenez, M.D. Scientist, Lecturer and Researcher

 Dr. Irvin Sahni, M.D. Lecturer and Scientist

 Paul Barattiero, C.Ped Hydration Specialist

 Dr. Robert Verkerk, Ph.D Executive Director of Alliance for Natural Health-International

 Bob Wright Author and Researcher, Founder of the AACI (American Anti-Cancer Institute)

 Dr. Galina Migalko, M.D., N.M.D World-renowned Expert in Cancer Diagnosis; Integrative Physician

 Dr. Bradford S. Weeks, M.D. Lecturer, Scientist and Researcher

 Dr. Patrick Vickers Founder - Northern Baja Gerson Center

 Cherie Calbom "The Juice Lady"

 Dr. Eric Zielinksi, D.C. Health Coach, Researcher, & Speaker

 Dr. Gaston Cornu-Labat, M.D. Author, Holistic Physician & Surgeon

 Dr. Gosia Kuszewski, N.D. Functional Medicine Naturopath & Medical Herbalist

 Dr. Henk Fransen, Ph.D Natural Healer, Speaker & Author

 Dr. Hila Cass, M.D. Integrative Medicine Physician, Author & Lecturer

A GLOBAL QUEST

PAGE 284

**Dr. Irina Kossovskaia,
M.D., Ph.D, N.M.D.**
Physician, Scientist, Professor,
Author & SCENAR expert

Dr. Ivars Kalvins, Ph.D
Scientist & Inventor,
Director - Latvian Institute
of Organic Synthesis

Dr. John Consemulder
Neuropsychologist, Author
& Healer

Dr. Jolly-Gabriel, Ph.D
Specialist in Hyperbaric
Oxygen Therapy

**Dr. Leonard Coldwell,
N.M.D., Ph.D**
Syndicated Radio Host and
Best-selling Author

Dr. Marcel Wolfe, W.L.Ed.
Wholistic Lifestyle Educator,
EMF & Frequency Expert

**Dr. Martin Bales, L.Ac.,
D.A.O.M.**
Certified Thermologist,
Licensed Acupuncturist

**Dr. Peteris Alberts,
M.D., Ph.D**
Head of Research & Development
- International Virotherapy Centre

Dr. Steven Klayman, D.C.
Holistic Chiropractor

**Dr. Subrata Chakravarty,
Ph.D.**
Chief Scientific Officer at Hope
4 Cancer Institute (Tijuana)

Dr. Suzanne Kim, M.D.
Integrative Medicine Physician -
Center for New Medicine
(California, USA)

Dr. Terry Harmon, D.C.
Chiropractor, Member of the
U.S. Wellness Advisory Council

**Dr. Thomas Lokensgard,
D.D.S., N.M.D.**
Holistic/Biological Dentist
& Naturopath

Dr. Xavier Curiel, M.D.
Integrative Medical
Director at Hope 4 Cancer
Institute (Tijuana)

**Dr. Robert Gorter,
M.D., Ph.D**
Director - Medical Center
Cologne (Germany)

Jefferey Jaxen
Author, Researcher &
Investigative Journalist

Jon Rappoport
Investigative Journalist
(30+ years), Nominated
for Pulitzer Prize

Laura Bond
Investigative Health Journalist
& Author

Liliana Partida, C.N.
Certified Nutritionist

Marcus Freudenmann
Author, Documentary
Film Director/Producer
& International Lecture

Tara Mann
Founder - Cancer Crackdown,
Former Big Pharma Sales Rep

Dr. Igor Smirnov, Ph.D
Inventor, Scientist, Radiation
Expert, Author & Speaker

Ard Pisa
Author, Researcher & Speaker

Dr. Raymond Hilu, M.D.
Founder and Medical Director -
The Hilu Institute (Spain)

Valerie Warwick, R.N.
Cancer Conqueror, Oncology
Nurse Specialist

Dr. Howard Fisher, D.C.
Anti-aging Expert, Lecturer
& Best-selling Author

**Dr. Manuela
Malaguti-Boyle, Ph.D, N.D.**

Dr. Kaspars Losans, M.D.
Oncologist, Medical Director -
International Virotherapy Centre

**Dr. Aleksandra Niedzwiecki,
Ph.D**
Director of Research - Dr. Rath
Research Institute (Netherlands)

**Dr. Garry F. Gordon,
M.D., D.O.**

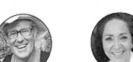

Joel Salatin
International Speaker,
Farmer & Best-selling Author

**Dr. Nalini Chilkov,
L.Ac., O.M.D.**
Author, Clinician
& Cellular Bilogist

Erin Elizabeth
Author, Researcher & Public
Speaker

Peter Starr
Documentary Film Maker
& Cancer Survivor

For more information about the experts who were interviewed in
THE TRUTH ABOUT CANCER: A GLOBAL QUEST
please visit the following website:

http://go2.thetruthaboutcancer.com/global-quest/experts-info-sheet/

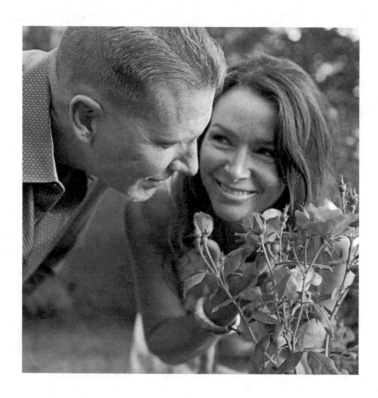